The Mind Matrix Model™

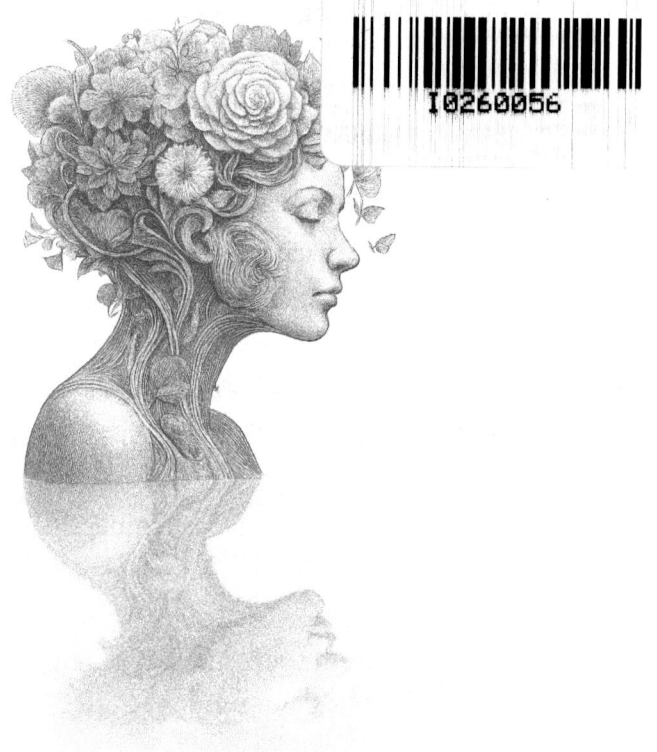

Sam McClellan

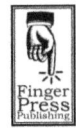

Finger Press Publishing
P.O. Box 10, Granby, MA 01033 USA
https://fingerpress.pub

Copyright © 2025 by Sam McClellan
All artwork and graphics
by Sam McClellan

All rights reserved. This book, or parts thereof, may not be reproduced in any form without written permission.

First edition: September 2025
v1.3

Published in the United States of America
ISBN: 979-8-9987884-0-6

Note that the techniques and suggestions in this book are not meant to replace professional, medical, or psychological treatment. The author and publisher are not responsible for any consequences of independent application of the advice herein.

Always consult a healthcare professional for any serious physical or mental health condition.

Contents

Introduction i

Section One—A Personalized Path to Balance vii

1. Welcome to the Mind Matrix Model 1
2. Meet the Three Selves of Your Mind 19
3. Monarch, Ministers & Scripts 29
4. Navigating the Mind Matrix Model 43
5. Stress, Anxiety & Depression in the Mind Matrix Model 65
6. Working with Stress, Anxiety and Depression 81
7. The Vital Self 95
8. Balancing the Vital Self 113
9. The Heart Self 141
10. Balancing the Heart Self 167
11. The Head Self 195
12. Balancing the Head Self 211
13. The State Axis 237
14. Working with State 257
15. Balance Between the Selves 287
16. Loops and Overrides 303
17. Symbols as the Architects of Perception 315
18. Self and Other 329
19. Setting Healthy Boundaries 357
20. Conclusion 375

Section Two—Next Steps 385
   Online Resources..388
   21. Blocks & Procrastination 389
   22. Dietary Guide..397
   23. Acupressure...405
   24. Essential Oils 411
   25. Homeopathy..415
   26. Nutritional Supplements & Adaptogens......................421
   27. Sleep Hygiene 431
   28. Meditation and Mindfulness 437
Annotated Bibliography 445
Index..457
About the Author 482

Introduction

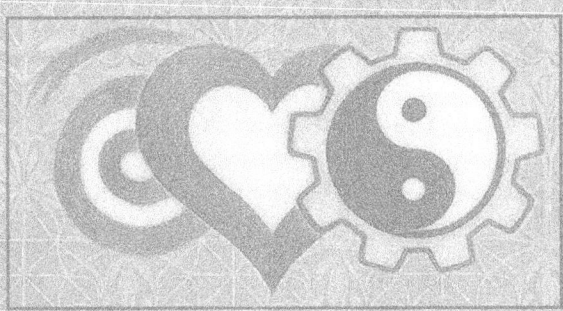

There was once a farmer in ancient China who owned a horse. "You are so lucky!" his neighbors told him, "to have a horse to pull the cart for you."
"Maybe," the farmer replied.

One day he didn't latch the gate properly and the horse ran off. "Oh no! This is terrible news!" his neighbors cried. "Such terrible misfortune!"
"Maybe," the farmer replied.

A few days later the horse returned, bringing with it six wild horses. "How fantastic! You are so lucky," his neighbors told him. "Now you are rich!"
"Maybe," the farmer replied.

The following week the farmer's son was breaking-in one of the wild horses when it kicked out and broke his leg.
"Oh no!" the neighbors cried, "such bad luck, all over again!"
"Maybe," the farmer replied.

The next day soldiers came and took away all the young men to fight in the war. The farmer's son was left behind.
"You are so lucky!" his neighbors cried.
"Maybe," the farmer replied.

The wisdom of this Daoist story lies in its simplicity. The farmer's calm acceptance of life's ups and downs reminds us that happiness doesn't come from controlling what happens, but from finding peace within it. This teaching speaks to the difference between seeking happiness and seeking equanimity—which we can define as calmness, composure, and a steady temper, especially in a difficult situation. Happiness is fleeting, tied to specific events or circumstances, but equanimity runs deeper.

The philosophy of Yin/Yang helps us see why this is so. It teaches us that opposites—joy and sadness, light and darkness, good fortune and bad—are inseparable. One cannot exist without the other. By embracing this truth, we can begin to find balance. When we stop resisting life's natural rhythm and learn to accept its dualities, we cultivate contentment—a state of mind that buffers us from life's inevitable ups and downs.

This mindset lies at the heart of the Mind Matrix Model. If you've ever felt overwhelmed by life's challenges or stuck in cycles of stress and anxiety, you're not alone. It's natural to seek a better way to live—a way to feel calmer, more balanced, and more connected to your true self. The Mind Matrix Model was created to help you achieve exactly that.

This framework doesn't just help you understand yourself; it gives you the tools to navigate the stresses of life, heal from past experiences, and find harmony across every area of your being. What sets the Model apart is its adaptability. It empowers you to identify your own patterns and provides personalized guidance to restore balance.

Whether you're seeking relief from stress, emotional stability, or clarity in your thoughts and decisions, this book offers a wide range of techniques to meet your unique needs. With the Mind Matrix Model, you'll discover how to cultivate contentment, work with your mind, and navigate life's constant changes with more resilience and grace.

The Empty Boat Parable

*If a man is crossing a river
and an empty boat collides with his own skiff,
even though he may be a bad-tempered man,
he will not become very angry.*

*But if he sees a man in the boat,
he will shout to him to steer clear.
If the other does not hear,
he will shout again, and yet again,
and begin cursing.*

And all because there is somebody in the boat.

*Yet if the boat were empty,
he would not be shouting and angry.*

~ Zhuangzi

What this story points out is that we are often triggered by people's actions, letting their actions upset us and thereby giving our power away and making us miserable. If we could just stay aware, we'd realize those choices set us up for suffering. How do we change that?

We need to change our reactive patterns, the unconscious reactions based on past experiences and/or old beliefs.

As you learn to recognize when you're triggered and get better at climbing your way out of the reactive state, you begin to see how, much of the time, we aren't making conscious choices. You begin seeing that we are surrounded by people who are lost in reactive states, constantly being triggered into fight, flight or freeze. *We don't need to join in their misery.*

If you allow triggered people to trigger you, it's kind of like a reactive pinball machine. So much easier if you can let things go.

Why This Book is Different

Many readers notice something early on as they move through this book: it does not read quickly.

This is not because the ideas are deliberately obscure, nor because the material is meant only for specialists. It is because this book is asking you to read in a way that most modern books—and most modern education—rarely require.

Most nonfiction is designed to be read primarily with the analytic mind. It presents ideas in a linear sequence, builds arguments step by step, and rewards speed, categorization, and summary. You can skim, underline key points, and move on with a sense that you have "got it."

This book works differently.

Rather than presenting a single idea or argument, it introduces a map—one that spans body, emotion, thought, development, and state. Understanding it does not come from memorizing definitions alone, but from seeing how patterns repeat across different layers of experience. That kind of understanding cannot be rushed. It emerges through integration.

As a result, you may find yourself reading more slowly than usual. You may reread a paragraph, pause unexpectedly, or feel the need to set the book down for a moment before continuing. For some readers, the material may even feel more like a textbook at times—not because it is academic, but because it is asking you to hold several perspectives at once.

This is intentional.

The Mind Matrix Model is not only something to be understood; it is something to be oriented within. As you read, you are not just absorbing concepts—you are quietly learning how to shift between different ways of perceiving: sensing, feeling, reflecting, and integrating. For many people, especially those accustomed to fast, analytic reading, this shift itself takes effort.

If you notice resistance, fatigue, or a sense of "this is taking longer than I expected," that does not mean you are doing anything wrong. In fact, it often means you are engaging with the material at the level it is meant to be engaged.

You do not need to read this book quickly. You do not need to remember everything on the first pass. And you do not need to fully understand each concept before moving forward. The structure of the book is recursive by design—ideas are revisited, deepened, and reframed as you go.

Think of this book less as something to get through, and more as something to spend time with. It is not designed to be "finished" in the usual sense. Instead, it is meant to function as a resource—one you can return to at different points in your life, in different states, and with different questions. What stands out on a first reading may recede into the background later, while something that once felt abstract may suddenly feel precise and practical.

You may find yourself revisiting certain chapters repeatedly, using them less as linear text and more as reference points—places to reorient when something feels off, confusing, or out of balance. That is part of how the model is meant to be used.

The Mind Matrix is not a sequence of ideas to master, but a framework to live with. Over time, its value comes less from remembering what it says, and more from recognizing where you are within it.

In the sections that follow, a framework will begin to take shape—one that is meant to support balance not only in theory, but in lived experience. Allow yourself the space to read in a way that matches that intention.

A Framework for Balance

At its core, the Mind Matrix is about helping you integrate the three essential aspects of yourself:

> **The Vital Self:** Your physical and energetic foundation. By working with this Self, you'll learn to feel less anxious and more grounded, calm, and physically in tune.
>
> **The Heart Self:** Your emotional and relational center. Balancing this Self helps you manage emotions, connect with others, and build meaningful relationships.
>
> **The Head Self:** Your mental and analytical capacity. Strengthening this Self supports clearer thinking, problem-solving, and decision-making.

Along with these is your **State**, or overall state of mind. We in the West tend to think we are victims of our state of mind, meaning that we don't have much control over whether we're in a more Positive or Negative State. However, regulating your State is a skill you can learn.

By bringing these aspects into harmony, you create a strong foundation for growth, resilience, and well-being.

Tools for Your Journey

No two people are alike, and neither are their paths to balance. That's why the Model integrates both Western and alternative approaches to well-being. You'll find guidance on exploring therapies, modalities, and lifestyle practices that can make a meaningful difference in your life. These include:

Therapies and Modalities: From talk therapy and mindfulness practices to acupressure, bodywork, and integrative psychology, the Mind Matrix Model offers insights into which approaches may work best for you.

- **Stress and Trauma Management:** Learn how to address challenges like stress, anxiety, and unresolved trauma in ways that feel empowering and manageable.
- **Holistic Approaches:** Discover the benefits of nutritional support, dietary changes, herbal remedies, acupressure, and other natural approaches to restoring balance.
- **Practical Steps for Transformation:** Explore actionable steps for building resilience, enhancing self-awareness, and creating a sense of harmony in your daily life.

These tools are not rigid prescriptions. Instead, they serve as options for you to explore, experiment with, and tailor to your own journey.

Website Resources

We'll be exploring the Mind Matrix Model website in more detail in Chapter Four: *Navigating the Mind Matrix Model*. The website is designed to extend the book's content—offering additional resources including additional Next Step chapters, a platform for discussion and connection, and access to both downloadable and interactive tools.

For those who would like a deeper understanding of the science and theory behind the Mind Matrix Model, including the neurological foundations and its integration with psychology and developmental theory, there are a number of resources in the Advanced section.

You can view it or download the PDF by scanning the QR code with your phone or tablet's camera, or by visiting the quick link:

https://mmm.tips/theory

mmm.tips/theory

Steps Toward a More Harmonious Life

The journey toward balance isn't about fixing what's broken. It's about nurturing what's already within you. The Mind Matrix Model offers a step-by-step approach that begins with self-awareness and unfolds through exploration and growth. Along the way, you'll learn how to:

- Identify where you feel out of sync and how to realign.
- Choose therapies and approaches that resonate with you.
- Create small, meaningful changes in your daily routines to support long-term balance over time.
- Build a toolkit of practices that help you handle stress, anxiety, and trauma in healthy, effective ways.

Your Journey Begins

This book is an invitation to take charge of your well-being, to explore new ways of thinking and being, and to create a life that feels more harmonious and fulfilling. Whether you're seeking relief from life's pressures or a deeper sense of connection and purpose, the Mind Matrix Model book was created to serve as a guide.

Special thanks to Sebern Fisher, whose explorations of the mind made this book possible. Warm thanks to my editor, Celia Jeffries, and to all of my very patient and wise readers. And to my lovely wife, Carrie, for her many contributions to this book, and to my life.

SECTION ONE

A Personalized Path to Balance

An overview of the Mind Matrix Model and how it can be used to understand your mind and improve your quality of life.

Chapter One
Welcome to the Mind Matrix Model

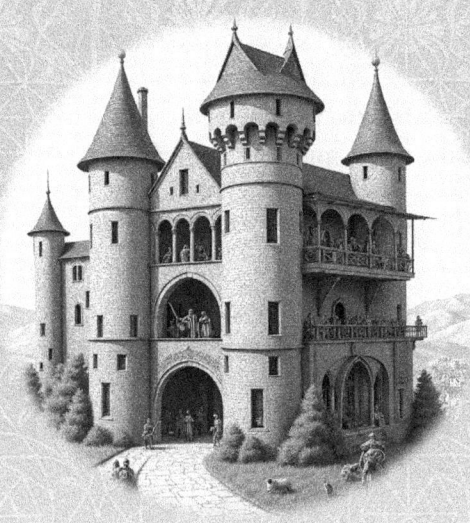

My mind to me a kingdom is;
Such present joys therein I find,
That it excels all other bliss
That earth affords or grows by kind:
Though much I want that most would have,
Yet still my mind forbids to crave.

~ Excerpt from My Mind to Me A Kingdom Is
  by Edward Dyer, 1588

Introduction: Your Mind as a Kingdom

The first stanza from this poem written by Edward Dyer in 1588 beautifully captures the essence of what we're about to explore together. Imagine your mind as a vast, intricate kingdom, filled with wonders and challenges, joys and struggles. This kingdom is where you experience life in all its complexity, and understanding it can be the key to unlocking a more fulfilling and balanced existence.

In this chapter, we'll introduce the core pieces of the Mind Matrix Model. It's a lot at once, and that's okay—it's not meant to all sink in right away. Throughout the book, we'll circle back to these ideas again and again, each time adding more depth and clarity. So if it feels a little overwhelming at first (or a lot), don't worry. The model is broad, but once you start to recognize the patterns, it becomes intuitive and easy to work with.

Have you ever wanted to understand yourself and others?

We all have ideas about who we are—our strengths, our weaknesses, the things we love and appreciate about ourselves, and the things we'd like to change. But have you ever stopped to consider how your mind operates? Why certain patterns repeat? Why some habits seem unchangeable? And why people (including you!) sometimes behave in ways that aren't entirely reasonable? You might find yourself asking:

"Why did I react that way?"

"Why can't I just let that go?"

The truth is, our minds and bodies are incredibly complex systems, often operating on automatic processes that may have served us in the past but no longer fit our current lives. These behavior patterns are deeply tied to the states of our bodies, emotions, and thoughts, and they can sometimes feel like they have a life of their own.

What would you change if you knew it was possible?

Many people feel stuck in what we can call *Loops*, where different facets of the mind, different *Selves*, trigger one another back and forth including emotional reactivity, procrastination, or cycles of anxiety. Some of these Loops are due to *State* instability (what people often call their mood but it's much deeper than that) where the mind struggles to balance itself. Others are deeply embedded survival responses, shaped by past traumas.

One key to changing these patterns lies in understanding the difference between these two.

> **Balance issues**, also called **regulation issues** (how the mind tries to maintain balance), occur when your system is out of sync but can be rebalanced with regulation techniques.
>
> **Trauma responses** run deeper, often overriding regulation (balance) strategies and requiring specific healing approaches and therapies.

This distinction is crucial, and later chapters will guide you through addressing both instability and unresolved trauma in ways that can restore clarity and resilience. But first, some clarifications.

Why The Mind Instead of The Brain?

One question that people often bring up is, why are you talking about the mind instead of the brain? For most people, the two are relatively interchangeable (although you might say *"I changed my mind"* but probably wouldn't say *"I changed my brain."*) The difference is that your brain is an organ in your head, whereas your mind is what you experience. It's the difference between having a car and being a driver. The brain is like the car—it provides the mechanics for thought and function. But in the Mind Matrix Model, the mind is the driver—the one making choices and guiding the way. You need a brain to think, but your mind is the thinker.

Another reason to speak of the mind instead of the brain is that humans have been studying the mind for eons. While neuroscience is a relatively recent field, humanity's interest in consciousness, thought, emotion, and selfhood stretches back thousands of years.

Ancient Indian texts such as the Upanishads and Buddhist Abhidharma explored attention, perception, suffering, and awareness long before cortical structures were mapped. Chinese medicine developed sophisticated models of spirit, emotion, and bodily energy, tracking how mental states affect the health of the whole body and mind system. Western philosophy, from Plato to Descartes to phenomenology, built frameworks for understanding the self and the mind's relationship to reality.

These diverse traditions did not require fMRI images of the brain to make insightful claims about attention, memory, emotion, or even trauma. Their knowledge was experiential, relational, and embodied.

By using the term "mind," the Mind Matrix Model consciously draws on this longer lineage. It makes room for insights from cultures and practices that never reduced consciousness to synapses. It honors the wisdom found in mindfulness, meditation, storytelling, symbolic rituals, bodywork, and direct lived experience, all of which remain central to healing and regulation (balancing) today.

Framing the Three Selves of the Mind Matrix Model as aspects of the mind rather than modules of the brain allows for a richer, more human view of inner life, one that resonates across time, geography, and culture.

Lastly, we focus on the mind because *who you are and your experience of life is based on more than your brain.* Your brain does not operate in isolation. It is part of the central nervous system (CNS), which also includes the spinal cord. It is deeply connected to and influenced by the peripheral nervous system (PNS) which includes the autonomic nervous system (ANS). The ANS is made up of the sympathetic nervous system (SNS) and the parasympathetic nervous system (also PNS, a bit confusingly), and also the enteric nervous system (ENS), often called the "gut brain."

Along with these parts of your nervous system is your embodied experience. Imagine how different you'd be if you never lived in a body experiencing the world.

Together, these systems create the full experience of mind, with thoughts, emotions, perceptions and actions emerging from the interplay between nervous system activity, the senses, and environmental interaction.

This all becomes very important when we're talking about how to understand yourself.

Utilizing Both Analytic and Holistic Thinking

The Mind Matrix Model recognizes two key modes of thought: Analytic Mode and Holistic Mode. These are often labeled "left brain" and "right brain" in popular culture. Analytic thinking breaks things down into parts, figures out how they work, and then considers how they might connect. It's like walking every street of a city to understand it.

Holistic thinking, on the other hand, starts with the big picture—overall functions, relationships, and patterns—and then ties those to specific elements. It's like using a map: you may not know each street, but you can navigate the whole system.

In a balanced mind, these two modes work together. But in our culture, Analytic Mode thinking often dominates, sidelining Holistic Mode intuition and relational insight. This has shaped how we study the brain itself, mapping its countless structures but often not seeing how the brain and other systems work together. Missing the forest for the trees.

The Mind Matrix Model takes a different approach. We start with a holistic understanding of how the mind functions overall, then bring in analytic insight to understand the parts well enough to take care of the system and know what to do when something goes wrong.

We'll begin with a simple map of the mind's three aspects—**Vital Self, Heart Self, and Head Self**—an idea echoed in many ancient systems. From there, we bring in insights from psychology, wellness, neurology, and the findings of ancient mindfulness traditions. The result is a clear and flexible framework that helps you actually use what you learn.

A Banana, a Mind, and a Model

Did you know you can separate a banana into three sections lengthwise just using one finger?

If you've never tried it, peel a ripe banana and look at the bottom. There may be a little plug there called the *style remnant* or the *floral end*, a leftover piece from the banana flower. It's edible, but most people remove it. Go ahead and take it off if it's there.

Next, gently wiggle your finger into the little opening left behind. With just a bit of pressure, the banana naturally separates into three segments.

It's a little surprising at first. Most people think of a banana as one thing. But when you look more closely, you can see it's made up of three sections.

In a way, the mind is just like that.

We experience ourselves as one thing—just *me*. But under the surface, the mind is built from three distinct yet interconnected aspects. And when you know how to look, those parts naturally reveal themselves.

The Vital Self, Heart Self, and Head Self are not just poetic metaphors, they reflect real, observable aspects of how your brain and nervous system function. They show up in how you move and react, how you connect with others, and how you think and make sense of the world. Understanding these Three Selves gives you a powerful model for navigating life with more clarity, regulation, and self-awareness.

A Pattern Through Time

The idea that the human mind is made up of three distinct but interconnected aspects isn't new. Throughout history, cultures have described this triadic structure in different ways:

- Greek philosophy spoke of the soma (body), psyche (soul or emotion), and nous (mind or intellect).
- In Christian theology, you'll find references to body, soul, and spirit, each playing a different role in the human experience.
- Indian philosophy, particularly in the Upanishads, speaks of annamaya (physical body), manomaya (mental-emotional body), and vijnanamaya (wisdom or discerning mind).
- In Islamic thought, the self is sometimes described as a balance of nafs (instinct/desire), qalb (heart), and aql (intellect).
- In modern psychology, we see the idea emerge in different forms: somatic therapies target body-based dysregulation, emotion-focused therapies center on relational wounds, and cognitive therapies engage thoughts and belief systems.
- In modern neuroscience, the Triune Brain model proposed by Paul MacLean in the 1960's divided the brain into three functional layers: the reptilian brain (instinct and arousal), limbic system (emotion and social bonding), and neocortex (thinking and reasoning).

Across time and culture, people have recognized that the mind isn't just one thing, it's a system with three interconnected aspects.

The Three Selves

The Mind Matrix Model builds on this deep lineage. It gives modern names and functional clarity to three core dimensions of the self.

The Vital Self

This is your body-centered Self. It governs survival instincts, energy regulation, sensory input, and energy level. The Vital Self is where you feel fatigue or restlessness, groundedness or activation. It handles patterns like fight, flight, or freeze. When your stomach clenches or your breath shortens, this is the Vital Self speaking. It communicates through sensation.

The Vital Self anchors your sense of physical safety. It's constantly asking: Am I safe? Am I okay? Do I have what I need right now?

Dysregulation (imbalance) here affects your whole system, because when the body doesn't feel safe, every other part of the mind is affected. We call that *State* in the Mind Matrix Model, but we'll get to that in a bit.

The Heart Self

This is your emotional and relational Self. It holds your capacity for feelings and connection, for empathy, love, grief, shame, and intimacy. The Heart Self is the part of you that longs to belong, that seeks connection, and that holds emotional wounds. It's also that aspect that seeks alone time to regulate and restore emotional balance, allowing you to reconnect with yourself so you can engage more authentically with others.

It governs how you perceive other people and how you interpret emotional cues. It's where attachment patterns live, and where you store relational memory. If you feel abandoned, adored, misunderstood, or emotionally safe, you're in the realm of the Heart Self.

When the Heart Self is balanced, it allows for mutual connection, vulnerability, and healthy boundaries. When it's dysregulated, it may trigger withdrawal, controlling behavior, or emotional volatility.

The Head Self

This is your cognitive Self. It organizes meaning, beliefs, problem-solving, plans, language, and internal narrative. It's the storyteller, the analyst, the meaning-maker. It creates your sense of reality. The Head Self can operate in two modes that we've already discussed: Analytic Mode (focused, linear, deductive) and Holistic Mode (big-picture, intuitive, symbolic).

The Head Self is always trying to answer: Why is this happening? What does it mean? What do I do next? When balanced, it brings reflection, creativity, and strategic thinking. When imbalanced, it can swing between overanalysis and overwhelm; rigid beliefs or spaciness.

> *Each Self has its own voice, priorities, and range of expression. Together, they form the terrain of the Mind Matrix Model: the internal space of your mind for sensing, feeling, and thinking.*

Learning to recognize which Self is active at a given moment helps you respond with more clarity, flexibility, and compassion. Like the banana that naturally separates into three parts, your mind already holds this structure. The Model simply gives you a way to see what was always there.

Three Selves, Three Axes

Each of the three aspects of the mind—Vital Self, Heart Self, and Head Self—can be seen as having a particular direction in the mind's inner space. Just as a compass helps you navigate the outer world, these directions help you map your inner world.

The Vital Self: Up and Down – Energy and Arousal

The Vital Self is your base layer, the part of you that manages physical energy, instinct, and survival. It moves up and down in a vertical axis of energy or activity level, or arousal as it's called in neurology.

When your Vital Self is in high gear, or high arousal, you might feel amped up: energetic, hyper-focused, tense, or ready for action. When it shifts downward, you might feel quiet, tired, or shut down. At its best, the Vital Self flows between these poles smoothly.

This vertical rhythm has deep cultural roots. We speak of someone being uplifted, in high spirits, or rising to the occasion. We also know what it feels like to crash, to feel low, or to be dragged down by life. Many meditation traditions speak of energy rising from the lower belly upward toward the heart or the head as part of spiritual development. In both biology and metaphor, the Vital Self flows vertically.

The Heart Self: Forward and Back – Self and Other

The Heart Self governs connection. It moves forward and back, like reaching out or pulling in. You can feel this axis whenever you decide whether to open up to someone or to withdraw or protect yourself.

Some people often lead with their hearts. They're expressive, social, warm. Others tend to hold back. They process their emotions inwardly, and prefer depth over breadth. In the Mind Matrix Model, we call this the introversive-extroversive spectrum. It's not just about being shy or outgoing, but about where emotion and connection move: inward or outward.

Culturally, this front-to-back movement carries rich symbolism. We "lean in" when we're interested or engaged. We "step back" when we need space or feel unsure. In Western cultures, facing forward is often associated with progress and strength, while turning your back can imply retreat or rejection.

The Heart Self asks: Am I moving toward or away? Reaching out or withdrawing inward?

The Head Self: Left and Right – Thinking and Meaning

The Head Self governs how we think and how we make sense of our world, form beliefs, tell stories, and imagine what's possible. It is the aspect that gives us our sense of reality. Its axis runs left to right, but not just in terms of left and right brain. This is about the left and right sides of the body, a distinction found in many traditions.

On the left side of the body, the Head Self leans toward holistic, intuitive, symbolic ways of understanding. This is where we grasp patterns, feel into meaning, and connect dots without needing to name every step. On the right side of the body, the Head Self shifts toward analytic, structured, verbal thinking—making lists, drawing lines, forming arguments, and defining categories.

Cultures throughout history have attached meaning to this left-right polarity:

- In Latin, dexter (right) became associated with skill, favor, and correctness—hence dexterity and right as both direction and righteousness. Sinister (left) came to mean unlucky or dangerous—not because of anything innate, but because of longstanding social bias.
- Similarly, in French, droit (right) means law, straightness, and correctness, while gauche (left) means awkward or clumsy.
- In Chinese medicine, the left side of the body is often linked with yin—receptive, intuitive, and interior—while the right is associated with yang—active, assertive, and exterior.
- In modern culture, political terms mirror thinking styles: liberals, who tend to favor Holistic Mode thinking, are referred to as the Left, while conservatives, who more often operate in Analytic Mode, are called the Right.

Even before neuroscience, people intuited that different sides of the body could express different kinds of mind. Modern neuroscience later discovered that these perceptions loosely track with crossed wiring in the brain: the left body connects to the right brain (which processes big-picture and intuitive functions), and the right body connects to the left brain (which handles more verbal and logical tasks).

So in the Mind Matrix Model, the Head Self axis runs:

Left Body → Holistic Mode (symbolic, spatial, emotional)

Right Body → Analytic Mode (verbal, logical, structured)

Both are essential. Trouble arises not when we favor one, but when we get stuck in either being rigidly analytic or floating in unfocused symbolism. Healing and clarity often come not from choosing a side, but from learning how to move between them gracefully.

So Why a Matrix?

In the Mind Matrix Model, the three axes of each Self form an underlying space that the mind functions within. You can picture this structure in three-dimensional space:

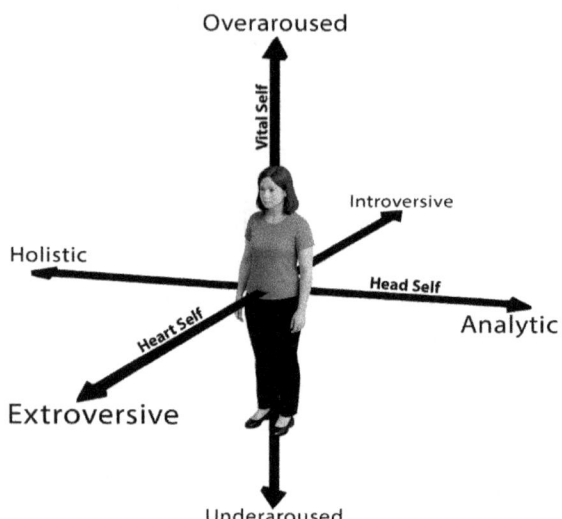

The Vital Self moves along a vertical axis, from Low Mode to High Mode, ranging from collapse to hyperarousal.

The Heart Self is oriented along a front-to-back axis, moving between being focused inward (internal emotion and self-awareness) or outward (connection to others and groups) We call these Introversive Mode and Extroversive Mode.

The Head Self is placed on a left-to-right axis. The left side of the body is traditionally associated with Holistic Mode—big picture and intuitive understanding; the right with Analytic Mode—logical and deductive thinking.

When we combine these three axes of movements—up and down (Vital Self), forward and back (Heart Self), and left and right (Head Self), we're not just describing tendencies. We're mapping a space.

Imagine standing in the center of a three-dimensional space. Your energy moves up or down depending on how activated or calm your body feels. Your emotions pull you forward or backward, reaching out or drawing in. And your thoughts drift left or right, between big picture and detailed logic.

The Oxford Dictionary defines a matrix as *"an environment or material in which something develops; a surrounding medium or structure."*

That's exactly what the Mind Matrix is: **the internal space in which your thoughts, feelings and sensations create your experience, your sense of self, and your relationships.**

This isn't just metaphor. Modern cognitive science describes the brain and nervous system along with the senses as a predictive modeling system, constantly constructing and refining an internal simulation of reality.

What does this mean?

We don't just perceive the world as it is; we experience a version of it, an internal model shaped by past experiences, sensory input, beliefs, and expectations.

That internal model is constantly updating, deeply influenced by our bodily state, our emotional landscape, and our thought patterns. What the Mind Matrix Model calls the Vital, Heart, and Head Selves.

Your Matrix is not passive. It determines what you notice, how you interpret it, how you respond, and even what you believe is possible.

State: The Ups and Downs Over Time

But just as in the outer world, along with these three dimensions there's one more dimension: time. That's where **State** comes in.

Your State—whether grounded or dysregulated, Positive or Negative—moves up and down over time and affects the entire Matrix. It's like being above water or below water, distinctly different experiences.

When your State is Positive, steady and regulated, everything feels easier and lighter. When it's Negative and dysregulated, everything feels harder and darker.

Think of State as a dimmer switch for the entire mind. It determines how brightly or dimly your mental kingdom is lit, shaping your perceptions, emotions, and thoughts.

These are the overall modes your mind operates in, which we can simply define as either Thrive Mode or Survive Mode.

State colors the entire system, influencing how each Self experiences and expresses itself. It determines how easily each Self moves between its two Modes, how they interact with each other, and thereby your overall regulation (balance) and mood.

State in the Mind Matrix Model

As we covered, State exists on a spectrum, from a very *Positive State* (clarity, openness, adaptability) to a very *Negative State* (reactivity, defensiveness, survival-focused).

While there is a spectrum between the Positive State and the Negative State, the transition between these States isn't gradual—*it's instant and often dramatic.*

One moment everything feels bright and manageable and your conscious mind is in the driver's seat. The next, a trigger plunges you into anxiety, anger, or shutdown and you become reactive. Your learned Scripts and your unconscious take over to one degree or another and your conscious mind is no longer running the show.

It's really like you are two different people sometimes, with different goals and a different view of the world. I'm sure you've had the experience of coming out of the Negative State and feeling bewildered, wondering what you were thinking, or feeling ashamed.

Your State affects how each Self functions:

Vital Self:
Positive State—Safe Mode. Balanced energy, well grounded.
Negative State—Threat Mode. Hypervigilance, hyperreactive, aggressive, or shut down.

Heart Self:
Positive State—Content Mode. Secure connections and a warm sense of yourself or positive self-esteem.
Negative State—Discontent Mode. Withdrawal, fear, or mistrust and a negative sense of yourself or negative self-esteem.

Head Self:
Positive State—Positive Mode. Flexible, clear thinking, generally optimistic. Reality looks overall positive.
Negative State—Negative Mode. Mental rigidity or chaos, generally pessimistic. Reality looks overall negative.

Here are some qualities of each State, compared to their related quality in the opposite State:

Positive/Balanced State (Thrive)	Negative/Reactive State (Survive)
Conscious, Centered	Reactive
Egalitarian	Hierarchical
Pleasure Seeking	Distraction/Relief Seeking
Creativity, Engagement	Reactive Actions
Focused on Positives	Focused on Negatives
Spectrum Viewpoint	Binary Viewpoint (ex. good/bad)
Thrive, Flourishing	Survival Orientation
Bountiful	Zero Sum, Never Enough
Awareness/Mindfulness	Vigilance
Discernment	Judgment
Agency, Empowerment	Victimhood
Gratitude	Focused on Lack
Contentment	Discontentment
Love	Fear

Other Aspects of the Mind Matrix Model

There are a number of other facets to the Model that we'll be going into. Here's a brief overview.

Dysregulation and Trauma

We've talked about regulation and mentioned dysregulation. Dysregulation means your system has lost its balance—it can't return to calm after stress. You may feel on edge, shut down, emotionally reactive, or just "off" without knowing why.

Trauma is what happens when an experience overwhelms your system's ability to cope. It leaves lasting imprints on the body and mind, either due to duration, intensity, or a combination of both, often locking in patterns of protection.

In the Mind Matrix, trauma and dysregulation are closely linked. Trauma causes dysregulation by trapping the system in the protective Negative State. Dysregulation makes you more vulnerable to trauma by narrowing your ability to adapt or recover. Most people carry some degree of both.

This book will help you recognize how trauma and dysregulation show up in your Vital, Heart, and Head Selves and how to work with both immediate symptoms and long-term healing.

Scripts, Triggers, and Sentries

Scripts are learned, automatic responses within each of the Selves, like programs running in the background taking care of everyday tasks, such as waking up and calming down (Vital Self), relating to others or managing your inner emotional state (Heart Self), and interpreting information or making decisions (Head Self).

Some Scripts are protective and reactive; these are called **Sentries**. They're often old strategies trying to keep you safe, even when the danger is no longer real. For example, getting defensive with a partner who reminds you of a critical parent.

A **trigger** is anything that reminds your system of past pain or threat and pulls you into a Negative State. This can activate a Sentry protective response like shutting down, lashing out, or people-pleasing. For example, the Vital Self might freeze or tense up; the Heart Self might become overly appeasing or controlling or withdrawn; and the Head Self might spiral into worst-case thinking, paranoia, or rigid mental Loops. Because triggers shift you into a Negative State, they often reduce or temporarily disable the conscious mind's ability to reflect, understand, or intervene.

These patterns aren't fixed. With awareness and the help of what in the Mind Matrix Model is called your **Reflective Catalyst** (your conscious ability to evaluate and redirect internal processes), you can change your Scripts and deactivate outdated Sentries.

Loops and Overrides

When Scripts or Sentries keep firing, your system can get stuck in a **Loop**—a repeating cycle that moves between the Selves. For example, an uncomfortable body reaction (Vital) sparks emotion (Heart), which fuels anxious thoughts (Head), which increases physical discomfort (Vital again), and so on.

The Mind Matrix offers **Override Strategies**, short-term fast techniques or long-term deep techniques that can interrupt Loops and restore balance. These can include things like grounding, breathwork, cognitive interrupts, journaling, or movement.

The goal isn't to control your system with force, it's to give your mind new, appropriate input it can use to change old patterns and beliefs. With practice, you'll learn to identify the Loop you're in, notice which Self or Selves are driving it, and apply a balancing Override.

How the Mind Learns to Be Itself

Where do our patterns come from—the ways we react, connect, or think? The way your Three Selves (Vital, Heart, and Head) function isn't random. It's shaped by a blend of **genetics** and **environment**. Genetics gives you the foundation of your sensitivity, temperament, and emotional wiring. But it's your early environment—including how you were held, soothed, touched, and related to—that teaches your system how to respond to the world.

Put simply: our early environment "teaches" the Three Selves how to operate.

This process unfolds in a sequence the Mind Matrix Model calls **Self-Other Development**: the growing ability to distinguish the difference between yourself and others. It forms the foundation for regulation, empathy, and clear thinking, and for your model of reality.

> **Vital Self (0–12 months)** Begins with awareness of the body, of self and others, and of the level of safety. The infant learns "I have a body, and I'm separate from the world." This stage builds trust, grounding, and a sense of physical comfort or, if disrupted, leaves the body bracing or shutting down.
>
> **Heart Self (9 months–3+ years)** Brings emotion and relationship online. The child begins feeling other people's emotions, testing boundaries (No!), and seeking connection. This stage wires the social brain, empathy, and self-worth.
>
> **Head Self (3–12+ years)** Adds thought and perspective. The child starts asking why, understanding that other people have their own thoughts and beliefs (called Theory of Mind in psychology), and forming belief systems. When earlier foundations are strong, the Head Self becomes open, flexible, and able to hold multiple truths. If not, it can become rigid, anxious, or overly dependent on others for clarity.

What Happens When Development Is Disrupted

When Self-Other Development is supported, the Selves become balanced and integrated. But trauma, neglect, or chronic stress can throw that balance off and deeply affect how you feel and interact. For example:

- Emotionally intense but easily overwhelmed = Heart Self imbalance
- Smart and reflective but disconnected from the body = Head Self dominant over Vital Self
- Restless or exhausted = Vital Self instability
- Withdrawn or flat = Vital and Heart Selves suppressed by prolonged stress.

These patterns aren't flaws, they're adaptations. Your system learned to survive in whatever conditions it was given. The Mind Matrix Model helps you understand your adaptive patterns, recognize where development got stuck, and find practical ways to restore flexibility and balance.

Understanding where your own development might have been supported or disrupted gives you the power to change. You can begin to notice your patterns, rework old Scripts, and build new ways of relating to yourself and others. That's the heart of the Mind Matrix Model.

The Emergent Properties of the Mind

The Mind Matrix Model is based on *emergent properties of the mind*—meaning that the whole is greater than the sum of its parts. It's like a symphony orchestra, where the music relies on each musician following the conductor, their music notes, and those around them. Otherwise, if everyone is playing different parts at different speeds, it would just be noise.

Your mind arises from the interaction of multiple systems, including your brain, your gut brain, your autonomic nervous system, your body, and your interactions with the world and others. These pieces aren't just separate—they're constantly working as a team:

- A relaxed nervous system (Vital Self) can make it easier to connect with others (Heart Self) or think clearly (Head Self).
- Strong relationships (Heart Self) can calm your body (Vital Self) and even help you see things more positively (Head Self).
- Spending time being creative or figuring things out (Head Self) can help you feel more relaxed (Vital Self) and happier (Heart Self).

The bigger picture: When these parts are in sync, you are in the Positive State. Life just feels better. You feel clearer, more grounded, and better able to handle whatever comes your way. Together, they create this amazing system that lets us grow, adapt, and thrive.

The Mind as a Kingdom

In the Mind Matrix Model, we use the analogy of a kingdom to describe how the mind works.

> The conscious mind is the **Monarch**, the ruler who holds the power to guide and direct.
>
> The unconscious aspects of each Self, the parts of our minds that we're not aware of or minimally aware of, are the **Ministers**, advisors and managers who carry out the Monarch's directives and manage their respective domains.

This kingdom analogy is not just about structure; it's about empowerment. Many of us feel like we aren't in control, that we are victims of our mind's reactions and habits.

As the Monarch, you have the ability to take charge of your state of mind, guiding your Three Ministers to work in harmony.

Regulation Before Awareness

While understanding your mind is important, State regulation comes first. You cannot think clearly or process emotions effectively if you are triggered and in the Negative State.

A central component of your State is anxiety, which I like to call ***the fire under the pot of your nervous system***. The higher the anxiety, the more likely you will be in the Negative State and the more likely your mind and body won't operate optimally. Over time, chronic anxiety can destroy your mental and physical health.

In today's world, most of us are carrying some level of anxiety, which means some level of dysregulation and vulnerability to triggers into the Negative State.

State regulation is best done from the bottom up—balancing the Vital Self in many cases is enough to lower anxiety and greatly improve the State of each Self, but it also makes it much easier to regulate the Heart and Head Selves.

Once we cover the Model in more detail, we're going to look into how to work with your anxiety, starting with *Chapter 5 - Stress and Anxiety in the Mind Matrix Model*, before we begin to work with your Three Selves.

Final Thoughts: The Journey to Balance

The Mind Matrix Model invites you on a journey of self-discovery, growth, and transformation. The goal is not just to understand your mind, although that by itself can be very helpful. The goal is also to learn practical ways to manage your State, work with your Selves, shift patterns, and heal deeply embedded survival responses.

> **First, focus on regulation.** Learn to stabilize your State so that awareness can be useful.
>
> **Then, explore balancing dysregulation and reprogramming Sentries.** If deeper issues persist, address them with targeted approaches.
>
> **Finally, cultivate Self-integration.** Align your Three Selves for clarity, adaptability, and well-being.

Your mind is not locked. Change is possible, not by trying to control your Selves but by learning to work with them. Working to restore balance and create a life that is more nourishing and sustainable.

You are the Monarch in your inner kingdom, and you have the ability to change.

The following chapters will guide you through the process, step by step.

Welcome to the Mind Matrix Model!

Chapter Two

Meet the Three Selves of Your Mind

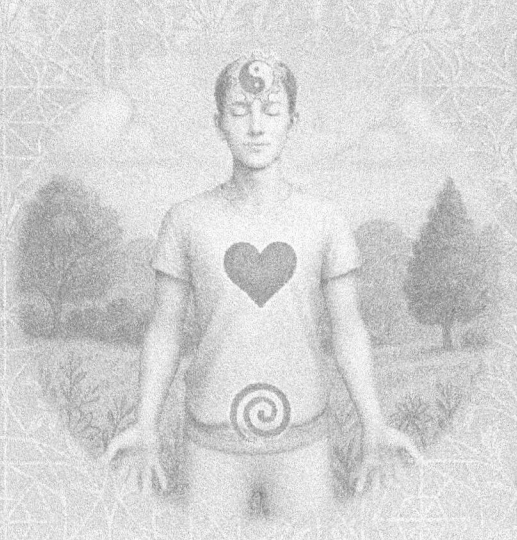

The Kingdom of the Mind

Once upon a time, in the vast Kingdom of the Mind, a great castle stood. This castle, known as the Castle of Selves, housed the three essential levels of the mind: the Vital Self, the Heart Self, and the Head Self. Each level had its unique functions and inhabitants, and all worked in harmony under the guidance of the Monarch, the conscious mind...

The Foundation: The Vital Level

The castle's first floor was where the stewards of the kingdom, guided by the Minister of the Vital Self, managed its foundational needs.

Engineers maintained the heating and plumbing systems, ensuring the castle was warm and comfortable. The kitchens were always alive with the aroma of hearty meals prepared to sustain the castle's inhabitants. In the gymnasium, knights trained diligently, keeping their bodies strong and agile. The clinic, with its expert physicians, oversaw the health and wellbeing of all the castle's inhabitants.

Down below, the stables housed magnificent horses, ready to carry the Monarch and knights into the surrounding countryside to gather resources, face external challenges, or explore the wonders of nature.

When the Monarch felt unwell or noticed dangers at the edges of the forest, her attention would naturally shift to this level. "The kingdom needs its strength," the Monarch would say, donning armor to join the knights in their exercises. She oversaw the stockpiling of food and the maintenance of defenses, ensuring that the castle's vital systems operated seamlessly.

The Heart Level

Above, on the second floor, a more serene environment awaited. Quiet rooms with warm sunlight streaming through stained glass windows offered spaces for poetry, music, and meditation. Artists and musicians as well as social planners lived here, crafting beauty and harmony to enrich the kingdom, guided by the Minister of the Heart. One special doorway opened to the village and community beyond the castle, where the Monarch would mingle with the townsfolk, engaging in conversations and sharing wisdom.

When a troubling feeling arose or a longing for connection was felt, the Monarch climbed to this level. She sat with poets to reflect on emotions, listened to musicians who transformed feelings into melodies, and penned letters to strengthen bonds with allies. Through the village door, she ventured out to connect with others, resolving disputes, fostering relationships, and celebrating shared joys.

The Summit: The Head Level

The topmost floor of the castle was a hub of intellect and governance. Here, the Monarch worked in a grand hall managed by the Minister of the Mind and their wise assistants, the mathematicians specializing in analytic thinking and the wizards specializing in holistic thinking. This was where decisions were made, plans were devised, and solutions to the kingdom's challenges were crafted. The wizards brought insights into the mysteries of the universe, while the mathematicians worked out elegant solutions for any problems faced by the Monarch.

When a complex challenge arose, the Monarch gathered these wise advisors to deliberate. They worked tirelessly even while the Monarch slept or was otherwise occupied, balancing analysis and intuition, detail and overview. She often consulted the artists and social planners of the second floor or the knights on the first floor for their perspectives. Together, they crafted innovative solutions and strategies for the kingdom's prosperity.

The Flow of Attention

The Monarch's attention flowed naturally between these levels, guided by the kingdom's needs. During times of illness or physical strain, her focus settled on the Vital level, addressing the physical needs of the kingdom and fortifying the castle's defenses. When emotions stirred or the call for connection grew loud, the Monarch would climb to the Heart level, engaging with the artists and social experts of the kingdom as well as with the people of the village. And when decisions needed clarity, or the kingdom faced intellectual challenges, she ascended to the Head level, working alongside her advisors.

This dynamic interplay ensured that the Kingdom of the Mind thrived, its castle standing as a testament to balance and integration. Through her attentive stewardship, the Monarch cultivated harmony, drawing strength from each level and weaving their contributions into a unified whole.

Thus, the Kingdom of the Mind remained resilient, healthy, creative, and full of life—a place of peace and prosperity under the guidance of the Monarch.

Welcome back to our journey through the Mind Matrix Model! In the last chapter, we introduced you to the idea of your mind as a kingdom, with you as the wise Monarch overseeing everything. Now, let's dive deeper into the three key players in this kingdom: the Three Selves. Each of these Selves represents a core part of who you are, and they all work together to help you navigate life. So, let's get to know them better!

The Vital Self: Your Body's Energy Manager

The Vital Self is all about keeping you alive and kicking. Think of it as your body's thermostat, determining how much energy is needed. It's what makes sure you wake up in the morning, get hungry at the right times, and respond to challenges when needed. It's responsible for:

> *Physical Energy:* Raising your thermostat to make sure you have the energy to get through your day, and lowering your thermostat when it's time to rest.
>
> *Survival Instincts:* Keeping you safe by managing your fight-or-flight response.
>
> *Thriving:* Helping you feel alive and ready to engage with the world.

How It Works

Think of your Vital Self as the backstage crew of your life—quietly keeping things running behind the scenes. It's what manages your energy, alertness, breathing, and basic body rhythms. You don't have to think about making your heart beat or digesting lunch—that's your Vital Self at work.

Here are the key systems it uses:

- **Brainstem & Reticular Activating System (RAS):** These control your alertness. If you're wide awake or deeply asleep, that's the RAS adjusting your internal "dimmer switch."

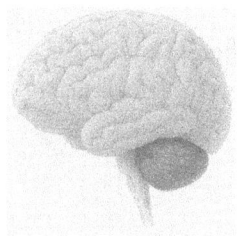

  - **Cerebellum:** Coordinates movement and stores muscle memory—like riding a bike or dancing without thinking. It also helps with emotional balance.

- **Autonomic Nervous System (ANS):** This system toggles between your "go mode" (Sympathetic Nervous System or SNS)—stress, action, alertness) and your "rest mode" (Parasympathetic Nervous System or PNS)—recovery, digestion, calm).
- **Enteric Nervous System (ENS):** Sometimes called your "second brain," it's the gut network that affects digestion, mood, and overall well-being.

These systems talk constantly with the rest of your body and brain, adjusting how energized or calm you feel. When in balance, your Vital Self helps you feel alive, steady, and ready to respond to the world. When off balance, you might feel anxious, exhausted, physically depressed, shut down, or all of these in a loop.

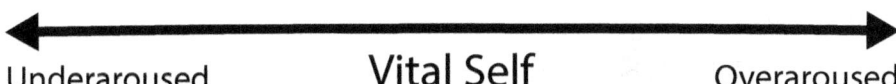

Underaroused   **Vital Self**   Overaroused

The Vital Self Axis: Arousal

The Vital Self operates along an arousal axis, ranging from lower to higher states of energy and engagement, called lower and higher arousal modes. Here's what that looks like:

Low Arousal: In this state, the body is relaxed, conserving energy, and focused on restoration. This can range from deep rest to a calm, reflective state, allowing for physical recovery and mental clarity. An example of lower activation is lying in a hammock, watching the clouds drift by, or simply sitting in quiet meditation.

High Arousal: Here, the body is mobilized for engagement, focus, and action. This can range from moderate alertness to intense physical exertion. Higher activation is essential for tasks requiring concentration, dynamic movement, or quick responses. It is especially active when you feel threatened, called "fight or flight." Examples of high arousal include feeling energized during an invigorating hike, delivering a speech, or preparing for an athletic competition.

Example

Imagine you're at a party. If you're in low arousal, you might want to find a quiet corner to recharge. If you're in high arousal, you're probably the life of the party, dancing and engaging with everyone.

The Heart Self: Your Relationship & Emotional Guide

The Heart Self is all about your connections with others and your inner emotional world. It's like your personal relationship counselor and emotional coach rolled into one. Here's what it does:

- **Emotional Awareness and Regulation:** Helps you feel, understand, and navigate your emotions, whether it's expressing joy, calming down when upset, or working through complex feelings.
- **Social Interactions**: Guides you in forming and maintaining relationships, from casual acquaintances to deep friendships.
- **Empathy**: Allows you to understand and share the feelings of others, fostering connection and compassion.

How It Works

The Heart Self is all about emotions, relationships, and making sense of your social world. At its heart is the limbic system, a network of brain structures in the *cerebrum* (the uppermost part of the brain) that handles feelings, emotional memories, and social interactions. Here are the key players:

- **Amygdala:** This almond-shaped structure in the temporal lobe of the cerebrum acts like your emotional alarm system, processing emotions like fear and anger, especially when survival instincts kick in.
- **Hippocampus:** Also found in the temporal lobe of the cerebrum, the hippocampus helps you form emotional memories, tying your feelings to specific experiences.
- **Thalamus:** Acts as a central relay station, filtering and forwarding sensory input to other parts of the brain, including the amygdala and cortex. It's critical for how emotional and social signals are prioritized.
- **Hypothalamus:** Regulates autonomic and endocrine responses tied to emotions and relationships — everything from stress hormones to bonding neurochemistry (like oxytocin). It's the key bridge between emotional experience and bodily state.

- **Anterior Cingulate Cortex (ACC):** Sitting in the frontal area of the cerebrum, the ACC helps you manage emotions and navigate social interactions, like handling conflicts or reading social cues.

These areas work together to process emotions and connect them with your relationships and memories, keeping your emotional world in balance.

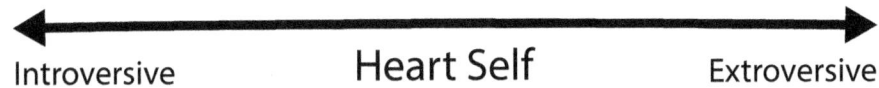

Introversive   **Heart Self**   Extroversive

The Heart Self Axis: Introversion to Extroversion

This Self operates along an axis from introversive to extroversive. This can be a short term change of focus based on what's currently going on, but it can also be an overall, long-term tendency. Here's what that means:

Introversive Mode: In the short term, you might feel the need to spend time alone or in small groups for some quiet time to recharge after social interactions, for example. Someone who generally feels more comfortable in solitude, one to one, or small groups leans toward being an introvert.

Extroversive Mode: In the shorter term, you might be feeling energized by being around others and engaging in social activities and in group settings. If you generally prefer engaging with others in social environments and feel drained if you have to spend too much time solo, you're most likely an extrovert.

Example

Picture yourself at a family gathering. If you're more introverted, you might enjoy chatting with a few close relatives but feel drained after a while. If you're more extroverted, you might thrive on the energy of the crowd and feel invigorated by the social interaction.

> *One of my more lighthearted observations, looking back at the COVID-19 pandemic of 2020-22, was that the introverts were generally happy to be isolated and stuck at home. Meanwhile, the extroverts were climbing the walls.*

The Head Self: Your Thinking & Problem-Solving

The Head Self is your thinking machine. It's all about processing information, solving problems, and making sense of the world. This Self is like your personal problem solver and strategist.

Your Head Self is the part of you that thinks, plans, solves problems, and makes sense of the world. It's based in your cerebral cortex—the brain's outer layer—but also involves deeper areas like the hippocampus (for memory), the thalamus (for filtering information), and the anterior cingulate (for focus and conflict resolution).

How It Works

The Head Self works in two main modes:

Analytic Mode is logical, detail-oriented, and step-by-step. It's what you use when doing math, writing a report, or fixing something.

Holistic Mode is intuitive and big-picture. It connects ideas, reads between the lines, and picks up on patterns—like when you're brainstorming or sensing the mood in a room.

You've probably heard about "left-brain" vs "right-brain" thinking—analytic vs creative—but in reality, your brain is always using both sides, with the two hemispheres constantly communicating. Most people lean more toward one mode than the other, but both are important.

When the Head Self is balanced, you can shift easily between logical thinking and creative insight. When out of balance, you might get stuck in overthinking or lose focus and drift. We'll explore how to bring these modes into better harmony in the Balancing the Head Self chapter.

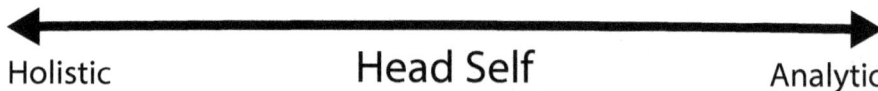

Holistic   **Head Self**   Analytic

The Head Self Axis: Analytic to Holistic Modes

This Self operates along an axis from Analytic to Holistic Modes. Here's what that looks like:

Analytic Mode: Breaking things down into smaller parts and analyzing them step by step. It's great for tasks like math problems or organizing information.

Holistic Mode: Seeing the whole picture and understanding how things fit together. It's excellent for creative projects or understanding complex systems.

Example

Think about solving a puzzle. If you're using Analytic Mode, you'll focus on the individual pieces and how they fit together. If you're using Holistic Mode, you'll look at the overall image and try to understand the pattern.

The Interplay of the Three Selves

These Three Selves are like a team, constantly interacting and influencing each other. For example:

- **Vital Self Boost:** When you're feeling energetic (Vital Self), it can boost your confidence and make you feel more social (Heart Self).
- **Stress Impact:** When you're stressed (Heart Self), it can make it harder to think clearly (Head Self).

By understanding these interactions, you can learn to create balance and harmony within your mind. As the Monarch of your mental kingdom, you have the power to guide the interplay of the Three Selves, ensuring they work together to support your well-being.

Conclusion: Embrace Your Inner Team

I hope this introduction to the Three Selves shows you that you're not just a collection of parts; your mind and body are a dynamic, interconnected system. By getting to know your Three Selves, you can better understand yourself and take charge of your mental and emotional health.

In the next chapter, we'll explore the roles of the Monarch, the Ministers of each of the Selves, and Scripts—the key players in orchestrating this system—so you can begin to unlock your mind's full potential.

So, embrace your inner team and start building the balanced, thriving life you deserve!

Chapter Three
Monarch, Ministers & Scripts

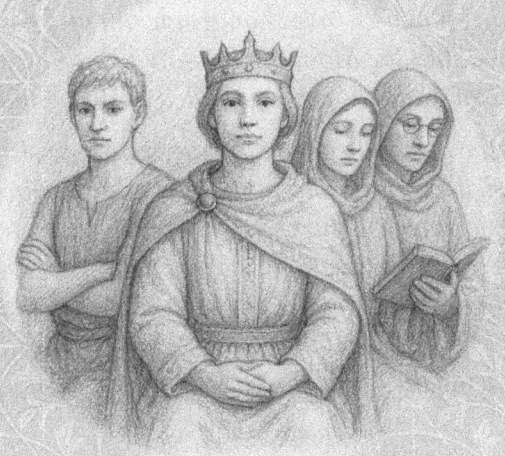

The Kingdom Under Siege: The Negative State

The Kingdom of the Mind was in turmoil. Trolls lurked at the edges of the countryside, lumbering toward the castle and venturing into the village to harass the villagers, their guttural grunts and heavy footsteps echoing through the night. Fear gripped the people, their murmurs swelling into angry accusations: "The Monarch has failed us!" they cried. "Where is the plan to protect us?"

Meanwhile, the wizards and mathematicians were locked in heated debate, their voices rising in frustration. The wizards spoke of casting great spells to drive the trolls away, but the mathematicians countered with calculations of risk and resource depletion. The halls of the Head Self level rang with discord, each argument pulling the Monarch in a different direction.

The Monarch wandered restlessly, moving from one level of the castle to another, seeking answers yet finding only conflict. On the Vital level, she consulted the knights, who sharpened their swords and pushed strongly for direct action. "We should ride out and confront the trolls!" they exclaimed. But the Monarch hesitated, for the knights could not guarantee victory and the cost of a failed battle would be catastrophic.

Throughout the castle, the Monarch faced the anguish of her people. Some wept, pleading for protection; others shouted in anger, blaming the Monarch for their plight. Overwhelmed by their sorrow and rage, the Monarch sought solace in the quiet meditation spaces and the soothing strains of music of the Heart Level. Yet even these could not ease the weight of responsibility. Sleep eluded her, and many nights were spent pacing the dimly lit corridors of the castle, pondering what to do.

A Gathering of Minds and Hearts
In the depths of this Negative State, the Monarch realized she could not solve this crisis alone. Summoning her courage, she sought the counsel of a few trusted advisors, whispering questions in the stillness of night. These hushed conversations brought a flicker of clarity.

"Bring the kingdom together," one advisor suggested. "We must unite our strengths."

And so, the Monarch issued a decree. All the inhabitants of the castle—knights, artists, social planners, musicians, mathematicians, and wizards—were called to assemble in the grand hall. The hall was adorned with candles, their warm light pushing back the shadows of fear.

When all were gathered, the Monarch stood at the center and spoke. "Our kingdom is threatened," she said, her voice steady despite the storm in her heart. "The trolls are encroaching, and fear has made us turn against one another. But we are stronger together. Tonight, let us speak, let us listen, and let us create something greater than our fear."

The Council of Integration

The knights shared their observations of the trolls' movements, speaking of their strength and cunning. The artists painted vivid images of the trolls, capturing both their menace and their odd, foolish nature, while the musicians composed haunting melodies that reflected the kingdom's collective anxiety.

The mathematicians presented detailed maps and calculations, suggesting defensive structures to protect the village. The wizards offered incantations that could amplify the villagers' courage and create illusions to confuse the trolls. The village elders shared stories of past trials, reminding everyone of their resilience and ingenuity. And the social planners spoke of a strategy to engage the villagers in defending the kingdom.

As the night wore on, the tension began to dissolve. The music swelled, and the people danced, their movements weaving a tapestry of unity and hope. The Monarch listened intently, her mind piecing together the insights of all who had spoken. Slowly, a plan began to take shape.

A Solution Emerges

The next morning, the Monarch called the kingdom to action. Guided by the collective wisdom of her people, she outlined a multifaceted plan:

Fortify the Village: *Under the mathematicians' guidance, the knights and villagers built sturdy fences and reinforced walls to keep the trolls at bay.*

Create a Sanctuary: *The wizards enchanted the meditation spaces to serve as sanctuaries, where the Monarch and her subjects could find solace and strength during moments of fear.*

Employ Illusions: *Using their art and magic, the artists and wizards created lifelike illusions of enormous stone giants—beings the trolls feared. These illusions were placed at the edges of the forest to deter the trolls.*

Build Connection: *The musicians organized communal gatherings, where villagers could sing, dance, and share their fears. These gatherings strengthened bonds and lifted spirits, making the community more resilient.*

Engage the Trolls: *The knights, guided by the wisdom of the wizards and mathematicians as well as the village elders, ventured cautiously into the forest. Rather than fighting, they left great cauldrons of food at a safe distance, gradually luring the trolls away from the castle and toward the mountains where they could feast in peace.*

Restoration and Renewal
In the days that followed, the kingdom began to heal. The trolls, distracted and frightened by the illusions and appeased by the offerings, moved further into the mountains. The villagers, once paralyzed by fear, found strength in their unity and the knowledge that their voices had shaped the solution. The castle's halls, once heavy with discord, now echoed with laughter and music.

The Monarch, though weary, felt a deep sense of peace. By embracing the collective wisdom of the kingdom, she had transformed a time of darkness into an opportunity for growth. And as she stood atop the castle, gazing out at the peaceful countryside, she knew the Kingdom of the Mind had emerged stronger than ever.

The Mind as a Kingdom, Part II

As I said in the last chapter, in the Mind Matrix Model we use the governance model of a kingdom or monarchy as an analogy or a model for how the mind works, with the conscious mind as the Monarch, the leader. The unconscious mind is divided among each of the Three Selves, and we call them Ministers—the Vital Minister, Heart Minister, and Head Minister. It's a helpful way of understanding the different levels of control and decision-making within your mind.

The Monarch: Your Conscious Mind

The Monarch represents your conscious mind in our kingdom of the mind, the part of you that is self-aware, deliberate, and responsible for making decisions such as what actions you should take or what you should focus on. Like a ruler overseeing the kingdom of the mind, the Monarch provides overall guidance and direction, ensuring that the different parts of the mind work together effectively. And like a ruler overseeing a kingdom, there are many things going on that the Monarch is unaware of.

The Monarch has partial awareness of all Three Selves:

- It senses physical energy and bodily awareness in the Vital Self.
- It observes emotional and relational dynamics in the Heart Self.
- It focuses on thoughts, logic, problems and decision-making in the Head Self.

But this awareness is only partial, because much of what happens within the Three Selves occurs at an unconscious level.

The Reflective Catalyst

In the Mind Matrix, the Monarch holds the role of the *Reflective Catalyst*, which is the ability to steer the course of the Self. It makes decisions and initiates actions which are then mostly carried out by the subconscious and unconscious parts of the mind. It has the power to change old patterns and Scripts and validate new ones, but only if they are brought to conscious awareness. This reflective oversight helps ensure that your interactions and responses are right for the present situations, rather than being driven by outdated learned behaviors or Scripts.

The Ministers: The Subconscious & Unconscious

The Monarch gives orders and initiates actions, but the vast majority of the "work" is done by the *Ministers*. The Ministers represent the *subconscious* (close to conscious) and *unconscious* (deeper, farther from conscious) aspects of the mind that operate outside of your awareness. They support the Monarch by handling routine processes, retrieving information, processing issues, and performing automatic functions, freeing the conscious mind to focus on bigger decisions and problems.

Think of how much of your daily life is carried out with little or no conscious effort: brushing your teeth, getting dressed, eating, or even driving. The Monarch can intervene when needed—like deciding to take a detour while driving—but it generally relies on the Ministers to handle these routine activities.

Now compare that to learning to drive for the first time. Every detail required your full attention: checking mirrors, steering, operating the accelerator, brake, or clutch. It was hard to imagine how at some point you could do all of that with little effort or thought, but within a short time you got the hang of it, thanks to those unconscious Ministers.

Without the Ministers managing routine tasks, we would need to consciously oversee everything we do, which would quickly become overwhelming.

Each Self has its own Minister, responsible for specific aspects of the mind's functioning:

> **The Minister of the Vital Self** manages regulation of physical energy and bodily processes and awareness. It keeps the body running smoothly, adjusting heart rate, breathing, and other systems as needed.
>
> For instance, when you as the Monarch decide to exercise, the Vital Minister ensures that your body responds appropriately by increasing blood flow, oxygen intake, and energy production. It also maintains balance by calming your body after a stress response, like releasing hormones to relax after being startled, or directing energy toward digestion after a meal.
>
> And it manages your *proprioceptive awareness*, your ability to tell where your body is in the space around you. It's the reason that a

gymnast can flip and twirl through space and land on their feet. It is also the repository of movement Scripts like driving a car or playing a piano. We'll talk more about Scripts later in this chapter.

The Minister of the Heart Self oversees your emotional responses and social awareness. This Minister retrieves relevant emotional memories, shapes your tone of voice, and adjusts your body language to match social situations.

For example, when you smile back at someone who smiles at you, it's often the Heart Minister acting before the Monarch has even consciously registered the interaction. It also helps the Monarch decide how to respond emotionally by drawing on past experiences.

However, for people on the autism spectrum, the automatic functions of this Minister may work differently, making it harder to recognize or respond to social cues.

In these cases, social interactions often require more conscious effort and cognitive thought, as though learning them for the first time each time, which can make these exchanges more challenging and effortful.

The Minister of the Head Self is responsible for processing and retrieving information, evaluating issues, solving problems, and connecting ideas. When you consciously work on a problem, for instance, it's the Head Minister that pulls up relevant knowledge from your memory and presents possible solutions to the Monarch. Similarly, when you suddenly recall a book title or have a creative idea, it's this Minister quietly doing the heavy lifting behind the scenes. It helps you when you regularly appear effortlessly insightful and intelligent, like you do, even though much of the work happens unconsciously.

The Ministers in the Negative State

When your mind is triggered into the *Negative State*, the Ministers shift into survival mode and take control, often bypassing the Monarch. This can happen partially—where the Monarch struggles to regain control—or completely, where the conscious mind essentially "checks out."

For example, during an accident or traumatic event, the Ministers may take over entirely, automatically guiding your body through fight-or-flight responses, such as jumping out of the way of danger.

As a result, you may later have little or no memory of the event because the Monarch wasn't fully present—or perhaps not present at all—a phenomenon known as *dissociation*.

The Ministers in the Negative State prioritize instinctive, automatic responses that are essential for survival, such as the fight-or-flight reaction. While these responses are necessary in moments of immediate danger, they can sometimes be too forceful, overriding your conscious mind in situations that don't warrant such extreme reactions. This can lead to inappropriate or exaggerated responses, like snapping at a loved one when feeling stressed.

The Balance Between Monarch and Ministers

Together, the Monarch and the Ministers show how different levels of your mind work together to manage conscious thought, routine functioning, and instinctual responses. While the Ministers handle the majority of mental and physical processes, the Monarch's function as the Reflective Catalyst makes sure that your decisions and actions are appropriate to the situation.

Understanding this dynamic framework helps us recognize when the Ministers might take over too much or when the Monarch needs to intervene more effectively. By cultivating a better balance between these levels of the mind, you can promote greater cooperation, flexibility, and overall well-being.

The metaphor of the Monarch and the Ministers reminds us that while your conscious mind may feel like the "driver," much of the mind's work happens below the surface. Learning to work with, rather than against, this dynamic system can help you navigate life with greater ease and adaptability.

Scripts in the Kingdom of the Mind

Scripts are pre-programmed patterns of behavior that allow your mind to function efficiently by automating routine tasks and responses. Ministers (the unconscious aspects of the Three Selves) often run on autopilot Scripts—routines they've learned—to keep the kingdom safe. They free the Monarch, your conscious mind, from micromanaging details and allow the Ministers, the subconscious and unconscious aspects of the mind, to manage their domains without constant oversight.

Scripts can range from deliberate actions, like deciding how to respond in a conversation without actually thinking about it, to automatic behaviors, like flinching at a loud noise or instinctively following social norms. By using Scripts, your mind conserves energy and increases its capacity to handle complex tasks. Scripts fall into two main categories:

- **Genetic Scripts** are innate, like reflexes or survival instincts. Humans have comparatively few of these compared to other animals.
- **Learned Scripts** are shaped by experience, education, and socialization.

Each Self in the Mind Matrix operates its own Scripts:

Vital Self Scripts manage bodily functions and physical responses, such as breathing, hunger cues, and reactions to threats such as pulling your hand away from a hot stove or fight, flight or freeze in reaction to an attacker. They also carry out learned actions, like jumping rope or hammering nails.

Heart Self Scripts guide emotional reactions, social interactions, and personality patterns, like automatically reaching out to embrace when greeted or comforting a friend.

Head Self Scripts influence thinking patterns, problem-solving strategies, and decision-making habits, such as doing a budget or creating a work of art.

Sentries: The Kingdom's Protectors

Sentries are specialized Scripts that activate in the Negative State to protect the mind from perceived threats. Sentries are like the castle guards, always on the lookout for danger, sometimes raising alarm even when the danger is long past.

Each Self has its own Sentries, which respond in three ways: *advance* (confront the threat), *recede* (withdraw from the threat), or *hold* (freeze in place).

Vital Self Sentries respond to physical threats with fight (advance), flight (recede), or freeze (hold).

- **Fight/Aggression (Advance):** Physically confronting danger, such as pushing back or bracing for action.

- **Flight (Recede):** Escaping danger, like running away or avoiding harm.
- **Freeze (Hold):** Remaining motionless to avoid detection or further harm.

Heart Self Sentries react to emotional or social threats, such as rejection or conflict.

- **Dominance (Advance):** Confronting a perceived threat, such as arguing or lashing out.
- **Withdrawal (Recede):** Retreating emotionally or socially to avoid pain or rejection.
- **Appeasement (Hold):** Trying to pacify or maintain harmony, even at personal cost. This can include what psychology refers to as *fawn*, a response where a person reacts to a perceived threat from another person by attempting to please or placate them. While fawn is traditionally grouped with fight, flight, and freeze responses in trauma psychology, it is an inherently relational response. Within the Mind Matrix, appeasement—and fawn specifically—are seen as behaviors of the Heart Self, reflecting its role in managing relationships and social dynamics.

Head Self Sentries address mental challenges or uncertainty.

Overthinking (Advance): Obsessing over details or trying to find meaning, often leading to analysis paralysis.

Distraction (Recede): Avoiding mental discomfort by focusing on trivial or unrelated activities.

Perseveration (Hold): Getting stuck in repetitive thought patterns without reaching a resolution.

While Sentries are essential for protection, they can become outdated or overly reactive, which can lead to reactions that are over the top or not appropriate. By recognizing your Script patterns, bringing them into conscious awareness, the Monarch can fulfill its role as the *Reflective Catalyst,* working to recalibrate them and to make sure that the mind's protective mechanisms align with the present.

How Sentries Speak To Us

Each Self has its own way of communicating—the Vital Self through sensation and bodily awareness, the Heart Self through feelings, and the Head Self through voices and thoughts. In the same way each Sentry "speaks" to us in their own way.

Vital Self Sentry

The Vital Self focuses on physical safety and bodily awareness. Vital Self Sentries manifest as bodily sensations and instinctual reactions meant to maintain physical and energetic safety. These may surface as persistent fatigue, anxiety, or physical discomfort with an underlying message "I'm not safe," "I'm overwhelmed," or "I can't handle this."

By prompting us to withdraw or avoid potentially stressful or harmful situations, these Scripts attempt to maintain physical security, though they can also hinder genuine engagement and exploration in life.

Heart Self Sentry

The Heart Self is deeply involved in our relational and emotional experiences. Heart Self Sentries typically emerge from experiences of emotional disconnection or rejection. These might manifest as "feeling" Scripts like "I'm not lovable," "I must earn love," or "I'm too much for others to handle."

One way Heart Self Sentries show up is by pushing you to distance from someone you're close to in order to keep you safe from being emotionally hurt. For example, that feeling that you would be happier on your own, or that your partner or friend isn't as good as they could be.

These Scripts protect us by discouraging emotional vulnerability and closeness to avoid potential pain or rejection.

Head Self Sentry

The Head Self is the Self that uses words, hence Head Self Sentries are the thoughts we have that are about self-protection.

Commonly, these are critical thoughts like "I'm not smart enough," or "I always mess things up."

They could also be ones pushing you to do more—"You should be better than this," "Don't let them see me fail," or "I'm the only competent one here."

While some Head Sentries attack the self to prevent risk or rejection, others inflate the self to maintain control or avoid vulnerability. Thoughts like "No one else gets it," "I have to fix everything," or "I'm the one who always knows best" may sound confident, but they often mask a fear of being exposed, dismissed, or dependent. Both forms—self-deprecating and self-inflating—serve the same purpose: to guard the system when it doesn't feel safe enough to be vulnerable.

You're probably used to thinking that the voices in your head are you talking to you, but that's not true. *The key to understanding Head Self Sentries is knowing that they speak as though they are you.* And the way to know if it's you or not you is that Head Self Sentries are always negative, always at the core talking about what you aren't doing to protect yourself. It takes a little while and some practice to really understand this.

Recognizing and understanding these Sentries can transform our relationship with self-esteem, shifting from a perspective of inherent deficiency to one of protective responses that, while misguided, stem from a fundamental drive to keep us safe. We assume that the thoughts and feelings we have are our own, but in fact often they are not.

As we talked about earlier, one of the roles of the Monarch, your conscious self, is the Reflective Catalyst—the ability to initiate change in our unconscious or learned patterns. By learning to recognize Sentries consciously and seeing the ways that they no longer serve you, your conscious mind can catalyze your Three Selves to change, allowing for healing, growth, and a more authentic sense of self-worth.

Bringing It Home

At this point, you have all the main pieces of the Mind Matrix Model:

- ▸ The Three Selves—Vital, Heart, and Head—each with their own Axis of Action: arousal, relational focus, and cognitive orientation.
- ▸ Each Self is managed by a Minister, an aspect of your unconscious mind, which handles automatic functions and day-to-day patterns beneath conscious awareness.

- The system runs on Scripts—learned patterns of activity or response, like subroutines. These can be activated consciously (e.g., driving a car, hosting a meeting) or unconsciously (e.g., how you respond to a raised voice or navigate a disagreement). Scripts are not inherently negative, they reduce cognitive load and help you function efficiently.
- But when you're under stress, and especially when you shift into a Negative State, your system may activate Sentries: Scripts that were built to protect you in past situations of danger, rejection, or overwhelm. While they may have once been necessary for survival, Sentries can be outdated, inflexible, and maladaptive in the present.
- All of this is overseen—at least ideally—by the Monarch, your conscious self. The Monarch is responsible for guiding choices, reflecting on experience, and integrating the voices of the Three Selves.

When you're in the Positive State, the Monarch can listen clearly, coordinate responses, and help you live in alignment with what matters. But when you shift into the Negative State, the Monarch often gets pushed aside, and the Ministers of your Selves may react automatically.

- The Vital Self might try to protect you through aggression, escaping, or freezing/checking out.
- The Heart Self might collapse into people-pleasing or lash out in blame.
- The Head Self might spin into obsessive thinking or get lost in indecision.

These responses aren't flaws—they're attempts to stay safe. But they often come from old maps: things that helped you survive the past, not necessarily thrive in the present.

The task of the Monarch is not to suppress or override the Selves, but to listen, to regulate State, and to help bring the system back into alignment.

That's the real power of the Mind Matrix: it doesn't just name what's wrong, it shows you how to work with each part of yourself in a clear, compassionate, and practical way.

This isn't about being perfect. It's about building enough awareness and flexibility to return to balance—again and again.

In the next chapter, Navigating the Mind Matrix Model, we'll go over how you can use the rest of this book. You can jump to specific areas based on your present needs, or just continue reading on through the chapters.

After that, we'll look more deeply at how to navigate the Matrix in real time—especially during stress, anxiety, or emotional overload. You'll learn how to recognize which Self is most active, how to shift your State, and how to bring your Monarch back online when things start to fall apart.

Your Selves aren't problems to solve. They're parts of *you* that you can learn to understand, care for, and coordinate. And your Monarch? That's the conscious part of you learning how to lead—not by control, but by connection.

Chapter 4

Navigating the Mind Matrix Model

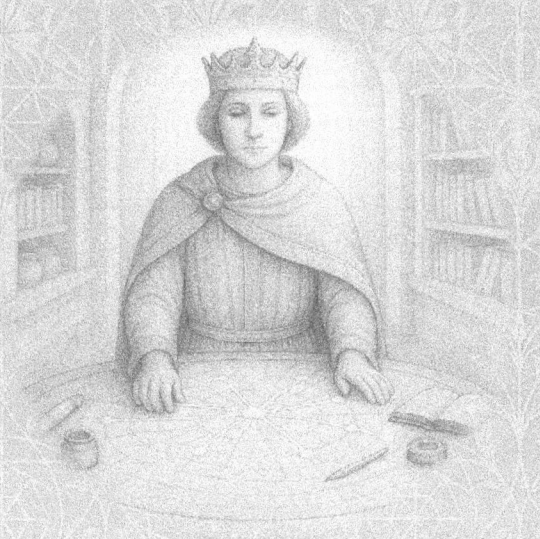

By now, you've encountered the core framework of the Mind Matrix Model—the Three Selves, State, and Self-Other along with each of their axes and how they interact. You also know about Scripts and their Negative State version, Sentries, which provide protective actions.

It's complex, and you most probably won't feel comfortable with it all on the first pass. That's okay, we're going to keep going over it as we go deeper, such that it becomes an integral part of how you view yourself and others. Just keep working on it.

This book is designed to meet you where you are. You're not expected to absorb everything in one reading. In fact, it's not that kind of book. The Mind Matrix is meant to be revisited, explored, and applied over time.

Tend Your Garden

The greatest benefits of this work come not from memorizing concepts, but from living with them and tending them like seeds. Some will take root quickly. Others may grow slowly, unfolding as your life brings new experiences, new challenges, and new insights.

Use this book as a guide along that path. The more consistently you engage with it—reading, reflecting, trying out practices—the more transformation becomes possible.

You don't have to go in order. You can start wherever your need is greatest.

A Flexible Path

If you're facing a pressing issue—anxiety, relationship conflict, emotional burnout—you can jump directly to those chapters. Each section is written to stand alone while connecting back to the full model. Wherever you begin, you'll find invitations to explore deeper.

You may also find it helpful to take multiple passes through the book:

> On your first pass, highlight what speaks to you.
>
> Try a few practices, skip around, take notes.
>
> On a second pass, drop what doesn't serve you and add what calls to you at that point.

We'll go into that more in the next section.

As well, rather than describing each modality or how to use each remedy in each chapter, I'm keeping those in the Next Steps section so you can refer to them separately once you know what specifically you need.

Let this be your healing journey—not a checklist, but a daily rhythm.

Choose Your Own Starting Point

Each chapter includes suggestions for how to engage with the material: questions to reflect on, strategies to try now, and deeper practices for sustained change. This is a book you return to—not one you finish and shelve.

Using Dynamic Reading

Books are usually linear, you start at the beginning and read one page after another to the end. But healing and self-discovery aren't always linear and each person has their own needs and their own way of learning. Each comes to this work with different needs, challenges, and priorities. Some may be looking for immediate relief from stress, while others want to explore deeper layers of personal transformation.

This chapter provides multiple ways to navigate The Mind Matrix Model Book based on what will serve you best right now. Think of it as an interactive roadmap—whether you want to read cover to cover or jump directly to the areas most relevant to you.

The idea is similar to a website's navigation bar and hyperlinks, so that you can link to different places and always make your way back to where you left off.

One necessary part of this for a physical book is bookmarks, a way to track the different paths and resources you are exploring. You can make your own, whether just using strips of torn paper that you add a name to, color coded or decorative ones on heavy paper or cardboard or cloth, or you can purchase ones. In any case, it's helpful if they have different names or colors or designs or all of these so that it's easy for you to jump to something you want to find.

Another part of dynamic reading that you may find helpful is to keep a notepad or use your journal to keep track of your information (the results of your questionnaires, what Self is most in need, what nutritionals to use, which acupressure points to press, etc.), to track your progress and perhaps to keep a record of your experiences and achievements. We'll talk about journals a little later in this chapter.

Tools, Not Overload

To keep the chapters focused, detailed instructions for therapies, supplements, acupressure points, and guided practices are included in the Next Steps section. Once you've identified what supports your system best, you can jump straight to those tools.

You don't have to do everything. You just have to start somewhere. And wherever you begin, the Model will meet you there.

So how do you actually begin using them? That's what we'll explore next.

Using the Tools: Acupressure, Essential Oils, and Homeopathy

The Mind Matrix Model includes a wide range of tools—acupressure, essential oils, homeopathy, and more—not because you need to use all of them, but because different systems respond to different supports.

You may find that one modality becomes a cornerstone for your healing while others play a supporting role. Some people respond most to physical interventions, others to symbolic or energetic ones. This is normal—and expected.

A Few Guidelines for Working with These Modalities:

Start small and be curious. You don't need to overhaul your whole life. Begin with one oil, one point, one remedy. Notice how it affects your State.

Consistency matters more than intensity. A few minutes of acupressure each day (on rising or going to bed, during lunchtime, etc.) will do more than an occasional 20-minute session. These tools work best as gentle, rhythmic signals to your nervous system.

Track your response. Many of these tools shift your State subtly. Keep a journal or jot down short notes: What shifted? What changed? Did it last? Did it open something new?

Combine with intention. Don't just press a point or apply a scent, invite your system into regulation. You are helping your Selves remember their natural rhythm.

You don't have to use everything that's listed. But if you use something, and do it with care and awareness, it will begin to change your State—and that changes everything.

For detailed instructions on how to use each tool, see the following chapters in the Next Steps section:

- ‣ Chapter 23 - Acupressure For Yourself & Others
- ‣ Chapter 24 - Essential Oils: History, Use, and Safety
- ‣ Chapter 25 - Homeopathy: Gentle Remedies for Balance & Health

Reflection Prompts: Using the Tools

Use these prompts to track how you are using the Mind Matrix Model, and how you might better use it.

> 1. What have I tried so far? Acupressure, oils, homeopathy, or something else? How did it affect my State, even subtly?
>
> 2. Do I feel drawn to certain tools or resistant to others? Why might that be?
>
> 3. When I use a tool slowly and with intention, what part of me responds? What changes in my body, heart, or mind?
>
> 4. How might I bring one small practice into my daily rhythm—not as a task, but as a kindness?

Pushback Means You're On the Path

As you start engaging with these practices, don't be surprised if part of you resists. That resistance isn't failure. It's feedback, and it often means you're moving in the right direction.

In the Mind Matrix Model, resistance comes from Sentries—protective Scripts shaped by past experience. Their job is to keep you from getting hurt again. But as your system begins to shift, those Sentries may activate to keep things "familiar."

Pushback by Self:

Vital Self Pushback:

You may feel restless, exhausted, or bored when trying to slow down and self-regulate. The body may crave sugar, screens, or constant motion.
Sentry message: "This isn't safe. Stillness is dangerous. Stay alert."
How to respond: Slow down gently. Do less, not more. Use grounding tools—like touch, breath, or scent—to send safety signals over time.

Heart Self Pushback:

You might feel shame, guilt, or even grief as you begin to claim your needs or set boundaries. Emotional habits like people-pleasing may flare.
Sentry message: "If you change, you'll lose connection. You'll be alone."
How to respond: Be compassionate with yourself. Let the Heart Self know it won't be abandoned. Seek co-regulation with safe people or nurturing environments.

Head Self Pushback:

You may hear mental chatter—"This is silly," "This won't work," or "You're just making things up." Or you may obsessively research instead of doing. Sentry message: "Don't surrender control. Stay in your head. If you feel, you'll fall apart."

How to respond:

Invite curiosity instead of certainty:

> *What if it's okay not to know? What if I just try this once, gently?*
>
> *I've tried that path, I want to try something new.*
>
> *That seems pretty fear-based, how about taking a risk?*

This Is Normal

Pushback is part of healing. You're changing your neural and emotional patterns. Old Scripts will test your commitment.

But with each override, each small act of presence, you teach your system something new:

> *"This is safe. I'm here. We can choose a different path."*

That's how regulation grows. That's how transformation begins.

Reflection Prompts: Working with Pushback

Use these prompts to bring unconscious Sentries to conscious awareness, where you can then decide what is useful and what is no longer relevant. This activates the Monarch's power of the Reflective Catalyst.

Vital Self

> *When I try to rest, slow down, or breathe deeply, what sensations or urges arise in my body?*
>
> *What does my body think it needs in those moments (e.g., food, escape, movement)? Could that be a Sentry strategy?*
>
> *How can I reassure my body that stillness or gentleness is safe, even for just one minute?*

Heart Self

> *When I begin to care for myself or say no to others, what feelings come up—guilt, sadness, fear of disconnection?*

Do I have a pattern of overgiving or staying silent to avoid conflict? How does that feel in my chest, my throat?

What would my Heart Self need to feel safe expressing itself more honestly?

Head Self

What kinds of thoughts show up when I try a new practice—doubt, judgment, distraction, minimization?

Is my Head Self trying to protect me from uncertainty, vulnerability, or emotional intensity?

Can I try softening those thoughts with curiosity instead of certainty? What if I just try without needing proof?

Watch for the responses you get, observing if they are Sentries (uncomfortable, fear-based, Negative State) or your own thoughts.

If you find one of these questions creates a lot of pushback or reactivity, try just repeating the question, waiting for the response, then just say:

Okay that's one layer of protection. What's under that?

In this way, you can make your way down through the layers until you get to the deeper feelings generating the pushback—fear, shame, hopelessness—then just sit with those feelings, breathing them out while breathing in light and positivity. Sticking with it in this way deeply engages the Reflective Catalyst, clearing out old Sentries and beliefs.

Journaling: A Mirror for the Monarch

It's very helpful to keep a journal while you're working with the Mind Matrix Model.

A journal is not just a notebook, it's a mirror, a container, a conversation between you and your Self. It gives the Monarch a place to reflect, review, and remember. And it becomes one of your most powerful tools for tracking change over time.

This isn't about keeping a perfect daily record. It's about creating a space where your thoughts, sensations, emotions, and insights can land without judgment.

Why Journal?

- To track your State and notice patterns across time.
- To observe your Three Selves—when each one is active, balanced, or in distress.
- To build awareness of what works and what doesn't as you experiment with new tools.
- To process emotions in a safe, contained space.
- To give your unconscious a place to speak and be seen.

What to Track

You can use your journal in a structured or freeform way. Here are some options for tracking your process:

1. State Check-Ins

At the end of the day, jot down:

> *What was my dominant State today—Positive, Negative, or somewhere in between?*
>
> *Which Self was most active?*
>
> *Did I experience a State Shift? What helped?*

2. Emotional Patterns

> *What emotions kept showing up today?*
>
> *Were they familiar or surprising?*
>
> *What triggered them?*
>
> *How did I respond?*

3. Sentry Activity

> *Did I notice a Script or Sentry pattern?*
>
> *What did it say? How did it try to protect me?*
>
> *Was I able to pause or respond differently?*

4. Override Strategy Notes

> *What tools did I use today?*
>
> *Did I try acupressure, breathwork, homeopathy, or something else?*

How did it affect my State or energy?

5. Reflections from Prompts

Use the journal prompts throughout this book (like the ones on pushback) to deepen your insight.

Creative Ways to Use Your Journal

Your journal doesn't have to be linear. It can be expressive, visual, and intuitive. Let it evolve with you.

- **Mind Matrix Maps:** Draw a diagram of your Vital, Heart, and Head Selves—note what each is feeling today.
- **Color-coded entries:** Use different ink or highlighters for each Self, or to mark State shifts.
- **Collage or symbols:** Use images to represent emotions, memories, or changes.
- **Write letters**: To your younger self, to a part of you that's hurting, to your Heart Self or Head Self.
- **Quotes and poems:** Include ones that resonate. Even a single line can anchor your day.
- **Audio or video journaling:** If writing isn't your thing, try voice memos on your phone to speak directly to your Selves.

Final Thought: Your Journal is a Witness

It doesn't need to be pretty. It doesn't need to be daily. It doesn't need to make sense. It just needs to be honest. Because the act of writing down what you feel, what you notice, and what you're learning can itself generate a State shift. It tells your nervous system:

I'm here. I'm listening. I'm with you.

Therapy and the Mind Matrix Model: Working Together

Sometimes, the most important step you can take on your healing path is asking someone to walk it with you.

Verbal therapy—especially with someone you can learn to trust—can be an essential foundation. A skilled therapist helps you feel seen, heard, and supported while gently inviting you into new patterns of awareness and relationship. For many people, this is the first place where their story is held with compassion, their defenses begin to soften, and their internal world becomes safer to explore.

This book is not meant to replace that kind of relationship, but it can be a powerful adjunct to it—a daily companion to deepen, extend, and personalize the work you're doing in therapy.

Therapy Is One Hour. Life Is the Rest.

Most therapy sessions happen once a week—maybe twice. But the mind, the body, and the emotions don't operate on a once-a-week schedule.

You need support in the in-between:

- When you wake up anxious.
- When you get triggered by something unexpected.
- When you're trying to reflect on a breakthrough—or survive a breakdown.

That's where the Mind Matrix Model comes in. It gives you a way to understand your internal experience in real time. It helps you track which Self is active, what kind of State you're in, and what kind of support you need. It offers immediate, practical tools—acupressure, breathwork, nutritionals, homeopathy, override strategies—for regulating your system between sessions.

It's not about "fixing" yourself on your own. It's about developing a language and toolkit that help you stay oriented, curious, and compassionate toward yourself—all week long.

When Therapy Needs Targeted Support

There are times when standard talk therapy may not reach the root of a struggle, especially when the nervous system is highly dysregulated, trauma is stored in the body, or thought loops won't resolve no matter how much insight you gain.

That's why this book includes a wide range of modality suggestions:

- Targeted therapies for the Vital Self
- Attachment-based and relational therapies for the Heart Self
- Cognitive and narrative approaches for the Head Self

Each modality listed is here not as a prescription, but as a possibility. If your therapist already works with one of these approaches, you may recognize it. If not, you might consider bringing what you've learned here into the room to discuss together. You may even discover that combining verbal therapy with bodywork, essential oils, or a movement practice unlocks something that wasn't accessible before.

Healing Happens in Layers

There is no single "right" path through this work. But one of the most powerful combinations is this:

A safe therapeutic relationship + a self-awareness framework you can carry with you.

Together, they create the conditions for lasting, sustainable change.

Whether you're new to therapy or decades in, the Mind Matrix Model is here to help you connect the dots between what you feel, how you function, and how you heal.

How to Bring the Mind Matrix Into Therapy

Your therapist doesn't need to know all about this model to support you in using it, but it would be helpful for them to have a basic understanding of the Mind Matrix Model terms. Below you'll see a Note to Therapists section that you can show them.

Think of the Mind Matrix Model as a translation tool—something that helps you describe your experience more clearly, notice patterns more quickly, and understand your internal shifts with greater nuance.

Here are some ways to bring it into your sessions:

Name which Self is struggling.

> "I think this is my Heart Self in a Negative State—it feels like shame, and I'm pulling away even though I want connection."

Use State language to track change.

> "I felt a State Shift after last session, but I couldn't hold it. Can we talk about what pulled me back into the Loop?"

Reflect on Self-Other patterns.

> "In this conflict with my partner, I was totally in an other-focused Heart mode—and I lost touch with what I actually needed."

Bring in tools you're trying.

"I tried one of the override strategies this week—acupressure and journaling helped more than I expected."

Track Sentries or Scripts.

"This feels like a Script I developed in childhood—my Head Self keeps taking over with old protective logic."

A Note for Therapists:

If you're reading this as a clinician, you can easily integrate the Mind Matrix Model into your existing framework. It pairs well with:

- Parts-based models like IFS
- Body-based modalities like Somatic Experiencing
- Cognitive therapies like CBT or DBT
- Attachment and trauma work of all kinds

It can also empower clients to take ownership of their healing between sessions—giving them a structured, compassionate way to notice what's happening, reflect on what's needed, and begin to respond with intentional support across the Three Selves.

Mini-Glossary: Core Terms in the Mind Matrix Model

The Monarch: The conscious mind—your reflective, aware self. The Monarch observes internal dynamics, makes intentional choices, and initiates Override Strategies. It plays a central role in coordinating the Three Selves and facilitating healing.

The Three Selves: The foundational triad of the mind in the Mind Matrix Model:

- **Vital Self:** Focuses on the balance between survival and thriving. Governs body awareness, energy (arousal) levels, and autonomic nervous system processes.
- **Heart Self:** Corresponds primarily with the limbic system. Manages emotions, attachment, relational dynamics, and the introversive/extroversive spectrum.
- **Head Self:** Involves the prefrontal cortex and upper brain functions. Responsible for thought, perception, planning, and cognitive processing.

Ministers: The unconscious or semi-conscious aspects of the Three Selves (Vital, Heart, Head) that run most daily patterns, behaviors, and automatic responses.

Script: A learned pattern of behavior, thought, or emotion—often adaptive, automatic, and efficient. Scripts help reduce cognitive load in familiar contexts.

Sentry: A specialized Script activated in the Negative State. Designed to protect against perceived threat, but often outdated or overly reactive.

Override Strategy: A conscious technique that helps shift State, interrupt Loops, or recalibrate one or more Selves. Can be fast (e.g., breath) or deep (e.g., therapy).

State or State Axis: The spectrum from Positive (Balanced, regulated) to Negative (Reactive, dysregulated) States. Determines how each Self is functioning at any moment.

Reminders and Rituals: Returning to Awareness

"The hardest part is remembering."

That sentence could begin almost any chapter in this book. How to integrate this all into your daily life. We need reminders to wake up and notice ourselves and the world around us. To remember to:

- Come back to awareness
- Shift your State
- Balance your Three Selves
- Notice your Sentries

And more. For me, I've often sort of looked up from what I was doing and asked myself, "Where have you been?" Sometimes weeks, months would go by without pausing to reflect and feel.

Shifting your State, moving yourself to a clearer and more conscious way of living, and continually clearing out your old patterns requires the conscious mind, the Monarch's Reflective Catalyst. So we need gentle, positive, non-punitive ways of reminding, waking.

Many religious practices incorporate this idea, such as the prayer beads of Christianity (rosary beads), Islam (tasbih beads) and Hinduism (japa mala beads).

In Judaism, the Mezuzah is a small case affixed to the doorposts of Jewish homes, containing a scroll with verses from Deuteronomy, including "You shall love the Lord your God..." Touching or kissing the mezuzah upon entering or exiting a room is a ritualized reminder of awareness, presence, and divine connection.

This section is about how to do that—how to build reminders into your day, not just as tasks or goals, but as rituals. Rituals are not about performance. They're about rhythm. They reconnect you to the present, and they give the Monarch a way to gather the Three Selves, even in chaos.

Why We Forget

We don't forget because we're lazy or undisciplined. We forget because the world is loud, fast, and immersive.

- You wake up and your Head Self is already Looping.
- Your Heart Self is scanning for emotional signals.
- Your Vital Self is reacting to light, noise, hunger, motion.
- Your Monarch isn't quite awake yet.

This is why we build rituals—not to fix ourselves, but to return to ourselves.

Tiny Rituals, Deep Reset

These practices don't require hours of time. They just require one breath of intention. Here are seven categories of micro-practices you can use to come back to awareness throughout the day.

1. Post-It Notes for the Soul

Get a pack of 1-inch sticky notes and place them:

- On your bathroom mirror
- On your steering wheel
- Near your phone charger
- On the inside of your laptop
- On the fridge or stove

Write short sensory cues:

"Feel your feet."
"Return to breath."
"Pause."
"You are not the Script."

Over time, your body will begin to associate those visual cues with a State shift.

2. The Bracelet Method

Wear a bracelet, ring, or band on your wrist, or an article of clothing like a scarf or sash—something tactile and neutral. Choose one you don't normally wear. Let it become your reminder. Every time you notice it:

Take a full inhale.

Drop your shoulders.

Ask, "Where am I right now?" Not physically—internally.

Which Self is active? Which one needs you?

This turns a passive object into an active override strategy.

3. Mindfulness Bell Apps

Technology doesn't have to pull you away from yourself—it can guide you back. There are several apps available on iOS and Android where you can set a bell to ring at specific intervals:

- Insight Timer App—Free with some in-app purchases.
- The Plum Village App—Free, look for the bell icon at the top right. You can also use it as a meditation timer. From Thich Nhat Hanh's Plum Village Zen Buddhist monastery.

Set for every 1/2 hour or hour, or whatever interval you prefer, and when it rings take three deep, slow breaths while focusing on relaxing your body. You can accompany this with a short affirmation:

"Monarch Check-in"

"Where is your breath?"

"Is this yours or someone else's?"

"Vital. Heart. Head. Who needs support?"

4. Transitional Micro-Practices

Every day has natural thresholds. Crossing them consciously helps regulate your State

Examples:

When you enter a room: pause, feel your feet, exhale slowly.

Before opening a door: gently push your awareness out to the room beyond.

Before speaking: inhale, soften your jaw, choose your tone.

When closing your laptop: "What needs to be left here?"

When brushing your teeth, look at yourself in the mirror. Consciously let go of any critical thoughts, and bring gratitude for your body.

These take less than 10 seconds and help de-script your automatic patterns.

5. Create a Ritual Corner

Dedicate a small space—on a desk, a shelf, a tray. Include:

- One grounding object (a stone, bowl, small sculpture)
- One symbolic item (a photo, poem, or meaningful object)
- One sensory cue (an oil, a feather, a soft cloth)

This is not an altar to something outside yourself. It is a place for your Three Selves to meet.

Stand or sit here for a few minutes or more daily. No agenda. Just presence.

6. Evening Transition

A mindful way to prepare for sleep. Before bed:

Place one hand on your heart and one on your belly.

Say to yourself, "Thank you for getting through today."

Ask, "Did I abandon myself today? Did I return?"

As much as you can with no judgment, just awareness and self-compassion.

Let this be the last thing you do before your body releases to sleep.

7. Create Your Own Cue Language

The unconscious responds best to repeated, body-based signals. Choose one simple phrase—what we might call a Monarch mantra—that cues awareness.

Examples:

> "Three Selves, One Breath."
>
> "Safe. Connected. Clear."
>
> "Pause the Script."

Repeat it often, especially when you feel flooded. Even silently, this acts as a cognitive Override Strategy to bring your Head Self back into coherence.

Why Ritual Works

Ritual doesn't try to change you. It reminds you that you're already whole.

> The Vital Self responds to rhythm and sensation.
>
> The Heart Self responds to emotional tone and familiarity.
>
> The Head Self responds to intentional meaning.

When you create rituals that engage all three, you are literally rewiring your State Range, giving your system the message: "It's safe to be here. You can let go of vigilance."

Awareness Is a Muscle

Awareness is not a permanent state. It's a practice. And like any muscle, it strengthens with use and fades with neglect.

So don't worry if you forget. Don't judge yourself if you loop.

> *Just return.*
>
> *And return again.*
>
> *And again.*

Because every time you do—even if it's just one breath—you are building a life that is not controlled by your past Scripts, but led by your conscious, awake, integrated Self.

Overview of Mind Matrix Techniques

The Mind Matrix Model includes a range of supportive techniques drawn from clinical, traditional, and somatic practices. You'll find these in the Working With chapters. Each one helps bring balance to your Vital, Heart, or Head Self and helps shift you toward a more Positive State. Here's a simplified, friendly overview of the most useful tools you can explore.

Acupressure

Acupressure is a gentle, powerful tool you can use with your fingers to calm your nervous system or help rebalance any of your Three Selves. You don't have to be exact to get benefits. Just find the general area of the point and gently press or massage it.

> **Point location:** Use your own finger-widths to measure from anatomical landmarks. For example, if the text says:
> *4 finger-widths from the wrist crease.*
> Start by placing your pinky finger on the wrist crease and measure to the tip of your index finger.

> **Don't worry about precision:** It's okay to work in a small area around the point.

> **Massage the area:** The pictures shown for each point include the meridian in that area. You can also massage the meridian or explore nearby points for tenderness.

> **Breathe while you do it:** Pairing acupressure with slow breathing, especially breathing out longer than breathing in, helps deepen the effect.

Breathwork

Breath is one of the quickest ways to regulate your State. Because it lies between conscious and unconscious control, it acts as a bridge between your Monarch (conscious awareness) and your Vital Self.

Try one of these anytime you feel anxious or stuck:

> **Coherent Breathing:** Inhale 5 seconds, exhale 5 seconds, repeat for 2–5 minutes.

> **Box Breathing:** Inhale 4s, hold 4s, exhale 4s, hold 4s.

- **Extended Exhale:** Inhale 4s, exhale 6–8s to activate calming.

"Every conscious breath is a handshake between the Monarch and the Vital Minister."

Essential Oils

Essential oils can calm the nervous system and help shift your State, especially through the Vital Self. But they must be used carefully:

- Never apply undiluted oils to the skin. Always mix with a carrier oil (like jojoba or almond).
- Be extremely careful not to get any in your eyes, for example rubbing your eyes when you have some oils on your fingers.
- Do not ingest unless under professional guidance.
- Use high-quality oils and avoid synthetic fragrance oils.

Ways to use:
- Inhale from the palms (dilute first).
- Diffuse in a room for ambient calming.
- Apply to pulse points (diluted) while breathing slowly.

Lavender, chamomile, and frankincense are great for calming. Peppermint and rosemary can be gently energizing. Trust your body's response—if a scent feels too strong, back off.

Homeopathy

Homeopathy works symbolically and somatically. While still debated in medical circles, many people find it deeply supportive, especially when emotional and physical symptoms are intertwined.

- Homeopathy may help with emotional overload, fatigue, or stuck patterns.
- Remedies are selected based on your whole pattern, not just symptoms.
- Can support all Three Selves through gentle stimulation and symbolic resonance.

Always choose remedies from a trusted source and follow instructions carefully. More is not better.

Guided Meditations

These help shift you into a calmer State by bringing your attention into the body. Mind Matrix meditations often focus on the Vital Self but can also help with emotional and cognitive patterns.

Try:

- Body and Breath Awareness
- Safe Place Visualization
- Descending Awareness (from head to belly)
- Titration (gently feeling something uncomfortable with support)

You can use these daily or anytime you feel dysregulated. Pair them with breath or essential oils for extra support.

Lifestyle Foundations

None of the above work well if your body isn't getting what it needs. These basics support all Three Selves:

Nutrition: Eat regularly, stay hydrated, and include calming nutrients like magnesium, omega-3s, and B vitamins. Be cautious with adaptogens—some are energizing (like Rhodiola), others calming (like Ashwagandha). *See Chapter 26 - Nutritional Supplements & Adaptogens in the Next Steps section.*

Movement: Gentle daily exercise and stretching helps regulate energy and mood.

Sleep: Try to sleep and wake at the same time daily, and avoid screens at night. *See Chapter 27 - Sleep Hygiene in the Next Steps section.*

Mindfulness and Meditation: Just a few minutes of daily presence builds resilience. *See Chapter 28 - Mindfulness & Meditation in the Next Steps section.*

All of these tools are optional. Start with what feels accessible. Your goal is not perfection—it's creating moments of safety, presence, and regulation throughout your day.

Website Resources

The website for the Mind Matrix Model is designed as an interactive companion to this book—a place where readers can go deeper, find updated resources, and connect with others working with the Model.

You can sign up for free access by scanning the QR code or visiting this short link:

mmm.tips/register

https://mmm.tips/register

Once inside, you'll find a growing set of resources, including:

> **Interactive forms:** These interactive forms for determining your balance in each of the Three Selves and State can be used to chart your progress over time, and each include many combination patterns that reveal more complex dynamics.
> **Document Library:** Downloadable worksheets, guided practices, diagnostic forms, and exercises that you can print, annotate, or complete online.
> **Discussion Forums:** Community spaces organized by topic (e.g., State regulation, Override Strategies, trauma recovery, the Three Selves). Ask questions, share experiences, and get support from other readers and practitioners.
> **Groups:** Specialized groups for readers, professionals, and practice partners—these allow more focused discussions and collaborative learning.
> **News Feed:** Updates, new releases, live event announcements, and community highlights in one central stream.
> **Video + Audio Resources:** Recordings of meditations, walk-throughs, and deeper dives into complex topics from the book.
> **Member Portal:** Each registered user has a private portal showing saved resources, recent activity, and personalized recommendations over time.

This platform will continue to grow, with additional features planned for the future—such as practice tracking tools, progress journals, and structured courses aligned with the book's chapters.

Final Thoughts

This book is designed to be as adaptive as your mind. Whether you're here for immediate tools or long-term transformation, the structure allows you to move freely between concepts without getting lost. As you read, take notes on what resonates, and use the references to deepen your understanding where needed.

Working with your own healing isn't always a straight line, it's typically more of a dynamic process. Hopefully this format will give you the opportunity to use the Mind Matrix Model book in a way that works best for you.

Chapter Five

Stress, Anxiety & Depression in the Mind Matrix Model

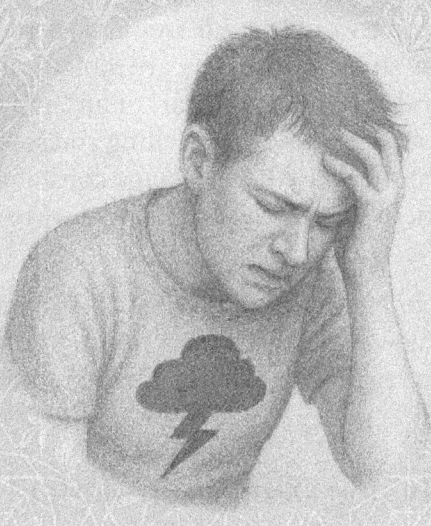

*When despair for the world grows in me
and I wake in the night at the least sound
in fear of what my life and my children's lives may be,
I go and lie down where the wood drake
rests in his beauty on the water, and the great heron feeds.
I come into the peace of wild things
who do not tax their lives with forethought
of grief. I come into the presence of still water.
And I feel above me the day-blind stars
waiting with their light. For a time
I rest in the grace of the world, and am free.*

~ The Peace of Wild Things
  by Wendell Berry

> *If you're currently feeling overwhelming anxiety, depression or despair and need quick relief, you might consider jumping ahead to* **Chapter Six: Working with Stress, Anxiety, and Depression** *for immediate strategies. You can always return here afterward for a deeper understanding.*

Stress, anxiety and depression are profoundly important and have a strong effect on every aspect of the Mind Matrix Model. They are also a great place to start our work together.

In our culture, most people would say life would be better without stress and anxiety. I would say stress and anxiety are profoundly misunderstood—stress is a natural and important part of life, and anxiety is a valuable signal from your mind and body telling you something critically important. The fact that they have both become constant experiences for so many people in modern life is a clear signal that we're all doing something wrong.

This chapter will help you to understand stress and anxiety, as well as depression, in a whole new light. You'll learn how they affect your Three Selves and learn how to regain balance when these responses to life's challenges become disruptive.

Why Stress, Anxiety, and Depression Matter

Stress, anxiety, and depression are often seen as separate problems. In the Mind Matrix Model, we view them as different faces of the same deeper imbalance. Each signals that your system is struggling to stay flexible, balanced, and connected across your Vital, Heart, and Head Selves. In essence, they're all *State issues*: they reflect a shift in your internal State from a Positive, regulated range into a Negative, dysregulated range.

Think of it this way:

> **Stress** is the beginning of the chain. It's the buildup of energy and tension when you face a challenge, whether positive or negative.
>
> **Anxiety** is what happens when that stressed energy doesn't get released properly—like an engine revving with nowhere to go, creating a Loop of worry and fear.
>
> **Depression** often comes later, when the system has been under strain for too long. It's what happens when that engine runs out of fuel entirely, leading to a collapse in energy, mood, and perspective.

In the Model's terms, stress, anxiety, and depression correspond to your system gradually sliding from a Positive State into a Negative State. If stress and anxiety are left unhealed or unreleased, they often cascade into depression over time.

Understanding how these feelings arise and how they affect your Three Selves is essential. It means you can respond to them not as random, separate "bad things" that happen to you, but as interconnected signals from your body, heart, and mind.

This chapter will help you see stress, anxiety, and depression in a new light—not as personal failures or permanent conditions, but as messages that something in your system needs care. You'll learn how each of the Three Selves (Vital, Heart, and Head) experiences these States, and why we're *not* meant to live in constant distress. By the end, you'll recognize that you're not alone or "broken" for feeling this way, and you'll be ready to learn how to regain balance when these responses become disruptive.

Stress: The First Shift

What *is* stress, really? Most people think of stress as an unhealthy reaction to too much pressure. Here, we'll define it a bit differently. *Stress is simply your body-mind's natural response to a challenge.* It's the activation of your nervous system when you need to rise to meet something—whether that "something" is as minor as getting out of a warm bed on a cold morning or as major as facing down a wild animal.

In small doses, stress can be helpful: it alerts and energizes you. In fact, a little positive stress (called **eustress**) keeps life exciting and helps you grow. It's what you feel when you're excited or motivated—like butterflies before a performance or the push to meet a deadline.

> *Maya, a passionate young musician, is gearing up for her first live performance. As showtime approaches, she feels her heart pounding a bit faster and a jittery buzz of energy. But she recognizes it as the good kind of rush—the excitement that means she cares about doing well. Instead of panicking, she channels that energy into focus. When she steps on stage under the bright lights, that nervous buzz turns into an electric mix of concentration and joy. She's not just anxious; she's alive and present. The crowd's energy lifts her higher with each note.*

> *In this case, **stress is working for her**, giving her the edge she needs to perform at her best.*

Stress becomes a problem when it's too intense, lasts too long, or stacks up without a break. This negative form of stress is often called **distress**. Distress is the feeling of being under siege by pressure. It's when challenges exceed your ability to cope or recover.

> *James has been carrying a lot on his shoulders: tight work deadlines, financial worries, family responsibilities piling up. Day after day, he grinds on without rest.*
>
> *After weeks of this, he starts waking up already exhausted, his body tense, his mind racing with "what ifs" about everything that could go wrong. Little problems start to set him off—he snaps at a coworker over a minor mistake. At night, he can't sleep; his thoughts won't shut off, and his body feels stuck in high gear with no off switch.*
>
> *What began as normal stress has tipped into **chronic distress**. James's system is telling him "Enough!" Even simple tasks feel overwhelming now. If he can't find a way to release or reduce this load, burnout (or worse) is around the corner.*

So, stress itself isn't "bad." It's a signal and a surge of energy. The issue is *what happens after the surge.* In healthy scenarios, after the challenge passes, your system should come back down to baseline and recover. Think of a steam train that needs to blow off steam after racing down the tracks. Our bodies have built-in ways to discharge stress too.

- Have you noticed how when a dog goes to lie down, they will spin around a few times (flattening the grass his ancestors slept on) and then a big sigh after they lie down? It's like they're deflating, letting go of the tension they just built up.

- Babies do something similar—after a big exciting event or when they're overtired, they might burst into tears before conking out. That crying is a baby's way of releasing stress.

- Even we adults have reflexes like this: sighing, deep breathing, yawning, laughing, even screaming into a pillow or having a good cry. These are all ways our Vital Self and nervous system try to reset and dump the excess energy.

And let's not forget physical activity. You've probably "blown off steam" by exercising, taking a walk, or even, as I like to joke, shaking your fists at the heavens in frustration. You might notice you often feel *better* after doing these things—maybe calmer or more clear-headed—though in the moment, it might not feel fun to, say, exercise when you're stressed.

The key point is, *stress needs an outlet*. If it gets one, your body and brain can return to a calm state. If it *doesn't*, that revved-up energy doesn't just vanish, it can start to cause problems.

> *One thing I like to remind myself and others is that stress is 1/10th what's happening to you, and 9/10ths how you interact with it. We can't always eliminate the sources of stress in our lives (I'm talking to you, parents with young kids!), but we can change the way we respond to it. And that change starts with truly understanding what stress actually is—a natural signal, not a personal failing.*

If stress keeps building without release, it's as if your system's stuck with the throttle on. Your Vital Self stays tense and hyper alert. Your Heart Self may feel emotionally raw or on edge. Your Head Self races to make sense of the discomfort.

In the Mind Matrix Model, we say that *unreleased stress pushes you out of the Positive State and locks you in a heightened Negative State*. Everything tightens up like a knot. You might even notice that when you finally *do* try to relax (say, at the end of a long week), you initially feel worse—edgy, restless, or emotionally turbulent. That's the built-up stress looking for a way out, and if you don't let it out, it will keep nagging you.

At some point, if stress isn't dealt with, it fuels the next stage of the process: anxiety. In other words, **when you don't (or can't) discharge stress, it transforms into anxiety.**

What is Fear?

While we're defining things, let's talk about fear. *Fear* is an easy one to define—it's the immediate reaction to something you see as a threat, either consciously or unconsciously. But fear looks a little different in the Mind Matrix Model. Each of the Three Selves perceives and responds to fear differently:

For the **Vital Self**, fear arises from a physical threat, such as an oncoming car or a predator.

For the **Heart Self**, fear emerges from social or emotional threats, like rejection, conflict, or betrayal.

For the **Head Self**, fear can come from a mental challenge, such as trying to solve an important problem or confronting an idea that shakes your sense of reality.

Typically, fear's effects ripple across the Three Selves. For instance, recognizing that you might lose your job (Head Self) could lead to concerns about losing social status (Heart Self) and trigger fears about physical survival due to financial insecurity (Vital Self). The Selves are always interconnected, amplifying and influencing one another in response to stress and fear.

Both stress and fear affect the Three Selves of the Model in unique ways, and how they manifest depends greatly on whether we are in the Positive State or have been triggered into the Negative State.

Anxiety: The Fire Under the Pot

Anxiety is what happens when stress gets *stuck*. It's as if your mind and body know something's wrong, but they can't quite resolve it, so they stay on high alert all the time.

One of my favorite sayings (as you may recall from the first chapter) is that *anxiety is like a fire under the pot of your nervous system.* The heat is always on, keeping everything at a constant simmer. The higher that flame, the more everything in you—your thoughts, your emotions, even your body—starts to boil over with exaggerated intensity.

You can see this in yourself, how when everything is fine you don't get phased by incidentals. But when you're stressed out, you experience every interruption, every miscalculation, every problem in an exaggerated way. You are more easily dysregulated when you are carrying a lot of stress.

In more everyday terms, anxiety is that uneasy, worried state that can descend on you even when there's no immediate threat in front of you. Unlike fear (which is an immediate "Uh oh, there's a threat right here, right now" reaction), anxiety is more of a lingering background buzz of *anticipation* and *dread*.

It's your system's way of saying, "Something *might* go wrong…what if…?" even when you can't pinpoint exactly what's triggering it.

It's stress that didn't get a clear off-ramp, it just keeps things simmering.

In a natural scenario, stress comes and then it goes. For example, animals in the wild don't stay anxious. A deer will run from a predator, and if it escapes, it will shake and tremble for a few minutes (releasing the stress), then go back to grazing as if nothing happened. Babies, too, will cry or giggle or wiggle to discharge energy and then calm down. Our ancestors were the same way, dealing with relatively short-term stressors and then discharging the stress around the campfire at night by talking or dancing.

But we modern human adults often short-circuit this process. We've been taught by our culture to suppress our natural release mechanisms, and unlike our ancestors, our society is based on long-term stressors. From high school on, we're thinking about college, then a job, then getting ahead or staying ahead of debt. There is no end to it.

On the other end, we often don't express our feelings because it's socially unacceptable. We hold in the tears, we stifle the screams, we "suck it up" and act composed. Even when we're alone. Our rational Head Self might override the Heart and Vital Selves, insisting, "I'm fine, it's fine, just keep going," even as tension is mounting inside. The result? The stress doesn't resolve; it accumulates in our system. We stay on alert internally, even if externally nothing obviously scary is happening. And that's anxiety.

Anxiety and The Three Selves

Anxiety manifests differently in each of the Three Selves:

Physically (Vital Self), it might be a racing heart, shallow breathing, a knotted stomach, jittery limbs, or an impending sense of doom or panic—the classic fight-or-flight activation symptoms that have nowhere to go.

Emotionally (Heart Self), anxiety often manifests as social fears or insecurity. You might constantly worry about losing relationships or being judged, or your internal judge or internal audience might be beating you up.

Mentally (Head Self), it shows up as racing thoughts, incessant what-ifs, and catastrophizing.

Your mind might spin scenarios of everything that could go wrong, or get stuck on an endless hamster wheel of overthinking. It's exhausting, but because the "fire under the pot" hasn't been put out, your system feels like it *has* to stay in overdrive.

Let's consider a real-life example.

> *A woman once came to me for acupressure therapy, desperate to find relief from her anxiety. During our sessions, she would relax a bit, even starting to feel some peace while on the table.*
>
> *But week after week, she'd come back saying the anxiety was as fierce as ever the moment she returned to her life. So I asked her about her daily routine. It turned out her days were a whirlwind: long, stressful work hours, taking care of her kids and an ill parent, barely any sleep, and unwinding each night with a couple of glasses of wine (hoping to numb the worry). No wonder the poor woman's system was on edge!*
>
> *We talked about how her body's stress responses couldn't fully calm down if every day she was lighting the fire again with more pressure (and even the alcohol, which might relax her briefly, was disturbing her sleep and balance). I encouraged her to make tiny changes outside of our sessions. Things like a short walk in the evenings, cutting down to one glass of wine or drinking herbal tea instead, and carving out even five minutes of quiet "me time" before bed.*
>
> *These were small steps, but they were aimed at helping her nervous system find moments of safety and release beyond the acupressure table. It wasn't an overnight miracle, but this insight was a vital first step. She began to realize that anxiety wasn't a monster that struck her out of nowhere; it was the product of an overtaxed system that hadn't been allowed to unwind. Slowly, as she made these adjustments, the constant fire under the pot began to cool.*

This story illustrates a key point: *anxiety isn't "all in your head."* It involves your whole being—your habits, your lifestyle, your body chemistry, your emotions. In Mind Matrix Model terms, it's your Vital, Heart, and Head Selves all stuck in a state of overactivation, a protective, high-alert mode, and can't find their way back to safety. If you're anxious, it's not because you're weak or crazy; it's because some part of you is *trying to protect you* by staying alert to possible threats. The problem is when that alert never turns off.

The Anxiety Loop

As I briefly mentioned in the first chapter, Loops occur when different parts of the mind—different Selves—trigger each other back and forth, creating cycles of emotional reactivity, procrastination, or anxiety. We'll explore Loops and Overrides in more detail in Chapter 13, but let's focus here on the most common one: the Vital Self–Head Self Anxiety Loop.

Once anxiety builds to a certain threshold—either gradually or suddenly due to the Vital Self being triggered into a Negative State—it sends alarm signals to the other Selves. The message is simple:
"I think there's a problem!"

The Head Self receives that signal and starts scanning for the cause. Because its job is to make sense of things, it inevitably finds something—internal or external:

"It's my job."

"It's the state of the world."

"It's money."

"It's my partner."

"It's... my anxiety."

I call this "the shelf." Anxiety is fear without a clearly identified reason, and the Head Self tries to resolve that by finding a reason to place on the shelf. Anything it finds gets added to the shelf and—because it feels real—confirms that there really is something wrong. And the shelf is expandable—the more anxiety, the bigger the shelf and the more fits on it.

This perceived threat then Loops back to the Vital Self, which responds with increased arousal:

"We have something to worry about!"

That, in turn, fuels more anxiety, tightening the cycle.

The way out is to recognize that you're in a Loop—not a real-time crisis—and consciously name the process as anxiety. Once named, you can begin to use the tools in the next chapter to calm and center yourself.

When you release the physiological stress, the anxious thoughts lose their fuel.

Depression: The Fire Gone Out

Chronic anxiety can be exhausting. Many people tell me they feel like they're "constantly bracing" for something, or that their mind won't stop racing. It's as if they're stuck revving high all day; by night, they're mentally and physically drained.

And ironically, that drained state can feed into the next phase: when their system just can't maintain this high alert anymore, it may shift into *shutdown*. That's where depression comes in.

If anxiety is an overactive alarm, depression is often what happens when the alarm has been blaring for too long and the batteries finally die. It's a state of *collapse*. In depression, the Vital Self loses its energy and motivation, the Heart Self loses its hope and capacity to feel positive emotions, and the Head Self loses perspective and flexibility. It's as if the constant strain burns you out from the inside, and you're left feeling empty, heavy, and disconnected.

Another way to think of depression is as a systemic shutdown. Earlier we used the analogy of a fire; here you might picture the fire has gone out. You don't just feel sad in one part of you, *every* part of you is affected. Your body feels drained of energy, your heart is weighed down or numb, and your mind is stuck in a Negative State Loop. No wonder even simple tasks, like getting out of bed or taking a shower, can start to feel impossibly hard when you're depressed. It's not "laziness" or "weakness." It's that your system has hit an overload point and crashed.

Depression can develop in different ways. Sometimes it's the aftermath of prolonged anxiety and stress. Imagine running your engine too hot for too long, eventually it burns out. If you've been anxious for months on end, your system might eventually hit a wall and shut down into depression as a kind of last-resort defense. Other times, depression can come more directly from a severe emotional blow or trauma, or a long-term debilitating illness or condition.

For example, a sudden loss, a major betrayal, or a period of intense hopelessness can send you into a depressive spiral even without a long anxious build-up. It can also result from physical depletion—say, a chronic illness or long-term exhaustion that just wears your Vital Self down to where you have no fuel left. And often, it's a mix of factors over time.

The Depression Loop

However it starts, depression usually involves a Negative State Loop between the Heart and Head Selves that pulls the whole system down. Here's what that Loop looks like: emotional pain or emptiness in the Heart Self fuels negative, bleak thoughts in the Head Self ("Nothing will ever get better…what's the point?"). Those thoughts, in turn, make you feel even more hopeless and emotionally raw, which then reinforces the Negative State. Around and around it goes, a vicious cycle.

While this Heart-Head Loop churns, the Vital Self steadily loses steam. Your physical energy drops, you want to sleep all the time or can't sleep at all, and your body might even start to feel heavy or numb. Even if the original trigger of the depression was, say, something physical, eventually your thoughts and feelings likely join the collapse; likewise, a primarily emotional depression will still leave you feeling tired and foggy-headed. The Three Selves will usually, or at least eventually, all get pulled in.

Depression as Healing

It's important to note that depression isn't always about what's happening *now*. Sometimes depression in the present is actually old pain surfacing. You might have been running on anxiety and overdrive for years, unknowingly trying to suppress some past trauma or deep hurt.

The emergence of depression can be either because you've started healing or simply because you're too exhausted to keep it up. In the former case, that often happens when you finally have some space in your life, or some safety. It can seem quite ironic, after the kids leave the house and you're an empty nester, or once you leave that high demand job, that you start having intense feelings.

When that constant anxiety finally settles, all the suppressed grief, fear, or shame underneath can come flooding back in. This can be terrifying. "Why am I feeling this *now*, when everything in my life is *technically* okay? What's wrong with me?" But it's not a setback or weird anomaly; it's actually a sign of healing.

In therapy, it's often the case that once you remove the frantic energy of anxiety, the deeper layers (often sadness or trauma) can emerge to be healed.

Depression may be your system's way of saying it's time to deal with these older wounds, albeit gently and slowly. It asks you to finally feel what you couldn't feel before, because back then it was too overwhelming or you were too involved with other things.

This is why people sometimes experience depression after a big positive change or once things "settle down." Your system finally has the space to unveil what's unprocessed. It's crucial to understand this so you don't beat yourself up for feeling depressed "for no reason." There *is* a reason; it just might be an old one.

Now, none of this means depression is a fate you have to accept. Far from it. It just helps to explain *why* it happens, so you can approach yourself with more compassion. You're not broken or failing because you're depressed. Often, it means you've been *too strong for too long*—carrying burdens solo that would have collapsed anyone eventually.

Depression is telling you, "You have carried too much for too long. It's time to rest and heal." In a way, depression forces a stop. It's your whole being saying "I can't keep going like this." And as painful as that stop is, it's also an opportunity to care for yourself in a new way.

To get a clearer picture, let's look at a quick example.

> *Mary, a single parent and full-time nurse, has spent years putting everyone else first—her kids, her patients, her aging parents. She rarely takes time for herself and tells herself she just has to keep going. But lately, everything feels heavy. Getting out of bed takes effort. She cries easily, feels exhausted all the time, and can't remember the last time she felt joy. Even simple tasks like answering texts or cooking dinner feel overwhelming.*
>
> *Her depression isn't coming out of nowhere—it's her system saying, "I've carried too much for too long. I can't do this like I used to." It's not failure. It's a signal. A forced pause. An invitation to rest, release what's too much, and find a new way forward.*

This is a portrait of Vital Self-oriented depression affecting the Vital and Head Selves. Mary is exhausted physically, and it's as if a dark cloud follows her everywhere now. Because of that, her Heart Self is depressed and her Head Self is filled with dark thoughts such as "What's the point of trying?" "Nobody cares about me."

Someone else's depression might start differently. Another person might slide into depression after months of high-pressure job stress that eventually burns them out, leading to a primarily Head Self-driven depression of mental overload and hopeless thoughts. Yet another might experience depression largely in their body, after a prolonged illness or fatigue, making them want to sleep all day and withdraw.

In all cases, though the entry points differ, the end state looks similar: Vitality drained, emotions flattened, thoughts darkened.

How the Three Selves Experience S, A, D

We've been talking about how stress, anxiety, and depression each affect your Three Selves. It may help to lay it out in a clear way. The table below summarizes how each Self responds under stress, anxiety, and depression:

Self	Under Stress (challenge response)	Under Anxiety (stuck on high alert)	Under Depression (collapsed state)
Vital Self Body	Tension, hyper-arousal, body primed for action; adrenaline pumping	"Fight or flight" symptoms: racing heart, butterflies, shaky or restless energy that can't settle	Exhaustion and shutdown: fatigue, low energy, heaviness, body wants to hibernate
Heart Self Emotions	Emotional intensity, irritability or excitement, feelings run high (both positive or negative)	Self-worth issues, social fears, feeling overwhelmed by feelings, or a constant need for reassurance and relational control	Numbness or deep sadness: a sense of disconnection, hopelessness, loneliness, difficulty feeling pleasure
Head Self Mind	Mental busyness, lots of thoughts about the challenge, can be focused or overwhelmed	Racing thoughts and worry loops, imagining worst-case scenarios, intrusive thoughts that won't quit	Cognitive shutdown: "brain fog," very negative outlook, thoughts of despair or nihilism ("Nothing matters")

Of course, in real life, you might not experience all those symptoms at once. But often, one will dominate. For instance, in anxiety, some people feel it mostly as physical symptoms, while others are consumed by worries, and others primarily feel it as emotional panic, although all three Selves are usually involved to some degree. What's important is that a problem that starts in one Self can ripple into the others.

- Let's say your Vital Self is chronically exhausted (Vital depression); that physical low can trigger Heart Self loneliness (because you don't have the energy to get together with friends) and Head-self negativity (your mind sinks into gloom).
- Or if your Heart Self is in pain from the end of a relationship, you might find your Vital energy drops (you lie in bed all day) and your Head Self gets stuck on thoughts of regret or low self-worth.
- A Head Self overload (like extreme job stress) can lead to feeling emotionally numb or defeated (Heart) and physically drained (Vital).

In short, each Self affects the others—they are deeply interconnected.

The good news is that this interconnectedness also means healing one Self can help heal the others. Just as the Selves can pull each other *down*, they can also pull each other *up*. If you support even one part of your system, the benefits will tend to spread.

For example, doing something that restores your Vital energy (like improving sleep or doing gentle exercise) can give your Heart Self a bit more resilience and your Head Self a bit more clarity. Or working on more positive thought patterns can calm your Heart's emotions and even ease your body's tension.

Final Thoughts

Before we move on to the next chapter (where we'll dive into working with stress, anxiety, and depression), remember this: these states are not your enemy. They're signals. Your job, starting now, is to listen to what they're signaling about your needs. Stress might be telling you "I need an outlet or a break." Anxiety might be saying "I'm overwhelmed, something in me doesn't feel safe." Depression might be saying "I've been running on empty, I need deep rest and care."

It might feel daunting, but you've already begun the healing process by learning about these patterns. Awareness is a powerful first step. Rather than seeing yourself as weak or victimized for feeling stressed, anxious, or depressed, you can start to see how strong you've had to be to endure these states—and that now, you can choose a different path that nurtures all parts of you.

In Chapter Six, we'll explore practical strategies to help each of your Three Selves regain balance, step by step. You'll learn how to release stress safely, how to calm anxiety, and how to gently rekindle hope and energy when depression has dimmed them.

You are not alone in this, and you are not broken. The journey forward isn't about *fighting* yourself. It's about *befriending* yourself—being your own best friend—while working *with* your mind, heart, and body. So take a deep breath. You've got this, and we'll take it one small step at a time.

Chapter Six

Working with Stress, Anxiety and Depression

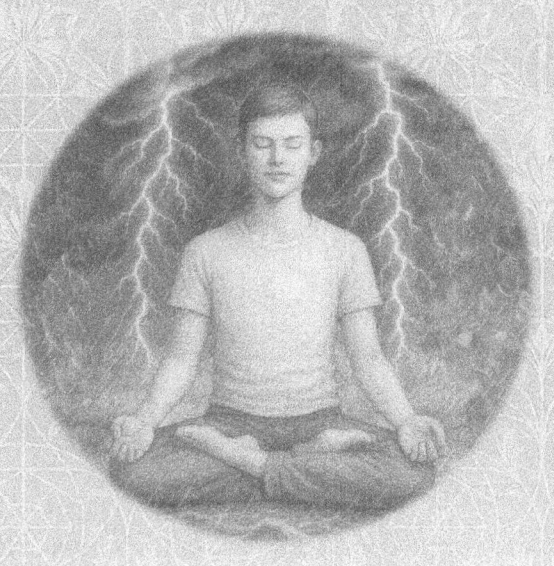

Let everything happen to you: beauty and terror.
Just keep going. No feeling is final.
Don't let yourself lose me.

Nearby is the country they call life.
You will know it by its seriousness.

Give me your hand.

~ Excerpt from Sonnets to Orpheus, Part Two, XII
  by Rainer Maria Rilke

> *Before we start, I want to make clear that these tools can be very useful but they are not a substitute for working with a therapist. If you are deeply suffering, such that your life feels out of control and you feel lost, you need to find a therapist who you can learn to trust and work with. This book can be a wonderful adjunct to that work.*

Stress, anxiety, and depression are different faces of the same deeper imbalance: a disruption in your system's ability to stay flexible, balanced, and connected across your Vital, Heart, and Head Selves. Each arises from stress that was too much to release easily:

Stress is the first shift—tension, pressure, activation.

Anxiety comes when the tension stays trapped and loops on itself.

Depression comes when the system can no longer hold the strain and collapses into shutdown.

Understanding how to work with them—gently, skillfully, and patiently—is essential for real healing. This chapter will give you a practical guide to:

- Choosing where and how to begin
- Matching your strategies to your current capacity
- Breaking cycles of overarousal and collapse safely
- Building a resilient, flexible State over time

Healing doesn't come from fighting harder. It comes from listening to where you are, and offering what your system can truly receive right now.

Choosing Your Starting Point

When you're overwhelmed by stress, caught in anxiety, or weighed down by depression, it's natural to want a clear path out, an escape route. The truth is, *there's no single "right" place to start.* The best entry point is the one your system can actually manage today.

Depending on how you're feeling right now:

- If you have *some* capacity at the moment – meaning you're anxious or low, but you can still muster a bit of focus or motivation – then you can likely engage directly with what you're feeling. You'll be able to do some exercises with your thoughts, emotions, or body sensations (we'll get to those in a moment).

> If you're *too* flooded by anxiety or *too* shut down by depression right now, then expecting yourself to "dive into healing" might be asking too much. And that's okay. In those cases, you may need to start with simple, soothing distractions just to get through the moment and calm down a notch. This isn't avoidance or failure, it's using a bridge to get yourself to a safer internal place.

The goal isn't to "fix" everything immediately. It's to find one small, real way to shift your State toward more regulation and resilience. Wherever you begin, the path is the same:

Regulate first. Reflect second. Heal steadily.

The Three Steps

Here is a poem inspired by the spirit of Portia Nelson's excellent (but copyrighted) poem, *An Autobiography in Five Chapters*:

The Path of Awareness

I walk down a street. There's a deep hole. I don't see it. I fall in. It hurts, and I don't know what happened. It's not my fault.

I walk down the same street. I see the hole, but I still fall in. It feels familiar. I blame the hole.

I walk down the same street. I know the hole is there. I fall in anyway. It is my fault. I climb out.

I walk down the same street. The hole is still there. This time, I walk around it.

I choose a different street.

This poem, like the original by Portia Nelson, offers a powerful metaphor for how we can work with triggers—familiar experiences that bring up old feelings and thoughts and plunge us into the Negative State and reactive patterns.

With time and awareness, we can begin to notice the hole, step around it, and eventually choose a different way forward.

The process of learning a new way of responding to a trigger over time in the Mind Matrix Model is threefold:

1. You get triggered because someone is mean, or you feel like you failed at something, or whatever. You lose yourself, lose awareness, and later on you kind of "wake up" and either the Sentries come in telling you it's your fault or that you've been victimized, or you realize you were triggered and you might have a strong emotional response.
2. You get triggered, and you watch yourself get triggered but can't stop it. Once it clears, you treat yourself with compassion and get back to center, then you review what happened.
3. You are in a triggering situation, but instead of being triggered you go into your breathing and your body sensations while still remaining attentive to the situation. Afterward you work to clear whatever activation or trauma is remaining.

This process takes time. You may need to walk down the same street and fall into the same hole so many times, but you can see your progress by how you respond. The key is compassion.

There are three parts to work with when triggered: *before, during and after.*

- **Before** is what we're doing right now, thinking about how to respond to triggers. Maybe reviewing some recent experiences of being triggered, and thinking about how you could have responded in ways that would care for yourself and be more appropriate.
- **During** is the hardest. Be patient with yourself, because it will take a while to get to the place where you can recognize you are in the middle of a triggering.
- **After** is how you ground yourself and care for yourself after the triggering has passed. You may just sort of "wake up" or you may have been conscious during but unable to avoid being triggered. As much as you can, drop into your breathing and your body awareness. Watch for the Sentry "voices" that will either guilt trip you or tell you that you're a victim.

First, learn how to come back from triggering with self-compassion and self-care. Think about what message you're sending to your unconscious when you come back to yourself. If you get upset, you're telling your unconscious that you don't like returning to awareness, basically giving it instructions not to "wake you up."

Instead, do some positive self-talk such as "Okay, I just got triggered and I'm letting it pass through me as I breathe and as I'm coming back into my body." At first, self-talk can seem a little silly (your Sentries pushing back) but over time it just becomes a way to interact with yourself kindly and positively.

The Three-Level Toolbox: Meeting Yourself Where You Are

Healing happens through small shifts—not by forcing, but by offering yourself the right kind of support for your current State. Depending on how activated, collapsed, or overwhelmed you are, you'll need different kinds of tools. Think of it like a toolbox with three parts:

Level 1: Mindful Engagement

If you have some stability, even a little, you can engage directly with your Vital, Heart, or Head Self.

Examples:

> **Vital Self (Body)**: Try a gentle movement or body-based calming activity. For example, take a walk around the block, do some light stretching or yoga, or simply practice deep breathing for a few minutes. Even something as basic as eating a healthy meal or drinking water can be a mindful body engagement (nourishing your body).
>
> **Heart Self (Emotions)**: Do something that helps you safely express or soothe your emotions. You might journal about what you're feeling, have a heart-to-heart talk with a trusted friend, or engage in a creative outlet like drawing or playing music that mirrors your mood.
>
> **Head Self (Mind)**: Use a cognitive or mindfulness technique. For instance, if anxious thoughts are racing, practice catching one or two of those thoughts and gently challenging them ("Is it absolutely true that everything will go wrong? Maybe not."). Or do a short mindfulness meditation to come back to the present moment.

Goal: Strengthen and stabilize your State directly.

Level 2: Good Distraction

If mindful engagement feels too hard and you're struggling with being in the Negative State, you may need temporary, healthy distractions that calm your system without overwhelming it.

Examples:

- Watching a comforting, funny or uplifting movie, show, or video (cat videos!), or reading a comfortable book.
- Listening to, or playing, calming or uplifting music.
- Doing a simple hobby (drawing, puzzles, crafts) or engaging with some task (housework, gardening, etc.)
- Sitting outside or going for a walk and noticing small sensory details (the sky, the breeze).
- Eating something enjoyable (mindfully if possible).
- Holding a warm cup of tea.
- Gentle sensory stimulation (soft blanket, hot shower, cuddling a pet).

Goal: Buy time and create a safer internal environment so deeper healing becomes possible later.

Level 3: Last-Resort Distraction (Mindfully)

When you are very dysregulated—caught in panic, despair, or shutdown—you may need something more suppressive to get through the moment. These will depend on your own lifestyle, but they involve the behaviors that you know "aren't right" and you're supposed to stop.

The defining characteristic of suppressive activities is that they allow you to escape, to dissociate, to separate from being consciously aware. The bowl of ice cream that is suddenly empty, the cigarette that is suddenly gone. Lost time. That's dissociation, separating from your body and your mind as a way to deal with suffering.

We're going to try to use these activities as tools to soften the suffering, rather than just checking out. The difference is to engage with them consciously, and to titrate (do a little bit and then stop) instead of falling into them. It's a challenge, and you may fail, but if you keep at it, you can change something that was all about avoidance into something that shows you what you've been avoiding in a way that, along with the other tools we're going to cover in this book, you can change things.

Examples:
- Junk food, sugar
- Smoking
- Alcohol or other recreational drugs
- Binge watching TV, or getting obsessed with something on the Internet
- Excessive work or activity

These will be different for everyone.

> ***Important: This is not an excuse to fall back into an addiction that you had already stopped, that's just going to complicate the issue.***

Choose something that you are struggling with or that you do now that you know isn't the best thing for you, but with a focus on titrating and staying conscious.

For example, if you struggle to get off sugar, you might normally pull out a quart of ice cream and a spoon, and a little while later you sort of "wake up" and notice that the quart is gone. That is pure distraction and suppression, but the relief is temporary.

Instead, get a small bowl and a teaspoon and put a few scoops in, a lot less than usual.

Before you start eating, take a slow, deep breath and breathe it out. If you can, take another one. Sometimes the impending relief is enough to help regulate you somewhat.

Take a bite and stay with it, savor it, and pause between bites to notice how it makes you feel. Notice why you like it—taste, sensation, the familiar ritual.

Slowing down the process and lowering the amount you eat allows your body to begin to feel the comforting effects of the sugar and fat without overdosing, whereas if you eat a lot quickly it just jacks up your sugar level and then when it crashes, you'll feel hypoglycemic and crave sugar again.

You can use this same technique with any substance or activity you've been using to suppress your feelings.

If you're smoking, take a puff/toke and put it out, and concentrate on feeling the effects in your body. Wait until you feel like the sensations have stabilized before you light up again.

If you're drinking, take a small glass and sip it. Take several slow deep breaths, watch to see how it makes you feel before your next sip. If there's something you really like about how it feels that's gotten lost in the usual distraction, find out what it is.

There's always a positive reason for these activities, hiding within the "bad." For most of us, these addictions are actually excuses to pause for a bit and relax, and they suppress the anxiety or depression we are trying to get away from. Over time, you'll be able to generate these feelings in more positive ways.

Continue taking bites slowly and with pauses as much as you can. Sometimes it becomes too much and you just have to dive in. That's okay, just do your best.

Next, instead of going to fill up the bowl again, go do something else, preferably something in level 2, distraction.

Important:
Use these consciously and compassionately—not to run away forever, but to create a bridge back toward regulation. They're tools to stabilize first, not avoid feeling forever.

> *You are not failing if you need Level 2 or Level 3 some days. Every moment you keep yourself safer, even imperfectly, you are building your capacity for deeper healing later.*

Healing is not about doing the "right" thing. It's about honoring where you are, having compassion for your own struggle and suffering, and moving one step closer to balance.

There will always be days when you fall into your feelings and can't stop yourself from doing "bad" or self-destructive behaviors. The idea is to bring your feelings to consciousness so that you can work with them in a way that doesn't overwhelm you.

To summarize the Three-Level Toolbox:

> **Level 1 (Engage)** when you can face things directly.

- **Level 2 (Distract)** when you need a break but want to stay in a healthy zone.
- **Level 3 (Suppress)** when you are at your limit and just need to survive the wave.

Creating Your Safe Place

If you are dealing with intense feelings and you find that the feelings are still too much and you can't settle, imagine being in a very safe, quiet place like in the woods, by a stream, on the beach, or in a field. You might also picture being with a very close friend or a beloved pet. You can also play soft music or nature sounds as you do this.

Close your eyes and try to really immerse yourself in seeing, feeling, hearing, even smelling the place. Feel yourself there in your body. The more real you can make it, the better. Allow yourself to relax and unwind, breathe slowly and deeply. Feel your muscles relax and your nervous system settling.

We call this Your Safe Place, and you can return to it as needed, any time you are triggered or if you are working through feelings and are getting overwhelmed.

Vital, Heart, and Head: Supporting Each Self

Each of your Three Selves experiences stress, anxiety, and depression differently. Healing happens when you support each one—not all at once, but gradually, according to what your system can handle. Here's how:

Vital Self: Rebuilding Energy and Grounding

When the Vital Self is stressed or anxious:

- Body is tense, restless, jumpy.
- Fight/flight energy feels stuck.

When the Vital Self is depressed:

- Body feels heavy, drained, or numb.
- Movement and motivation are hard to access.

Support the Vital Self with:

- Gentle movement (walk, stretch, slow dance)

- Deep, slow breathing (especially exhale-focused breathing)
- Warmth and soothing (blankets, baths, sunlight)
- Nourishing food and hydration
- Acupressure points for energy and grounding (*see Chapter 8 - Balancing the Vital Self for more*)

Vital Self healing principle:

Move slowly. Nourish first. Build capacity gently.

Heart Self: Feeling Safe and Reconnecting

When the Heart Self is stressed or anxious:

Emotions flood in waves—fear, anger, sadness.

When the Heart Self is depressed:

Emotions flatten—sadness, numbness, loneliness.

Support the Heart Self with:

- Expressing feelings in safe ways (journaling, art, talking)
- Gentle co-regulation (spending time with safe, calming people)
- Listening to music that matches or gently lifts your mood
- Allowing small doses of emotion (titrated feeling, not overwhelming yourself)
- Soothing aromatherapy (rose, lavender, bergamot oils)

Heart Self healing principle:

Allow feelings to arise slowly, in safe doses. Connection heals.

Head Self: Calming Loops and Restoring Hope

When the Head Self is stressed or anxious:

Thoughts race, catastrophize, spiral.

When the Head Self is depressed:

Thoughts freeze, collapse, or turn hopeless.

Support the Head Self with:

- Mindfulness (coming back to the present moment)

- Gentle thought reframing (challenging "all or nothing" beliefs)
- Breaking tasks into tiny, manageable steps
- Using soothing routines (schedules, planners, visual lists)
- Light mental engagement (simple games, puzzles, short reading)

Head Self healing principle:

Interrupt loops gently. Rebuild hope one small proof at a time.

> *Important:*
>
> *You don't have to work with all three Selves at once. Often, strengthening even one Self begins to lift the others.*
>
> *Start where it feels most possible today. Often that means starting with the Vital Self.*

Healing Mindset Principles

Healing stress, anxiety, and depression isn't about battling yourself. It's about learning to work with your system, patiently and skillfully. Here are some guiding principles:

1. Start Where You Are

Don't wait to feel "ready." Begin with whatever tiny step feels possible today—even if that's just drinking a glass of water, or sitting outside for a minute.

2. Regulate First, Reflect Later

You can't think or feel clearly when you're too activated or collapsed. Focus first on calming and stabilizing your State—then explore feelings or patterns.

3. Feelings Are Not the Enemy

Many of us were taught to fear our own feelings. But avoiding them keeps the loop alive.

Healing depression and anxiety often means *feeling what was once too much to feel*—slowly, safely, without force.

4. Healing Must Be Titrated

You don't have to (and shouldn't) feel everything all at once. Healing happens in small, manageable doses, especially in the beginning. A little bit of sadness processed. A little bit of anxiety calmed. A little bit of hope restored. If you feel like it's spinning out of control, use the Toolbox in this chapter to slow things down.

5. Beware the Hamster Wheel

Trying to "outrun" depression with frantic activity doesn't work, it increases anxiety and deepens exhaustion. Real recovery begins when you step off the wheel and listen to your system's true needs.

6. Anxiety Can Clear and Reveal Depression

As you heal anxiety and chronic stress, it's common for depression to surface. This is not a setback—it's a deeper layer coming into view for healing.

7. Building Capacity Takes Time

You're not weak because you can't "snap out of it." It's normal to have periods where you get lost in depression or anxiety. You're building skills to create awareness and support your Vital, Heart, and Head Selves—slowly, steadily. Each moment of patience and care rewires your system toward resilience.

8. Don't Reset the Counter

When you "fall off the wagon," there's often a delightful little Head Self Sentry voice that comes in saying, "Oh well, we blew it. I guess we're back to zero again." This voice can be so depressing that it can lead to falling back into addictions or behaviors you've been trying to leave behind.

Instead, count the days or achievements continuously, don't reset. It is a normal thing to relapse, and the last thing you want to do is to turn the picture over to a Sentry. So just keep counting.

There is nothing wrong with you because you are struggling. Stress, anxiety, and depression are not signs of personal failure. They are signs that your system—your Vital Self, your Heart Self, your Head Self—has carried too much, for too long, without enough space to recover.

The way forward is not to fight harder, it is to listen more kindly. To regulate when you can, to feel safe when you can. To build small bridges back toward hope, energy, and connection that over time get stronger.

Some days, the bridge might be just taking a slow walk. Some days, it might be texting a friend. Some days, it might simply be getting out of bed and breathing deeply for a few minutes.

Each act of care—no matter how small—is a seed of healing.

You don't have to race to the finish line. You don't have to be fearless. You don't have to heal perfectly.

You just have to keep meeting yourself with compassion…step by step…breath by breath.

Trust that your system knows how to heal if you give it the space and time it needs.

You are not broken. You are in the process of healing.

The Journey Ahead

These two chapters have offered new ways of understanding and working with stress, anxiety, and depression. I've chosen to start here because the tools introduced are immediately useful for almost everyone—and they create a strong foundation for everything that follows.

In the upcoming chapters, we'll explore each of the Three Selves in depth, how to work with your State, and much more. You'll find practical steps not only for short-term relief and greater balance, but also for lasting change. These include therapeutic approaches, movement practices, cognitive exercises, meditations, and self-care techniques like acupressure, nutrition and herbs, homeopathy, and essential oils.

Each strategy is tailored to your unique needs and patterns, many of which you'll come to recognize and understand more clearly as we go.

What comes next is the unfolding of your own map: a deeper understanding of your mind, and the tools and supports you can use to improve your quality of life.

Chapter Seven

The Vital Self

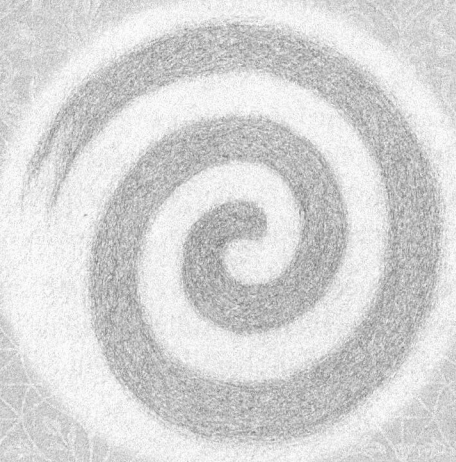

*Packed in my mind lie all the clothes
  Which outward nature wears,
And in its fashion's hourly change
  It all things else repairs.*

*In vain I look for change abroad,
  And can no difference find,
Till some new ray of peace uncalled
  Illumes my inmost mind...*

*Lo, when the sun streams through the wood,
  Upon a winter's morn,
Where'er his silent beams intrude
  The murky night is gone.*

~ Excerpt from The Inward Morning
  by Henry David Thoreau

Introduction: The Core of Survival and Thriving

Take a moment to think about your relationship with your day to day energy and state of mind, two things very much related to your Vital Self. Do you generally feel energized and responsive, easily adapting to life's demands, or do you often find yourself feeling tense, fatigued, or overwhelmed?

The Vital Self forms the essential foundation of your Mind Matrix, overseeing your body and its relationship to the space it lives and moves in. Unlike your Heart Self and Head Self, which process emotions and thoughts in nuanced ways, your Vital Self operates through direct physiological mechanisms. It's at the core of homeostasis, the function of keeping all of your systems in balance. It is in charge of energy regulation, physical survival, instinctual and reflexive responses, and bodily awareness.

Most of these things are either unconscious or something you take for granted, but it becomes very—even painfully—obvious how much we depend on our Vital Self when it's not working right.

How the Vital Self Speaks

The Vital Self communicates mostly through sensations. The body rush of excitement, the stomach tightening of fear, the dizziness of overstimulation, the heaviness of your body when you are tired. It communicates with you and with the unconscious of your other two Selves.

When balanced, your Vital Self allows you to adapt fluidly to internal signals and external demands, effortlessly shifting between states of rest, alertness, and action. But when it becomes dysregulated, you may experience chronic hypervigilance and tension (over-arousal), or fatigue and shutdown (under-arousal), disrupting your natural adaptability and leading to instability and unhealthy patterns.

In short, the Vital Self has earned its Mind Matrix Model name, being both essential (vital), and being the source of your vitality.

In this chapter, you'll explore your Vital Self's core mechanisms, learn how to recognize signs of dysregulation and imbalance, understand their root causes, and discover effective strategies for restoring balance. You'll learn how somatic and other therapies and holistic interventions can help you regain equilibrium, enhancing your overall well-being and resilience.

The Vital Self

The word "vital" has two meanings: it means both vitality or full of life and essential or absolutely necessary, and both of these meanings apply to the Vital Self. This part of you manages your energy, keeps your body alive, and helps you respond to the world through movement, instinct, and survival. It's the part of your system that takes care of your most basic needs—like breathing, heart rate, temperature, and whether you feel safe enough to rest or need to run. Without the Vital Self, nothing else can work properly. It's your foundation.

The Vital Self is mostly found in the deeper parts of your brain and your peripheral nervous system. It is the part of you that connects directly to your body, taking care of your basic needs and standing guard on the lookout for threats. It's like your internal caretaker and guard, constantly working to keep you balanced and appropriately energized, handling everything from hunger and thirst to sleep and movement, ensuring you're well-nourished, rested, and ready for action.

Although people often refer to these deeper, bodily processes as part of the "lower" or "primitive" brain, they are anything but that. In reality, these systems have evolved in tandem with the brain's higher cognitive functions, creating a network that is elegantly simple, extremely fast compared to the rest of the brain, and capable of governing a vast array of physical and sensory responses.

The Vital Self manages basic automatic processes like keeping you breathing and your heart pumping. It orchestrates reflexes such as pulling away from pain, and it's constantly monitoring the body's internal balance so you can respond fluidly to whatever arises internally or externally. It keeps track of how your body's doing overall, so you can respond smoothly to whatever's happening inside you or around you.

Another function of the Vital Self is filtering incoming sensory information through the brainstem and lower brain regions. The nervous system is constantly bombarded with input, but over 99% of that information is filtered out before reaching conscious awareness. This filtering helps protect the system from overload and allows you to focus on what seems most relevant or threatening in the moment.

However, when the Vital Self is dysregulated, it may either overfilter (numbing, dissociation) or underfilter (sensory overwhelm, hypervigilance)—shaping how you experience the world before thought or emotion even begin.

Because the Vital Self works so quickly and relies on instincts rather than careful thought, it can sometimes feel confusing or even alarming when it fires off strong reactions.

For example, it's behind the flash of anger when you feel threatened, the recoil of disgust when something seems harmful or gross, the pull of attraction toward what might be beneficial, or the feeling of "enough" that helps you stop eating when you're full.

While these gut-level impulses might clash with our more reflective or moral thinking, they serve an important role: keeping us safe, healthy, and alive. Recognizing these responses as coming from a deeply tuned survival system—not just a "less evolved" part of ourselves—helps us work with them rather than fighting against them.

But the Vital Self isn't only about survival. It manages *movement memory*, the ability to remember physical skills like riding a bike, swimming, or playing an instrument. Once you've practiced these skills, the Vital Self allows you to perform them smoothly and automatically, without having to consciously think about each step.

Remember the first time you drove a car, trying to pay attention to the road, the steering wheel, mirrors, accelerator and brake at the same time your mom or dad was yelling "Watch out for that tree!" But after a few tries, it got easier and now you hardly have to think about it. This ability takes a huge amount of work off of your conscious mind and the more strategic part of your unconscious we call the Head Self.

In a closely related way, it also handles your built-in sense of body awareness—where each part is in the space around you—called *proprioception*. That's why you can walk in the dark without tripping over your own feet or reach out and catch a ball without staring at your hand the whole time. If you've ever watched a gymnast flip and twist through the air, then land perfectly on their feet, you've seen an impressive example of how finely tuned our proprioception can be.

When the Vital Self's sense of proprioception is disrupted—due to fatigue, stress, or injury—you may feel clumsy, off-balance, or less aware of your physical boundaries. By practicing regular movement, mindfulness, and ensuring adequate rest, you can enhance your proprioceptive sense, leading to greater physical stability and confidence.

The Vital Self also sends out signals like pain, comfort, and fatigue. It communicates through sensations in your body, not with words or emotions. You know the sensations that say to you, "Take a break," "Stretch your legs," or "You need to rest now," feelings that clearly communicate its message without words.

If you listen to it, the Vital Self can help you to balance activity and rest, keep you resilient and prevent burnout. When you do listen to its messages and take care of yourself, everything can be in sync—feeling steady, energetic, and capable.

You've probably had the experience of being really in tune with your body, maybe when you've been exercising a lot or when you finally get the hang of a dance routine or dunking a basketball. It's exhilarating.

It can take a little detective work to figure out what exactly the Vital Self is trying to tell you.

› If you feel sluggish and low energy with difficulty getting moving, you may need more rest or you may be getting sick, or there could be emotional issues.

› If you feel too revved up, restless, have trouble sleeping, or even get physical symptoms like a racing heart or nonstop hunger, perhaps you're anxious and need to spend some time calming things down (or you're drinking too much coffee!)

Take the time to listen to your body, the messages the Vital Self is sending you. By tuning into these cues and responding appropriately, you can gain insight into your overall vitality and make choices that can help you feel more balanced, energized, and at home in your body.

The Neurological Basis of the Vital Self

You don't need a degree in neuroscience to appreciate how your body works—think of this next section as meeting the friendly team working quietly behind the scenes to keep you balanced and energized. Let's briefly meet each of these vital players and understand how they collaborate to keep you feeling stable and grounded.

Several key players in your brain and nervous system support the Vital Self:

- **Brainstem and Cerebellum**: The core of the Vital Self, these handle automatic functions like breathing and balance.
- **Amygdala**: Helps detect and respond to emotional and physical threats. It works with both the Vital Self and Heart Self.
- **Autonomic Nervous System (ANS)**: Manages your energy through two complementary systems—guided in part by the **reticular activating system (RAS)** in the brainstem —one for action (sympathetic nervous system) and one for relaxation (parasympathetic nervous system). The RAS is like the thermostat of the brain, determining how energized or calm you are in reaction to things around you and inside of you.
- **Enteric Nervous System (ENS)**: Often called your "gut brain," it's an entire brain in itself (about the size of a cat's brain) spread out through your digestive system which can strongly affect your digestion, your mood, and your stress levels.
  You've probably been hearing about the **gut biome**, the massive community of bacteria in your digestive system and how important it is. A healthy gut biome is a huge part of whether the ENS functions well, and therefore how you feel and how healthy you are.

Vaguely Nervous? No, Vagus Nerve!

One of the key players in maintaining balance for the Vital Self is the *vagus nerve*, which primarily activates your calming parasympathetic nervous system (PNS) to lower stress and help you relax. Interestingly, it sends most of its signals from the ENS, the gut brain, to the brain—letting your mind know what's going on in your body. It plays a big part in digestion, heart rate, and even emotional states, acting like a bridge between physical and emotional well-being.

While the vagus nerve helps you to relax, unwind and recover, if it is overactivated by severe stress or pain, overheating, or triggers like seeing blood, it can cause problems including a sudden and severe lightheadedness or fainting, as well as nausea or even vomiting. All in all, very unpleasant.

Simple strategies like deep breathing, gentle stretching, and humming (the vagus nerve goes right past the vocal cords) can help "tone" the vagus nerve, promoting a sense of calm and resilience. We'll be exploring more about the vagus nerve and these techniques in later chapters, so you can discover additional ways to tap into its calming power.

Things Gone Awry: Imbalances in the Vital Self

Each of your Three Selves can face challenges that throw them off, sometimes briefly and other times lasting far longer than you'd prefer.

For the Vital Self, these disruptions often stem from either imbalances or trauma. Imbalances might arise from something as straightforward as dietary choices, allergies, or sensitivities—like feeling sluggish after eating certain foods or restless after too much caffeine.

They can also come from environmental factors such as exposure to toxins, excessive noise, or even a stressful job that keeps your nervous system stuck in high gear. Genetics play a role as well, influencing how easily your system finds and maintains balance.

When the Vital Self becomes imbalanced, you might find yourself bouncing between feeling jittery, anxious, or restless (a sign of over-arousal) and feeling tired, lethargic, or emotionally flat (indicating under-arousal).

> *Jason, a software developer, frequently experienced high levels of stress at work, oscillating between restlessness and profound fatigue. By incorporating daily mindfulness and adjusting his diet to include adaptogenic herbs, he gradually stabilized his energy and improved overall resilience.*

You might notice that these states don't always match what's going on around you—they can seem random or even mysterious. Over time or with more severe issues, persistent imbalance can make it difficult to engage fully with life, leaving you feeling like you can't rally your energy or focus, or you're fighting your own body just to get through the day.

The good news is, once you start to understand your Vital Self signals, you can use the tools we're going to cover so that you can shift your State and improve your Vital Self balance. Whether it's adjusting your diet, managing environmental factors, or making lifestyle changes to reduce stress, there are many practical steps you can take to restore balance.

Additionally, interventions such as neurofeedback, mindfulness practices, gentle movement, and somatic therapies can directly support your nervous system, guiding it back toward stability and resilience.

As you become more aware of your Vital Self's patterns, you'll develop the skills to recognize when you're heading toward imbalance—and you'll have the tools to gently steer yourself back to a state of equilibrium and ease.

Dysregulation: The Vital Self Out of Balance

Your Vital Self is built to help you survive—and thrive—by constantly adapting to both internal conditions and external demands. But sometimes, those demands become too much, too fast, or go on for too long.

When that happens, the Vital Self can become chronically dysregulated: stuck in patterns of hyperarousal (agitation, tension, anxiety), hypoarousal (fatigue, numbness, fog), or bouncing chaotically between both. While trauma is a well-known cause of dysregulation, it is far from the only one.

Chronic dysregulation of the Vital Self can come from many sources, often layered together over time. These include:

Developmental Imbalance

When a child's early physical or sensory needs are met inconsistently—or the environment is overstimulating, chaotic, or neglectful—the nervous system adapts by becoming overly reactive or shutting down. Even without overt trauma, an infant who doesn't feel "held" by their environment may wire for tension, dissociation, or shallow breathing as a baseline.

Trauma and Stored Survival Responses

Trauma—especially physical trauma or threats to bodily integrity—can leave imprints in the brainstem and autonomic nervous system. This includes not only direct harm (accidents, violence, invasive medical procedures) but also long-term activation from growing up in a household that felt unsafe. The Vital Self doesn't need a "reason" to stay on guard; it simply learns what it was taught to expect.

Genetic and Constitutional Sensitivity

Some people are born with highly sensitive nervous systems. This may be experienced as neurodivergence (such as autism or ADHD), sensory processing sensitivity, or simply a naturally high reactivity to stimulation. These traits are not flaws, but they do mean that the system is more easily pushed out of balance by environmental stressors or internal depletion.

Chronic Illness and Inflammation

Any long-term health condition that affects energy, immunity, or inflammation—such as autoimmune disorders, hormonal imbalances, digestive issues, or persistent infections—can disrupt the Vital Self. This happens not just through symptoms, but through the constant strain on the system's ability to recover and self-regulate.

Environmental and Sensory Stressors

Noisy, crowded, artificial, or chemically toxic environments wear down the Vital Self over time. Poor lighting, lack of access to nature, exposure to screens and EMFs, even clutter or disorganization in the home can subtly and chronically tax the nervous system, leaving it more vulnerable to burnout and collapse.

Lifestyle Depletion

Sleep deprivation, poor diet, insufficient hydration, excessive stimulant use (caffeine, sugar), and lack of physical movement all impact the regulation capacity of the Vital Self. When the body doesn't get what it needs to function well, the system becomes more volatile and less resilient, even if there's no single "traumatic" event behind it.

Symbolic and Cultural Imprints

The Vital Self responds not just to physical reality, but to symbolic threat—images of violence, social comparison, and media saturation. Repeated exposure to fear-based messaging (news, social media, disaster narratives) keeps the body in low-level activation even when nothing dangerous is happening. This is especially true for highly sensitive or empathic people.

Structural Oppression and Economic Insecurity

Living in a society where your safety, resources, or worth are constantly questioned—due to discrimination, poverty, disability, or other systemic stressors—can keep the Vital Self on alert indefinitely. Even "coping" with this through numbness or hyperfunctioning is a form of dysregulation the body must pay for over time.

When the Vital Self becomes chronically dysregulated, your entire system loses flexibility. You may find it difficult to rest even when you're tired, to energize even when motivated, or to feel present in your own body. But this isn't a flaw, it's your body's attempt to adapt to overwhelming demands. With awareness and consistent support, it's possible to rebuild your State Range, restore trust in your body, and reestablish the deep foundation of regulation the Vital Self is meant to provide.

Trauma and the Vital Self

The Vital Self is the foundation of your survival system. It's the first to develop in infancy and the most deeply tied to your physical body. Because of this, trauma that affects the Vital Self can leave especially primal, lasting imprints, often without words or conscious memory.

What does Vital Self trauma look like?

It might not always be obvious. While people often associate trauma with major, dramatic events, the Vital Self is shaped just as profoundly by what was missing: warmth, attunement, predictable care. If the body didn't feel safe in the earliest months and years of life, the system may have adapted by becoming tense, hyper-alert, disconnected, or numb.

Common roots of Vital Self trauma include:

- Early medical trauma (NICU stays, surgeries, invasive procedures)
- Neglect or inconsistent caregiving in infancy
- Unsafe or chaotic home environments (unpredictability, tension)
- Physical abuse or rough handling
- Chronic illness or physical pain in childhood
- Overstimulation or sensory overwhelm with no ability to regulate
- Trauma stored in the body, even without physical harm

Even events that seemed minor to others—like being left to cry alone, being scolded for bodily needs, or being forced to perform before your system was ready—can wire the Vital Self to believe the world is not a safe place to rest, feel, or exist.

How does Vital Self trauma show up now?

You may not remember the source, but your body does. Vital trauma can manifest in both overactivation and shutdown:

- Chronic tension, shallow breathing, or hypervigilance
- Sleep difficulties, digestive issues, or sensory overwhelm
- Feeling "revved up" or stuck in fight-or-flight mode
- A sense of disconnection from your body, or difficulty feeling physical sensations
- A baseline belief that it's not safe to relax or let your guard down

In some cases, trauma to the Vital Self shows up as an inability to feel safe even in safety. The body may remain on alert, or collapse into fatigue, even when the present moment offers no threat. This is not a failure—it's the legacy of a system that had to adapt without help.

What heals Vital Self trauma?

Healing begins with safety—not by reliving the trauma, but by creating new experiences that contradict its message. That might include:

- Feeling your breath deepen while lying on the earth
- Being gently held by someone safe
- Swaying, rocking, or walking in rhythm
- Tending to basic needs with care—food, warmth, sleep
- Using acupressure, somatic practices, or trauma-informed bodywork

You don't have to understand the trauma cognitively for your body to begin releasing it. The Monarch—the conscious part of you—can help by witnessing gently, staying present, and creating environments that invite the body to soften, one moment at a time.

The Vital Self and Early Trauma

The Vital Self is all about survival and feeling safe. For a baby, that sense of safety comes from the people who care for them. When caregivers are consistent and nurturing, the baby starts to trust that the world is a secure place. But if a baby's basic needs for comfort and security aren't met—whether through neglect, trauma, or inconsistent care—this can feel like a threat to survival, even when there's no direct physical harm.

In these situations, the Vital Self can get temporarily triggered, or even get stuck, in the Negative State. We talked about this in the first chapter—the Negative State can trigger the body and mind to remain on high alert, constantly scanning for danger. The baby learns to expect the worst, developing patterns of fear, hypervigilance, or emotional disconnection that can carry over into adulthood.

As adults, people who grew up with an unstable sense of safety might feel anxious, distrustful, or perpetually "on guard," even when things are objectively safe. They may find it difficult to relax or feel stuck between states of high stress and withdrawal. This can strongly interfere with feeling secure in relationships or within the world at large.

In short, early trauma or neglect can result in either being easily triggered into the Negative State, or create a lasting Negative State activation in the Vital Self—one rooted in fear and insecurity that impacts stress management, self-confidence, and overall well-being.

It can also affect their foundational development, particularly their ability to clearly distinguish between their own needs and others, what in the Mind Matrix Model is called *Self-Other Differentiation* which we'll talk about more in chapter eighteen.

Older kids or even adults with this imbalanced sense of self, along with being easily triggered, may end up being afraid that they aren't safe unless the people or things around them are okay. Or they may swing to the other side and be insensitive and unaware of the needs of others because they are too busy fending off the fear of not having enough.

The good news is that, with self-understanding, some good support, and often the appropriate therapies and modalities, it is possible to bring the Vital Self into more balance and greatly improve how you feel and your quality of life. Techniques like mindfulness and grounding exercises can help the Vital Self learn new patterns of safety.

In later chapters, we'll explore practical ways to work with trauma, heal these deep-rooted fears, and restore a greater sense of calm and resilience.

The Vital Self Axis: Balancing Arousal Levels

The Vital Self operates along a spectrum of arousal—from high-energy, active states to calm, restful states. As I mentioned above, this balance is managed by the *Reticular Activating System* (RAS), a network in the brainstem that regulates alertness and energy.

Low Arousal (Calm States): In restful states, the RAS slows down, promoting relaxation and recovery. It engages the calming parasympathetic system, allowing the body to recharge. This low activity level helps:

> **Relaxation and Physical Recovery**: The brainstem and hypothalamus lower heart rate and relax muscles, supporting physical healing and energy restoration. The hypothalamus acts like your body's internal thermostat and master regulator, adjusting hormones, temperature, and essential rhythms to keep your body balanced and comfortable.
>
> **Memory and Learning**: When the brain is less active, the hippocampus organizes and stores information from the day, strengthening your memory and enhancing learning. It acts as your mind's librarian, sorting through daily events, deciding what's important to keep, and helping you create meaningful connections between past and present experiences. All of this consolidation of memory lowers your stress level.
>
> **Emotional Balance**: Lower arousal calms the amygdala, reducing stress and helping the prefrontal cortex process emotions. The amygdala is like your internal alarm system, helping detect emotional significance and potential threats. When balanced, it stays calm, helping your prefrontal cortex manage and regulate your emotions smoothly, instead of triggering reactive or defensive responses.
>
> **Creativity and Reflection**: The Default Mode Network (DMN) activates, supporting creative thinking, problem-solving, and reflection. The DMN is a brain network that becomes active when you're resting or daydreaming, allowing your mind to integrate experiences, imagine future scenarios, and generate new ideas by connecting past experiences with present challenges.

High Arousal (Alert States): In high-energy states, the RAS increases activity, preparing you to face challenges by engaging the sympathetic (activating) system. It directs energy to specific areas based on need:

> **Sensory Focus**: It enhances sensory processing, helping you focus on important information.
>
> **Emotional Response**: The amygdala becomes more sensitive, heightening your emotional response to potential threats.
>
> **Decision-Making**: The prefrontal cortex boosts problem-solving and executive control.
>
> **Physical Readiness**: The motor cortex and basal ganglia prepare the body for quick, coordinated action. The basal ganglia, together with the cerebellum, act like your body's skilled choreographer, smoothly coordinating movement patterns, automating routine behaviors, and helping you perform familiar tasks efficiently and effortlessly.

By carefully adjusting arousal levels, the Reticular Activating System (RAS) keeps the Vital Self balanced, ensuring we're ready for action when needed but able to relax and recharge when it's time. This balance between high and low arousal is essential for both short-term survival and long-term health. However, the RAS can become imbalanced in a few different ways:

> **Overactivated** (High Arousal): When the RAS is running in overdrive, we may feel anxious, restless, or tense. We might also seek out riskier activities in an attempt to manage or release this high energy. In its most severe form, this overactivation can manifest as mania, where someone experiences extreme restlessness, impulsivity, and a reduced need for sleep.
>
> **Underactivated** (Low Arousal): On the other end of the spectrum, an underactive RAS can leave us feeling fatigued, sluggish, or unmotivated. This low-energy state can sometimes contribute to depressive feelings, making it tough to get up, move, or engage with daily life.
>
> **Instability** (Swinging Between the Two): Some people experience rapid shifts between high and low arousal—one moment feeling wired and restless, the next feeling drained or detached. These swings can be emotionally and physically exhausting, and they often disrupt routines and relationships.

The good news is that there are ways to help regulate your RAS and bring it back into balance. Regular exercise, for example, can channel excess energy and support a more stable arousal state. Consistent sleep schedules, relaxation techniques like deep breathing or gentle stretching, and a balanced diet can also help prevent big ups and downs.

The Vital Self and the State Axis

The Vital Self is deeply entwined with your State—it is both the messenger and the responder. When something shifts in your environment, your Vital Self is the first to register it: a tightening in your belly, a catch in your breath, a spark of energy or sudden fatigue. These physiological shifts are not just random—they're clues that your system is moving along the **State Axis**, from calm and regulated to reactive and overwhelmed, or back again.

Below you can see a diagram of the Vital Self axis interacting with State.

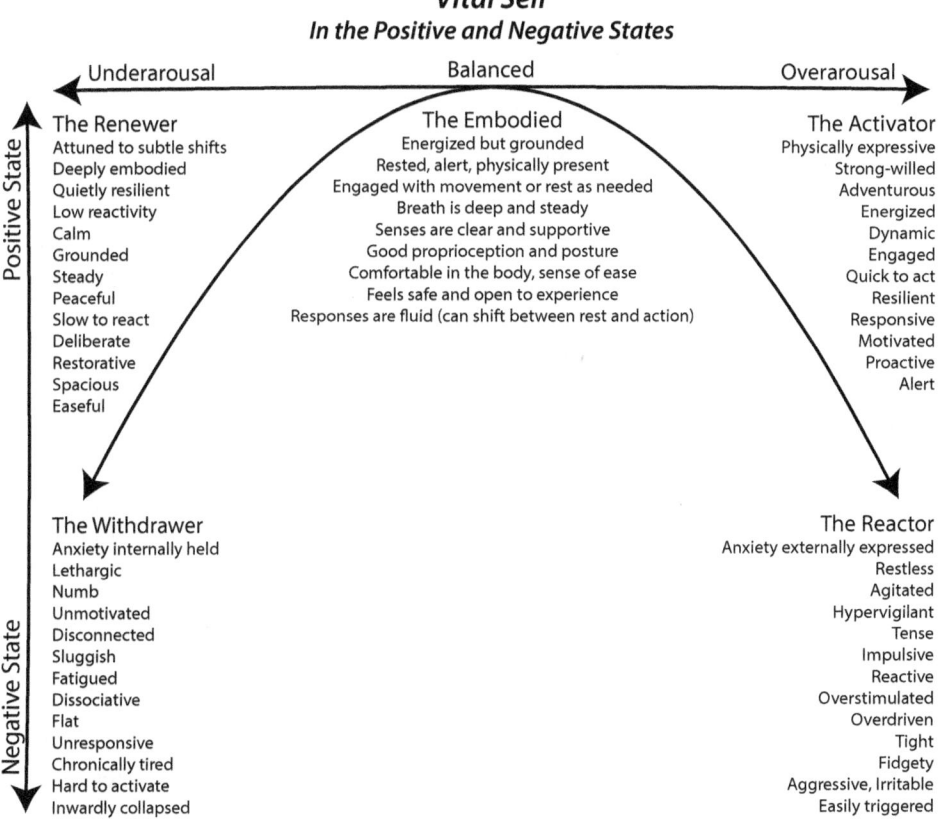

The vertical State arrow reflects how a Positive State evokes a grounded sense of self, a well regulated body, and supports calm breathing, steady heart rhythm, and a felt sense of safety. This, in turn, feeds upward into a healthy Heart Self and clear Head Self, sustaining your presence in the Positive State.

Think of the Vital Self as the body's ambassador to your overall State. It senses threat or safety first, sending signals that either keep you in the **Positive State**—centered, empowered, and adaptable—or push you into the **Negative State**, where survival mechanisms override reflection.

But when the Vital Self becomes dysregulated toward the Negative State—whether through tension, exhaustion, poor sleep, or chronic stress—it can pull the rest of the system down with it.

This is especially true when the Vital Self stays stuck in a **Loop**. For example, chronic stress might keep your sympathetic nervous system in overdrive (fight/flight), even when no danger is present. Over time, this can narrow your **State Range**—the territory in which you feel "okay." You might find yourself constantly on edge, reactive, or emotionally numb. And because the Vital Self reacts faster than the conscious mind, your State can shift before you even realize what's happening.

The good news is that the Vital Self is also the fastest route back into balance. Breath, movement, grounding, and touch all offer powerful ways to shift your physiology and reclaim your State. When your body calms, your thoughts often follow. When your breath slows, your heart softens. And when your Vital Self feels safe, the rest of the Mind Matrix can function as intended: clear, connected, and in flow.

Self-Other Development in the Vital Self

Self-Other Development begins with embodiment. As infants, we don't yet know that our body is "ours"—we cry, we move, we feel, but it takes time to understand that we are separate from the environment.

The Vital Self learns this through sensation, rhythm, and regulation. If our cries are answered, if we are held, seen, and soothed, we begin to sense our own boundaries. But if our needs are ignored or overstimulated, our bodies may learn to tune out or signal loudly to survive. This sets the foundation for how we orient toward self or other in all that follows.

Final Thoughts

The Vital Self is a powerful force in your life, guiding everything from your survival instincts to the energy that fuels creativity and joy. By understanding how it works and finding ways to keep it balanced, you can enhance your ability to truly thrive.

Whether through mindfulness, therapy, lifestyle changes, mindful eating, or using herbs, nutraceuticals (nutritional supplements), and other remedies, there are many ways to support a life full of vitality, resilience, and fulfillment. Learning to manage and balance your Vital Self strengthens the foundation for all the central nervous system's functions, leading to a healthier, more vibrant life.

Chapter Eight
Balancing the Vital Self

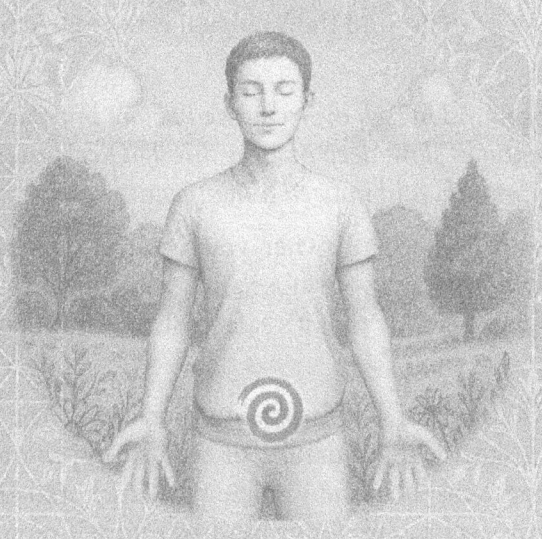

*Return to your breath
  to quiet the mind,
  to listen to the body.*

*Return to your feet
  to stand still,
  to know where you are.*

*You don't need to fight or run or hide.
You don't need to be different than you are.
  Only find your breath,
  only feel your body,
  only find your ground.*

*~ Return to Your Breath
  by Sam McClellan*

Grounding the Vital Self

For the Vital Self, stability comes from balancing movement with rest. Repetitive, familiar activities—like walking, stretching, making tea, or practicing a favorite skill—help us feel grounded and let go of tension. Whether you're running old football drills, playing the piano, or cooking a well-loved recipe, these comfortable routines keep the body centered and prepared for action.

Another helpful way to ground the Vital Self is through conscious breathing.

> *When Callie found herself overwhelmed before important meetings, she adopted a habit of slow, deep breaths through her nose, exhaling softly through her mouth, and noticed a significant decrease in anxiety.*

Slow, steady breaths—especially when you focus on the sensation of breathing deeply through your nose and gently out through your mouth—can signal the body that it's safe, easing tension and promoting resilience.

Environment also matters: simply placing your feet on the floor or ground, taking a short walk in nature, or even sitting comfortably in a calm, familiar space can help the Vital Self feel anchored and supported. We'll explore more techniques for grounding and self-regulation in later chapters, giving you practical tools to maintain this crucial balance.

At the same time, deep rest—including good sleep and mindful relaxation—is just as crucial. These quiet moments allow the body to recharge and process both physical and emotional experiences. By cycling between activity and rest, the Vital Self stays balanced, adapts more easily to stress, and supports the rest of our mind and body in meeting life's demands.

> *Please note that those with a body-based trauma background may find it very challenging initially to ground in the body or breath. In this case, grounding in the feel of gravity and the space around you should work well.*

We'll go into more ways to ground and balance the Vital Self later in this chapter and in related chapters.

Regulating Across the Vital Self Axis

The Vital Self operates along a spectrum of arousal—from low energy (hypoarousal, shutdown) to high energy (hyperarousal, fight/flight). Many people fluctuate between these poles, especially under chronic stress. Others tend to stay stuck on one side. For a better idea of where you fall, complete the following questionnaire.

Vital Self Questionnaire

This self-assessment helps you explore how your body and energy system—your Vital Self—responds to daily life. It identifies patterns of underactivation (hypoarousal), overactivation (hyperarousal), balance, or instability. Your results guide specific practices in the Mind Matrix Model to support regulation and vitality.

You can also access a downloadable PDF version of the form as well as an interactive version by visiting the Mind Matrix Model website. You'll need to register if you haven't yet. You can sign up for free access by scanning the QR code or visiting this short link:

mmm.tips/vitalform

https://mmm.tips/vitalform

The interactive form can be used to chart your progress over time, and includes many combination patterns that reveal more complex dynamics.

Instructions

For each question, choose the option (Rarely true, Sometimes true, Often true, Very true) that best describes your typical experience—not what you wish were true. Don't overthink it. Go with your first honest reaction.

Use a journal, notes app, or form field to track your responses.

If you are keeping a journal, this is a good time to write your responses down so you can check up on how you're doing later. Otherwise just grab a piece of paper or a screen device to track your answers.

> **Note:** *This is not a medical test, but a self-reflection tool designed to help you explore approaches for improving your quality of life. If you have any concerns, consider consulting a healthcare professional or therapist for personalized guidance.*

1. Energy and Alertness

A) I often feel drained or sluggish, even without much effort.
○ Rarely true=1 ○ Sometimes true=2 ○ Often true=3 ○ Very true=4

B) I generally have steady, consistent energy throughout the day.
○ Rarely true=1 ○ Sometimes true=2 ○ Often true=3 ○ Very true=4

C) I feel overly energized, jittery, or restless, especially under pressure.
○ Rarely true=1 ○ Sometimes true=2 ○ Often true=3 ○ Very true=4

D) I swing between exhaustion and being wired or overstimulated.
○ Rarely true=1 ○ Sometimes true=2 ○ Often true=3 ○ Very true=4

2. Sleep Patterns

A) I sleep a lot but rarely feel rested.
○ Rarely true=1 ○ Sometimes true=2 ○ Often true=3 ○ Very true=4

B) I sleep well most nights and usually wake up feeling refreshed.
○ Rarely true=1 ○ Sometimes true=2 ○ Often true=3 ○ Very true=4

C) I have trouble falling asleep or wake up feeling tense or on alert.
○ Rarely true=1 ○ Sometimes true=2 ○ Often true=3 ○ Very true=4

D) My sleep is inconsistent—some nights I oversleep, others I can't sleep at all.
○ Rarely true=1 ○ Sometimes true=2 ○ Often true=3 ○ Very true=4

3. Eating and Appetite

A) I frequently have low appetite or forget to eat.
○ Rarely true=1 ○ Sometimes true=2 ○ Often true=3 ○ Very true=4

B) I eat regularly and feel nourished by meals.
○ Rarely true=1 ○ Sometimes true=2 ○ Often true=3 ○ Very true=4

C) I crave food constantly, especially when stressed or overwhelmed.
○ Rarely true=1 ○ Sometimes true=2 ○ Often true=3 ○ Very true=4

D) I alternate between little appetite and overeating.
○ Rarely true=1 ○ Sometimes true=2 ○ Often true=3 ○ Very true=4

4. Physical Movement

A) I often feel heavy, slow or unmotivated to move.

○ Rarely true=1   ○ Sometimes true=2   ○ Often true=3   ○ Very true=4

B) I engage in regular activity and feel good moving or resting.

○ Rarely true=1   ○ Sometimes true=2   ○ Often true=3   ○ Very true=4

C) I feel a constant need to move or fidget, even when I'm tired.

○ Rarely true=1   ○ Sometimes true=2   ○ Often true=3   ○ Very true=4

D) I swing between long periods of inactivity and bursts of high energy.

○ Rarely true=1   ○ Sometimes true=2   ○ Often true=3   ○ Very true=4

5. Breathing

A) I forget to breathe deeply or feel like my breath is flat or stuck.

○ Rarely true=1   ○ Sometimes true=2   ○ Often true=3   ○ Very true=4

B) My breath is usually steady and helps me feel centered.

○ Rarely true=1   ○ Sometimes true=2   ○ Often true=3   ○ Very true=4

C) My breathing is fast or shallow, especially under stress.

○ Rarely true=1   ○ Sometimes true=2   ○ Often true=3   ○ Very true=4

D) I go from shallow breathing to big sighs or suddenly gasping.

○ Rarely true=1   ○ Sometimes true=2   ○ Often true=3   ○ Very true=4

6. Body Awareness

A) I often feel disconnected from my body or unaware of how it feels.

○ Rarely true=1   ○ Sometimes true=2   ○ Often true=3   ○ Very true=4

B) I'm generally aware of how my body feels and what it needs.

○ Rarely true=1   ○ Sometimes true=2   ○ Often true=3   ○ Very true=4

C) I notice a lot of tension or overstimulation in my body.

○ Rarely true=1   ○ Sometimes true=2   ○ Often true=3   ○ Very true=4

D) I shift between being numb and being overly sensation sensitive.

○ Rarely true=1   ○ Sometimes true=2   ○ Often true=3   ○ Very true=4

7. Stress Response

A) I tend to freeze, go blank, or zone out when stressed.

○ Rarely true=1   ○ Sometimes true=2   ○ Often true=3   ○ Very true=4

B) I can respond to stress and return to calm fairly easily.

○ Rarely true=1   ○ Sometimes true=2   ○ Often true=3   ○ Very true=4

C) I get easily agitated or overreact to small stressors.

○ Rarely true=1   ○ Sometimes true=2   ○ Often true=3   ○ Very true=4

D) I flip between shutting down and getting worked up quickly.

○ Rarely true=1   ○ Sometimes true=2   ○ Often true=3   ○ Very true=4

8. Daily Rhythm

A) I often feel like I'm dragging through the day and just getting by.

○ Rarely true=1   ○ Sometimes true=2   ○ Often true=3   ○ Very true=4

B) My energy rises and falls naturally throughout the day.

○ Rarely true=1   ○ Sometimes true=2   ○ Often true=3   ○ Very true=4

C) I feel constantly activated or busy with little downtime.

○ Rarely true=1   ○ Sometimes true=2   ○ Often true=3   ○ Very true=4

D) My days are unpredictable—some are slow and foggy, others are hyperactive and overwhelming.

○ Rarely true=1   ○ Sometimes true=2   ○ Often true=3   ○ Very true=4

9. Mental Clarity

A) My thinking feels foggy or slow much of the time.

○ Rarely true=1   ○ Sometimes true=2   ○ Often true=3   ○ Very true=4

B) My thinking is generally clear, even under mild stress.

○ Rarely true=1   ○ Sometimes true=2   ○ Often true=3   ○ Very true=4

C) My mind races or feels overstimulated, especially under pressure.

○ Rarely true=1   ○ Sometimes true=2   ○ Often true=3   ○ Very true=4

D) I swing between mental fog and overthinking.

○ Rarely true=1   ○ Sometimes true=2   ○ Often true=3   ○ Very true=4

10. Body Temperature and Sensation

A) I feel cold or numb often, especially in my hands and feet.
○ Rarely true=1   ○ Sometimes true=2   ○ Often true=3   ○ Very true=4

B) I generally feel comfortable with my body temperature.
○ Rarely true=1   ○ Sometimes true=2   ○ Often true=3   ○ Very true=4

C) I feel overheated or too activated, like my system is revved up.
○ Rarely true=1   ○ Sometimes true=2   ○ Often true=3   ○ Very true=4

D) I experience sharp swings—sweaty and hot one moment, chilled or flat the next.
○ Rarely true=1   ○ Sometimes true=2   ○ Often true=3   ○ Very true=4

How to Score Your Vital Self Axis Questionnaire

Step 1: Tally Your Scores

> Go through your answers and total the points for each letter:

Each time you rated an A, add the point value you selected (1 = Rarely True, 4 = Very True) to your A total.

> Do the same for B, C, and D responses. For example, if you answered Rarely true eight times, that would total 8, Sometimes true eight times would be 16, Often true eight times = 24, Very true eight times = 32.

Best to add this up on a separate piece of paper or in your journal.

Each letter will have a total between 10 (lowest) and 40 (highest).

Your Scores:

A =   B =   C =   D =

Each letter represents a type of Vital Self pattern:

A = Hypoaroused Vital Self - Low energy, shutdown, fatigue, or numbness.

B = Balanced Vital Self - Stable, resilient energy regulation.

C = Hyperaroused Vital Self - Overdrive, tension, restlessness, or constant activation.

D = Unstable Vital Self - Swings between extremes.

Step 2: Interpretation

Find which pattern below matches your scores.

A=30 or more - Hypoaroused Vital Self (Underactive)

Your system may be operating in chronic low energy—shutdown, fatigue, or numbness. This often develops from burnout, long-term stress, or trauma that led your system to give up on mobilizing.

What to support: Gentle reactivation through rhythmic movement, grounding, and Vital Self-oriented Override Strategies that restore trust in action and sensation.

Read: Ch. 7: The Vital Self; Ch. 8: Balancing the Vital Self

B=30 or more - Balanced Vital Self (Regulated & Resilient)

You appear to have stable energy regulation. You can respond to physical and emotional demands without collapsing or overreacting. Your system knows how to reset.

What to support: Maintain steady routines, sleep rhythm, nutrition, and joyful movement. Leverage your stability to support Heart and Head regulation when needed.

Read: Ch. 7: The Vital Self; Ch. 8: Balancing the Vital Self

C=30 or more - Hyperaroused Vital Self (Overactive)

Your system may be running hot—always on guard, tense, or easily overstimulated. Even rest may feel unreachable or guilt-inducing. This often reflects unprocessed urgency in the body.

What to support: Calming, deceleration, and practices that downshift the nervous system (e.g., exhale-focused breathing, movement, touch).

Read: Ch. 7: The Vital Self; Ch. 8: Balancing the Vital Self

D=25 or more - Unstable Vital Self (Swinging / Fragmented)

You may be swinging between highs and lows—wired one moment, shut down the next. This points to a fragile rhythm system, often shaped by trauma or overwhelm.

What to support: Safety, predictability, rhythm. Prioritize containment and co-regulation, and avoid extremes like overstimulation or collapse.

Read: Ch. 7: The Vital Self; Ch. 8: Balancing the Vital Self

If none of your scores is 30 or more, choose the one that is the highest score. This indicates that you could have a more complex pattern that the interactive form on the website would reveal.

Follow-Up Reflection (Optional)

These can go in a journal:

"When do I feel most alive and grounded?"

"When do I notice my body starts to check out or race?"

"What helps me feel calm but alert?"

"What does my body need more of—movement, stillness, rhythm, or nourishment?"

Next Steps

Look for the sections in this chapter that correspond to your results:

- If you scored mostly A, read: Approaches to Balancing Underactive Vital Self
- If you scored mostly C, read: Approaches to Balancing Overactive Vital Self
- If you scored mostly D, or a mix of A and C, read: Approaches to Stabilizing the Vital Self

These sections include grounding practices, movement-based strategies, breathwork, nutrition and herbs, homeopathy, and trauma-informed somatic tools—all selected to help restore your energy system.

If you have ongoing health or emotional concerns, consider talking with a trusted healthcare professional who can give tailored advice. You might also ask a friend or family member to fill this questionnaire out about you for extra insight, since our own perspectives can sometimes be biased.

Therapies

These are therapies that can be specifically helpful for dysregulation in the Vital Self:

Neurofeedback

What It Is: A therapy that uses real-time monitoring of the activity of your brainwaves (using an EEG, or electroencephalograph) to teach your brain how to self-regulate and promote stable arousal levels.

How It Helps: Neurofeedback can be useful for many conditions including ADHD, anxiety, and insomnia by giving your brain immediate feedback to learn healthier patterns. It specifically addresses hypoarousal and hyperarousal.

EMDR (Eye Movement Desensitization and Reprocessing)

What It Is: A trauma-focused therapy that uses bilateral stimulation (such as eye movements, tapping, or tones) while recalling distressing experiences, allowing the brain and nervous system to reprocess and release stored emotional and physiological charge.

How It Helps: EMDR is especially effective for trauma-based dysregulation that lives in the Vital Self—flashbacks, freeze states, and chronic tension patterns. By targeting unresolved survival responses held in the body, EMDR helps the nervous system return to a more stable baseline. It can also support emotional integration across the Heart and Head Selves.

Mindfulness-Based Stress Reduction (MBSR)

What It Is: MBSR combines mindfulness meditation, gentle yoga, and body awareness exercises.

How It Helps: This structured program helps reduce stress, balance arousal levels, and enhance emotional stability. It's widely studied and often recommended by healthcare providers.

The following therapies are specifically helpful for Vital Self trauma, and also address Vital Self dysregulation.

Deep Brain Reorienting (DBR)

What It Is: DBR focuses on deep brain structures involved in threat and trauma responses, specifically in the brainstem which most other therapies can't reach directly.

How It Helps: By addressing the deep areas of the brain, DBR helps release deeply rooted emotional responses connected to early trauma or overwhelming experiences. Over time, it aims to reorganize how your nervous system reacts to stress, leading to a more grounded, stable sense of self.

Somatic Experiencing

What It Is: A body-focused therapy that helps you become aware of and release stored trauma through sensation-based work. It is one of the few therapies that is acknowledged to address brainstem-level trauma.

How It Helps: By paying attention to how stress and trauma live in the body, you can gradually resolve physical manifestations of stress and restore a more balanced arousal level.

Nutritional Strategies and Supplements

Your body needs the right nutrients to stay balanced. While individual needs vary, some people find benefit in focusing on:

- **Omega-3 Fatty Acids:** Found in fish oil or flaxseeds, omega-3s support brain health and may help regulate mood.
- **Magnesium:** Known as the "relaxation" mineral, it can help with sleep and stress management. The best forms are magnesium glycinate or magnesium l-threonate, avoid magnesium oxide as it's poorly absorbed and can build up in your system.
- **B Vitamins:** Important for energy and a healthy nervous system.
- **Adaptogens:** Herbs thought to help the body adapt to stress, though responses can differ from person to person. These include:

    Ashwagandha, which promotes relaxation, improves resilience, and balances adrenal function

    Holy basil (Tulsi), which calms anxiety and regulates cortisol levels

    Rhodiola rosea, known for combating fatigue and supporting energy

Asian ginseng (panax ginseng or siberian ginseng), known to boost energy and mental clarity

American ginseng (panax quinquefolius), a gentler option that helps balance the nervous system, offering calming effects suitable even for those sensitive to overstimulation.

See *Chapter 26 - Nutritional Supplements & Adaptogens* for more.

Note: Some adaptogens, like rhodiola and Asian ginseng, can be stimulating and may cause agitation or restlessness, especially if you're prone to high anxiety, heat sensations, or overstimulation. Gentler adaptogens like ashwagandha and holy basil tend to be more calming and balancing. Always start with smaller doses and pay close attention to how your body responds, adjusting accordingly.

Always consider checking with a healthcare professional before adding new supplements, especially if you take medications or have underlying health issues.

Lifestyle Changes: A Foundation for Your Vital Self

Healthy daily habits are crucial for establishing and maintaining a stable Vital Self, helping you remain balanced, energized, and resilient to life's challenges. Integrating these habits consistently into your routine creates lasting positive effects on your physical, emotional, and mental health.

Regular Exercise: Channeling and Balancing Your Energy

Physical movement is essential not just for fitness but for the overall regulation of your Vital Self. Exercise helps channel energy constructively, releasing built-up stress and tension while promoting healthy circulation, metabolism, and mood stabilization.

Daily Movement: Aim for at least 20-30 minutes of moderate physical activity daily. Walking, biking, or yoga are excellent choices.

Mindful Movement: Practices like yoga, Tai Chi, or Qigong not only provide physical benefits but also cultivate mindfulness and body awareness, further supporting your Vital Self's balance.

Gentle Exercise: Incorporate gentle stretching or yoga for at least 10–20 minutes, 3–4 times weekly, daily if stress levels are high.

Balanced Nutrition

The food you consume directly impacts your energy levels, mood, and overall health. A balanced diet provides consistent energy and reduces the likelihood of inflammation or digestive issues that disrupt your vitality.

Generally speaking, there are two kinds of diets - those that emphasize protein and those that emphasize complex carbohydrates. The Mediterranean diet is a good diet to start with, then add in more protein or more complex carbs as needed.

- **Balanced Meals**: Incorporate protein, healthy fats, complex carbohydrates, and plenty of vegetables into each meal. See the **Dietary Guidelines** chapter in the Next Steps section for more
- **Dietary Changes:** Introduce adaptogenic herbs gradually, taking recommended dosages consistently for at least 6–8 weeks to notice improvements.
- **Mindful Eating**: Eat slowly and with awareness, noting how different foods affect your energy and mood.
- **Hydration**: Stay well-hydrated throughout the day, drinking water regularly rather than waiting until you're thirsty.

Consistent Sleep Patterns

Consistent sleep is foundational for emotional, cognitive, and physical health. Good sleep hygiene helps regulate your body's internal rhythms, enhancing overall resilience.

Regular Sleep Schedule:

- Aim for consistent sleep and wake times, even on weekends.
- Try not to stay up past 11pm.
- Develop a relaxing bedtime routine to signal your body it's time to unwind, such as reading, meditation, or gentle stretching.

See *Chapter 27 - Sleep Hygiene – Your Guide to Restful Sleep* in the Next Steps section for more.

Regular Mindfulness and Meditation

Mindfulness practices reduce anxiety, improve emotional regulation, and help you remain grounded amid stress.

Aim for 5–10 minutes of mindfulness or meditation 2 or 3 times per day, ideally at regular intervals (e.g., morning, midday, and evening) and work up to 20-30 minutes if that works for you.

> **Short Mindfulness Breaks**: Take short mindfulness pauses during your day to breathe deeply, relax your body, and reset your state.
>
> **Dedicated Meditation Practice**: Engage in regular meditation sessions, such as Vipassana or guided mindfulness meditation, to build deeper resilience and awareness.

See *Chapter 28 - Meditation and Mindfulness* in the Next Steps section for techniques and practices.

Creating a Supportive Environment

Your environment significantly impacts your Vital Self's balance. Creating calming, supportive spaces can make your daily life more harmonious and less stressful.

> **Personal Space**: Keep your home and workspace comfortable and something that feels good to return to. Decorations that you love, meaningful objects and photographs, and any other ways to make your space feel nurturing and safe.
>
> **Nature Exposure**: Regularly spend time in nature, as natural environments have proven calming effects, lowering stress levels and enhancing mood.

Regular Check-ins and Self-Reflection

Take moments throughout the day to "check-in" with yourself, noticing your physical sensations, emotions, and energy levels. Couple this with a ritual for extra effect, such as lighting a candle, making tea in a very mindful way with a special cup or burning incense, etc.

> **Daily Reflection**: Briefly reflect at the end of the day on what felt nourishing and what might need adjustment.
>
> **Mindful Transitions**: Insert moments throughout your day—alarms or visual reminders—to pause, breathe, and reconnect with your body.

Incorporating these lifestyle changes into your daily routines can profoundly stabilize and strengthen your Vital Self, supporting your overall well-being and resilience.

Essential Oils for the Vital Self Axis

Essential oils offer a way to gently shift arousal states through scent. While scientific evidence varies, many people find them soothing or energizing. If you have allergies, respiratory conditions, or other health concerns, approach essential oils with caution and consider consulting an aromatherapy practitioner.

Each of these oils can be used in a diffuser, diluted for topical use (e.g., over the chest or wrists), or simply inhaled from the palms for a quick reset. For more information on using essential oils, see *Chapter 24 - Essential Oils—History, Use, and Safety* in the Next Steps section.

Underactive Vital Self (Low Energy)

Peppermint: Invigorates and clears mental fog.

Rosemary: Supports mental clarity and circulation.

Ginger: Warming and stimulating, helps revitalize a sluggish state.

Balanced Vital Self

Lavender: Calms while maintaining a sense of steady energy.

Frankincense: Grounding and centering, for overall balance.

Geranium: Helps stabilize mood and energy levels.

Overactive Vital Self (High Energy/Tension)

Chamomile: Soothes nervous tension and hyperactivity.

Ylang-Ylang: Reduces stress and helps calm the mind.

Sandalwood: Grounding, helping ease excessive energy.

Vital Self Instability (Fluctuating States)

Bergamot: Gently uplifts, smoothing out emotional highs and lows.

Patchouli: Grounds scattered energy, promoting stability.

Clary Sage: Regulates emotional and hormonal fluctuations, encouraging balance.

Using Essential Oils

Diffusion: A gentle, longer-lasting effect throughout a room. You'll need to purchase an essential oil diffuser.

Direct Inhalation: Quick and concentrated—great for immediate relief.

Diluted on Pulse Points: Offers a slow-release effect when combined with a carrier oil (like jojoba or almond).

Bathing: Adding essential oils diluted with bath salts or carrier oils into warm baths promotes relaxation, reduces stress, and can ease muscle tension.

Homeopathic Remedies for the Vital Self Axis

Here's a list of carefully selected homeopathic remedies that support Vital Self balance, especially around themes of inward and outward emotional regulation. These can be helpful for emotional sensitivity, relational overwhelm, boundary collapse, and suppressed or frozen feelings—key patterns often seen in Vital Self imbalance within the Mind Matrix Model.

A common starting dose is **30c potency, taken 3–4 times per day**. If you notice clear improvement, you may shift to **a single dose of 200c** for deeper, longer-lasting support. For more guidance, see the appendix chapter *Homeopathy: Gentle Remedies for Balance and Health*.

Underactive Vital Self

Phosphoricum Acidum: For mental and physical exhaustion after stress or illness.

Calcarea Carbonica: For sluggishness, low stamina, and potential weight gain.

Gelsemium: For overall heaviness and fatigue, often with anticipatory anxiety.

Balanced Vital Self

Sulphur: Helps maintain vitality, especially if there's irritability or heat-related issues.

Pulsatilla: Promotes emotional and physical balance, helpful for mood fluctuations.

Natrum Muriaticum: Encourages stability and resilience, especially for those who prefer emotional control.

Overactive Vital Self

Nux Vomica: Addresses overstimulation, irritability, and stress-related digestive issues.

Aconitum Napellus: For sudden restlessness and anxiety after shocks or jolts.

Argentum Nitricum: Reduces nervous agitation and impulsive behavior.

Vital Self Instability

Ignatia Amara: Helps stabilize mood swings and inner tension.

Lycopodium Clavatum: Boosts self-confidence and balances energy swings.

Sepia: Useful for hormonal imbalances, irritability, and oscillations between apathy and restlessness.

Acupressure for Balancing the Vital Self

Acupressure is a powerful component of Traditional Chinese Medicine (TCM), using finger pressure on specific points to harmonize the body's energy (Qi). It's particularly beneficial for stabilizing the Vital Self by addressing low and high arousal states through balancing Kidney Yin and Kidney Yang.

For detailed instructions on technique, timing, and best practices, see the Next Steps *Chapter 23 - Acupressure For Yourself and Others.*

> **Kidney Yin and Yang: The Vital Foundation**
>
> *In TCM (Traditional Chinese Medicine), the Kidney system—comprised of the Kidney and Bladder meridians—is foundational for the Vital Self, influencing how your body manages energy, rest, and activity.*
>
> *Think of this system as your body's battery, storing energy (Kidney Yin) and activating energy when needed (Kidney Yang).*
>
> *Proper balance between Kidney Yin and Kidney Yang allows your Vital Self to maintain resilience, effectively responding to different states of arousal.*

Kidney Yin: *Cooling, nourishing, and calming functions*

Associated With: *Parasympathetic Nervous System (PNS)—active during rest, relaxation, and recovery.*

When Kidney Yin is sufficient, your body's restorative processes function optimally. You experience deep rest, emotional calmness, and ample energy reserves.

Signs of Kidney Yin Imbalance (Low Yin, High Arousal):

Restlessness or insomnia (difficulty calming down)

Irritability or anxiety (feeling emotionally "hot")

Night sweats or dryness (mouth, skin, eyes)

Difficulty recovering from stress or exertion

From the TCM perspective, Kidney Yin deficiency can feel like constantly "burning the candle at both ends," leaving you depleted, overheated, or overly tense.

Kidney Yang: *Warming, Energizing, and Activating*

Associated With: *Sympathetic Nervous System (SNS)—prepares your body for action, activity, and responsiveness.*

Adequate Kidney Yang provides the internal warmth and energy necessary for motivation, movement, and facing life's challenges effectively.

Signs of Kidney Yang Imbalance (Low Yang, Low Arousal):

Chronic fatigue, especially noticeable in the morning

Sensitivity to cold, particularly in feet or lower back

Low libido, motivation, or "spark"

Difficulty initiating action or coping with physical exertion

Weak Kidney Yang often manifests as overall coldness, diminished stamina, and inconsistent energy throughout the day.

Points for Increasing Low Energy/Arousal

Low arousal can manifest as fatigue, low motivation, poor ability to concentrate or fucus,or an inability to activate energy when needed.

The following points are helpful for gently stimulating the system and supporting Kidney Yang.

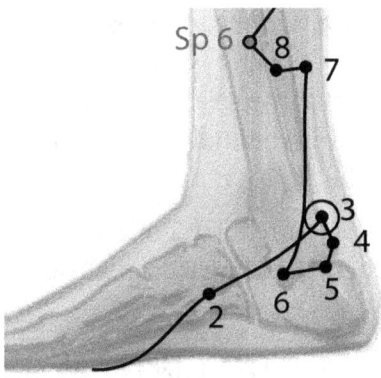

Kidney 3 (Taixi or Great Stream)

Purpose: Ki 3 is the source point for the Kidney meridian, providing overall balance and stability to Kidney Yin and Yang.

Location: On the inside of the ankle, midway between the high point of the medial malleolus (the inner ankle bone) and the Achilles tendon.

How to Use: Apply gentle, steady pressure with your thumb or finger for 1-2 minutes. Ki 3 harmonizes both Kidney Yin and Yang, helping to stabilize energy levels and prevent extreme highs or lows.

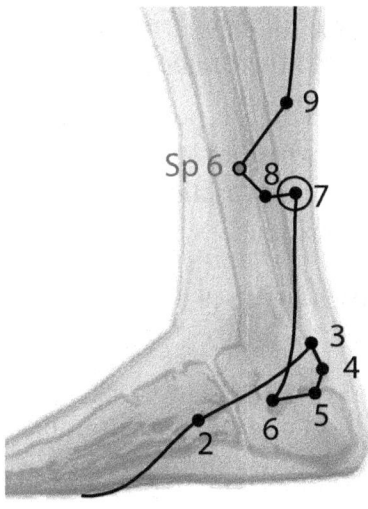

Kidney 7 (Fuliu or Returning Current)

Purpose: Ki 7 is a tonification point for Kidney Yang, helping to increase warmth, energy, and resilience.

Location: Five finger-widths above Ki 3, two finger-widths behind the shin bone.

How to Use: Apply gentle pressure with your thumb or finger, holding for 1-2 minutes. This point helps lift energy without overstimulation, providing a slow, steady boost.

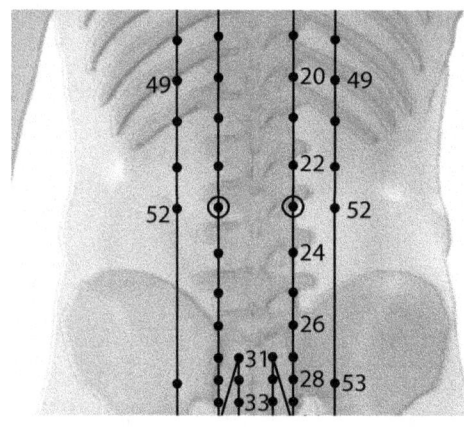

Bladder 23 (Shenshu or Kidney Shu)

Purpose: Bl 23 strengthens Kidney energy and tonifies Yang, providing resilience and warmth to combat low arousal.

Location: On the lower back, about three finger-widths out from the spine at the level of the second lumbar vertebra (aligned with the waistline).

How to Use: Use your thumbs to apply firm pressure for 1-2 minutes on each side. This point reinforces Kidney energy, adding a deep, steady boost to vitality.

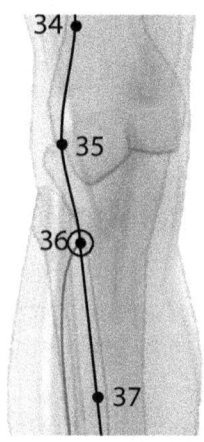

Stomach 36 (Zusanli or Leg Three Miles)

Purpose: St 36 is well known to boost overall energy, vitality, and immunity, helping to alleviate fatigue and improve mental clarity.

Location: Six finger-widths below the kneecap, one finger-width lateral to the shinbone.

How to Use: Press and hold this point for 1-2 minutes on each leg. It provides a sustained increase in energy and can be particularly helpful for physical and mental fatigue.

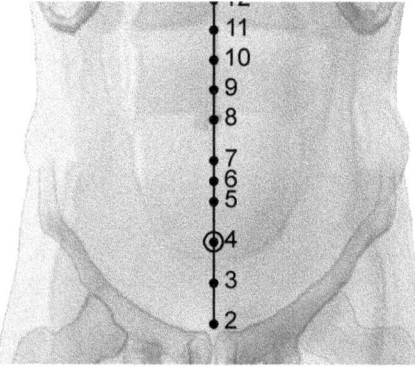

Conception Vessel 4 (Guanyuan or Gate of Origin)

Purpose: CV 4 tonifies Kidney Essence (Jing) and supports overall energy levels, providing grounding and balance.

Location: On the midline of the lower abdomen, about five finger-widths below the navel (start with your finger in the navel, go to the pinky then one more).

How to Use: Apply gentle but steady pressure for 1-2 minutes. Ren 4 is ideal for replenishing core energy, which can feel uplifting and revitalizing.

Points for Calming High Anxiety/Arousal

High arousal, or hyperarousal, can present as anxiety, irritability, racing thoughts, or overstimulation. The following points help calm the system and build Kidney Yin, grounding and relaxing the body and mind.

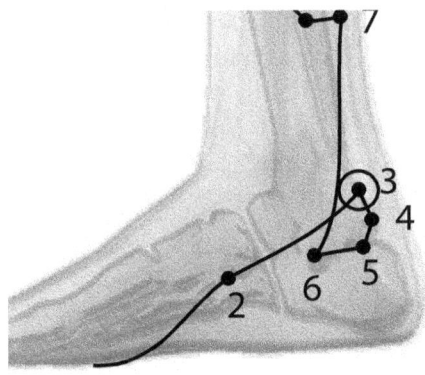

Kidney 3 (Taixi or Great Stream)

Purpose: Ki 3 is the source point for the Kidney meridian, providing overall balance and stability to Kidney Yin and Yang.

Location: On the inside of the ankle, midway between the high point of the medial malleolus (the inner ankle bone) and the Achilles tendon.

How to Use: Apply gentle, steady pressure with your thumb or finger for 1-2 minutes. Ki 3 harmonizes both yin and yang, helping to stabilize energy levels and prevent extreme highs or lows.

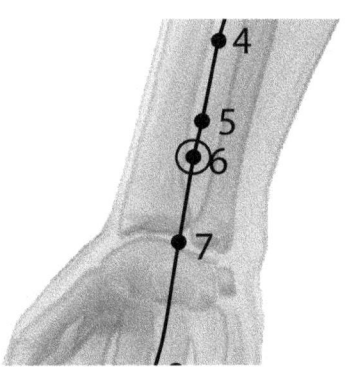

Pericardium 6 (Neiguan or Inner Gate)

Purpose: Pc 6 calms the mind, relieves anxiety, and reduces physical symptoms of stress such as palpitations.

Location: On the inner forearm, four finger-widths above the wrist crease, between the tendons.

How to Use: Apply steady pressure for 1-2 minutes. This point helps activate the parasympathetic nervous system, supporting Kidney Yin by promoting relaxation and emotional calm.

Kidney 1 (Yongquan or Gushing Spring)

Purpose: Ki 1 is the sedation point for the Kidney meridian. It grounds excess energy, drawing it down and helping to calm both the body and mind.

Location: On the sole of the foot, about one-third down from the base of the toes, between the ball of the foot and the center of the heel in the soft area.

How to Use: Apply gentle but firm pressure with your thumb for 1 minute on each foot. This point can be highly effective for calming a racing mind, particularly when paired with Ki 3 for balanced stimulation.

Heart 7 (Shenmen or Spirit Gate)

Purpose: Ht 7 calms the mind, soothes irritability, and reduces emotional agitation, especially during periods of high arousal.

Location: On the inner wrist crease, to the side of the tendon (flexor carpi ulnaris) toward the middle of the wrist.

How to Use: Apply gentle pressure with your thumb or fingertip, holding for 1-2 minutes on each wrist. This point helps ease mental tension and supports emotional stability.

Spleen 6 (Sanyinjiao or Three Yin Intersection)

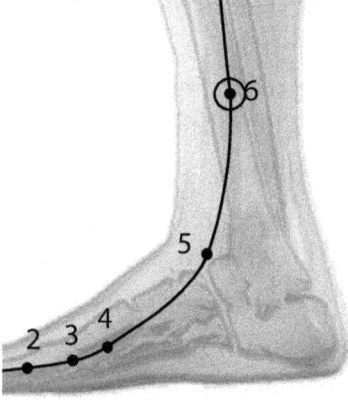

Purpose: Sp 6 relieves stress and promotes emotional grounding, helping to prevent overactivation and reducing high energy states.

Location: On the inner side of the lower leg, about six finger-widths above the medial malleolus (the inner bump of the ankle, behind the shinbone).

How to Use: Apply steady pressure for 1-2 minutes on each leg. Sp 6 has a calming effect and helps support Kidney Yin by grounding excessive energy.

Points for Balancing Instability

Fluctuations Between Low and High Arousal

Instability or fluctuations in arousal may feel like cycles of hyperactivity followed by fatigue, difficulty maintaining energy, or unpredictability in mood and energy levels. The following points help balance these extremes, promoting resilience and stabilizing the Vital Self.

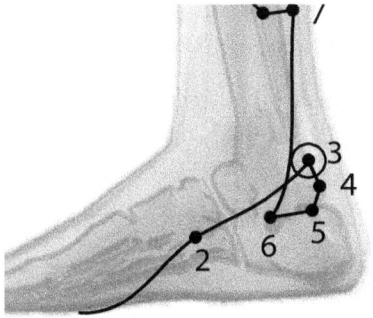

Kidney 3 (Taixi or Great Stream)

Purpose: Ki 3 is the source point for the Kidney meridian, providing overall balance and stability to Kidney Yin and Yang.

Location: On the inside of the ankle, midway between the high point of the medial malleolus (the inner ankle bone) and the Achilles tendon.

How to Use: Apply gentle, steady pressure with your thumb or finger for 1-2 minutes. Ki 3 harmonizes both yin and yang, helping to stabilize energy levels and prevent extreme highs or lows.

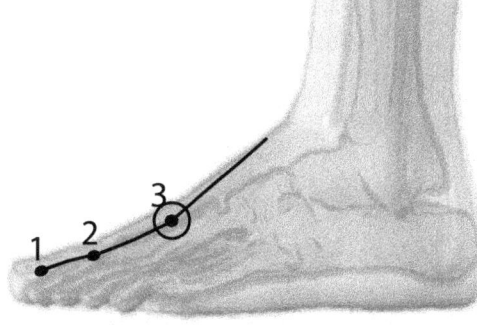

Liver 3 (Taichong or Great Surge)

Purpose: Li 3 regulates energy flow, supporting emotional and physical stability and preventing extreme fluctuations.

Location: On the top of the foot, in the webbing between the big toe and the second toe, about four finger-widths back from the toes.

How to Use: Press and hold this point for 1-2 minutes on each foot. Li 3 relieves pent-up tension, which can ease fluctuations and promote a stable baseline.

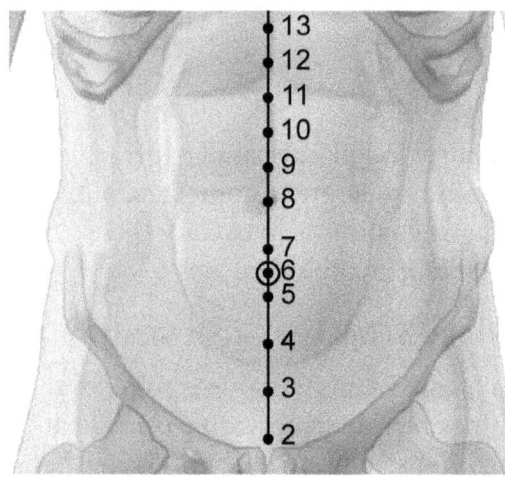

Conception Vessel 6 (Qihai or Sea of Qi)

Purpose: CV 6 supports grounding, stability, and balanced energy flow, helping to prevent highs and lows.

Location: On the midline of the abdomen, four fingers below the navel.

How to Use: Apply steady, gentle pressure for 1-2 minutes. This point strengthens the body's core energy, supporting a consistent and resilient Vital Self.

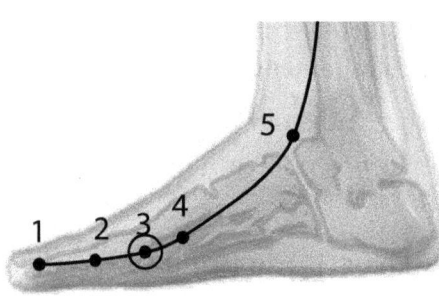

Spleen 3 (Taibai or Supreme White)

Purpose: Sp 3 stabilizes energy, supports digestion, and helps maintain a steady flow of Qi, which can prevent fluctuations.

Location: On the inner side of the foot under the bone, in the depression just behind the base of the big toe.

How to Use: Apply moderate pressure with your thumb, holding for 1-2 minutes on each foot. Sp 3 helps create a balanced flow of energy, reducing both excess and deficiency.

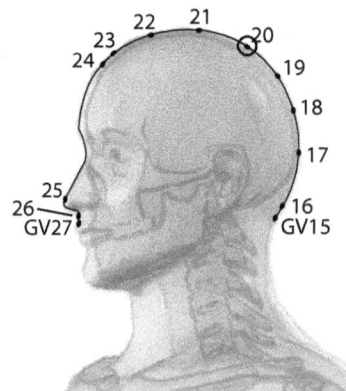

Governing Vessel 20 (Baihui or Hundred Meetings)

Purpose: GV 20 balances Yang energy in the body, helping stabilize both mental and physical energy levels.

Location: On the top of the head, along the midline. Go straight up from the tops of both ears to the center of the head. You'll feel a soft spot.

How to Use: Apply gentle pressure with your fingertips or palm, holding for 1-2 minutes. This point helps bring clarity and stability, especially useful for balancing energy fluctuations.

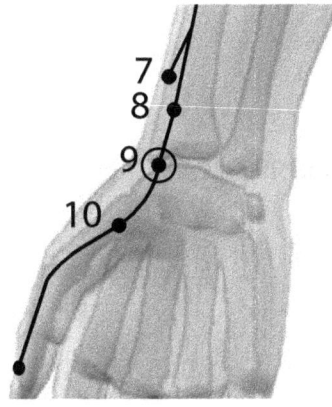

Lung 9 (Taiyuan or Great Abyss)

Purpose: Lu 9 nourishes Lung and Kidney energy, supports the flow of Qi, and provides stability, which is helpful for consistent energy levels.

Location: On the wrist crease, in the depression on the radial artery (you'll feel a pulse).

How to Use: Apply gentle pressure with your thumb, holding for 1 minute on each wrist. Lu 9 reinforces the connection between breath and energy flow, promoting steadiness and resilience.

Vital Self Fast Reset Meditation

Use this when you're overwhelmed, scattered, or overstimulated.

Length: ~2–3 minutes
Posture: Seated or standing. Feet flat on the floor, hands resting gently on thighs or at your sides.

Take a deep breath in through your nose.
Hold it for just a moment
Now exhale slowly through your mouth.

Let your shoulders drop.
Let your jaw soften.
Let your belly move freely with your breath.

Bring your awareness down.
Out of your head.
Down into your body.

Feel your feet on the ground.
Wiggle your toes.
Feel the contact—solid, steady, dependable.

Now notice your breath again.
Don't change it—just feel it.
Inhale
Exhale

Let the breath move through you like a gentle wave.
Let the breath *find you*.

Now, bring your awareness to your spine.
Imagine your spine lengthening upward as if someone's gently lifting the crown of your head.
And at the same time, feel your tailbone anchoring you down.

This is your **Vital Center**—present, steady, alive.

Take one more full breath.
Inhale through the nose.
Exhale through the mouth.

And when you're ready, open your eyes or return to what you were doing, a little more *here*, a little more *you*.

Affirmation: Say quietly to yourself:

> *I am safe*
> *I am well*
> *I am grounded in my body.*

Vital Self Daily Ritual Meditation

A grounding and energizing morning or mid-day practice.

Length: ~5–8 minutes
Posture: Seated on the floor or a firm chair; or standing, relaxed posture.

Close your eyes.
Bring one hand to your heart and one hand to your belly.
Feel the movement of your breath beneath your hands.

Let your breath deepen.
Let it slow, but don't force it.
Let your body find its rhythm.

Now imagine the breath flowing through your whole body.
Down to your toes.
Out through your fingers.

Into your spine.
Bathing every cell.

With each inhale, invite in energy.
With each exhale, let go of tension, stiffness, stagnation.

Now, feel into your Vital Self.
Ask gently: *How am I feeling, physically, right now?*
Tired? Restless? Strong? Numb? Tight?

There's no need to fix—just feel.

Place your attention on your lower belly.
This is your **Vital Center**.
Imagine a warm golden light glowing there.

With each breath, the light grows—filling your belly, your pelvis, your legs, your feet.
You are rooted.
You are present.
You are alive.

Let this golden energy spiral upward—
through your torso, chest, shoulders, arms, and finally your head.

Let it swirl, then settle—gathering back in the belly.
One simple, pulsing flame.

Affirmation: Say quietly to yourself:

> *I am here.*
> *I am safe.*
> *I am vital.*

Take one last breath in.
Stretch or move if it feels right.
And when you're ready, gently open your eyes.

Final Thoughts

Each of these therapies and modalities has its own strengths, and not every approach will appeal to everyone. Feel free to experiment safely with what resonates for you—perhaps combining a few practices, like mindfulness and acupressure, or looking into homeopathy or neurofeedback if you're curious. Above all, keep in mind:

> **Consultation:** If you have ongoing or significant mental/physical health concerns, it's wise to consult a qualified healthcare provider.

> **Consistency:** Most of these modalities are most effective when practiced regularly.

> **Trial:** You may need to try a number of modalities and therapies to find ones that are a good fit for you. Also, it's possible that your needs will change over time so if you don't feel like something is helping you, notice what you are attracted to. And of course, you can always come back to this chapter and try something else.

> **Self-Compassion:** Listen to your body. Give yourself grace if it takes time to find the right balance or combination of techniques.

Learning to care for your Vital Self is a journey. With patience and the right tools, you can create a more balanced, energized, and resilient foundation for your entire well-being.

Chapter Nine

The Heart Self

Spend all you have for loveliness,
  Buy it and never count the cost;
For one white singing hour of peace
  Count many a year of strife well lost,
And for a breath of ecstasy
Give all you have been, or could be.

~ Excerpt from Barter
  by Sara Teasdale

Introduction to the Heart Self

The Heart Self is all about how you connect with others and manage your emotional world. It is the part of you that feels. It moves in waves—connecting, retreating, reaching again. This part of you guides you in building friendships, managing emotions, and responding and adapting to social situations in thoughtful, appropriate ways.

Thanks to the Heart Self, you can experience empathy, form bonds, and read social cues—all essential skills for creating and sustaining meaningful relationships. It also keeps track of your emotional state, letting you know when you need more "me" time or more social time.

The Neurological Basis of the Heart Self

At the center of the Heart Self is the limbic system, a network of brain structures that link feelings, memories, and social interactions.

- Amygdala: This almond-shaped structure in the temporal lobe acts like your emotional alarm system, processing emotions such as fear and anger, especially when survival instincts are engaged.
- Hippocampus: Also in the temporal lobe, the hippocampus helps form emotional memories, tying your feelings to specific experiences.
- Anterior Cingulate Cortex (ACC): Located in the frontal region, the ACC supports emotional regulation and social navigation, such as handling conflicts or reading social cues.
- Thalamus: Serving as the brain's relay station, the thalamus filters and directs sensory input, helping emotional and social signals reach the right areas for processing.
- Hypothalamus: A vital regulator of hormones and autonomic functions, the hypothalamus connects emotional experience with the body's responses, from stress reactions to bonding hormones like oxytocin.
- Insula: This region integrates awareness of the body's internal state with empathy and emotional awareness.
- Orbitofrontal Cortex (OFC): Plays a key role in evaluating emotional and social information, guiding choices in relationships.
- Septal Nuclei: Linked with bonding, attachment, and feelings of warmth and connection.

Together, these structures form the core circuitry of the Heart Self, allowing you to feel emotions, connect with others, and weave your relationships into memory.

Focus vs. Directed

In the Mind Matrix Model, the Heart Self spans an axis, or spectrum, from introverts who are more self-focused and more other-directed, to extroverts who are more other-focused and more self-directed, with balance in the middle. Understanding where you naturally fall on this spectrum can help you understand your social habits, how you process emotions, and how you relate to others.

Introverts generally need a fair amount of quiet, self-focused reflective time by themselves to recharge and balance. They are typically more comfortable one-on-one; otherwise, they can start getting anxious. At the same time, they are often keenly aware of social dynamics and very sensitive to the feelings of others (other-directed). In fact, they can often neglect their own needs while taking care of the needs or wants of others.

Conversely, extroverts love to socialize and are more comfortable and recharge in groups (other-focused). If they don't get enough social time, they start getting more anxious and restless. However they tend to be very self-directed and focused on their own needs and wants and can be less aware or insensitive to the needs and feelings of others (self-directed).

Clearly there is a spectrum here, relatively few people are at the extreme and plenty of people are more towards the middle, where they need quiet time but also need social interaction, and where they aren't either largely self- or other-directed.

It's normal and healthy to have a tendency one way or the other, but it's not great for your mental health and relationships to be overly tilted to one side to the extent that you're inflexible or too flexible, it causes problems socially.

A healthy Heart Self helps you to strike an appropriate, healthy balance between connecting with others and connecting with yourself.

> *Julia, naturally introverted, realized she was consistently avoiding social interactions to the point of isolation. With gentle encouragement and structured exposure, she learned to balance solitude with intentional social engagements, greatly enhancing her emotional well-being.*

Introversion, Extroversion and Ambiversion

Your Heart Self affects you in many ways, from your approach to socializing to how you manage stress. Finding a healthy balance between these traits helps build strong relationships with yourself and with others.

The Heart Self functions along an introversion-extroversion spectrum, shaping how you balance self-reflection with social engagement.

> **Introverts** recharge with solitude and deeper personal reflection, tending to be highly sensitive to social dynamics but quickly overstimulated by groups.
>
> **Extroverts** recharge through social interaction and group engagement, thriving in active environments but sometimes neglecting their own emotional boundaries.

Understanding your natural tendencies helps in cultivating balanced relationships and emotional health.

Introverts: The Reflective Observer

Self-focused people often prefer calm environments, reflection, and deep one-on-one connections rather than large gatherings. They tend to be introspective and emotionally sensitive, enjoying time spent in thought.

> *Sarah is a writer who spends much of her time working alone. She enjoys solitary walks in nature, where she can reflect on her thoughts and emotions.*
>
> *Sarah is deeply introspective, valuing quality over quantity in her relationships. She recharges by spending time alone, journaling, or engaging in creative activities.*

Strengths: Inward-focused individuals excel at introspection, creativity, and forming deep bonds, with a rich inner life and strong self-awareness. They often have a grasp on the complex emotional dynamics of a person or group.

Challenges: They may find it difficult to assert themselves or remain in touch with their own opinions when with others or especially in groups. They may feel isolated or lonely if they lean too heavily on solitude.

Extroverts: The Engaged Socializer

Other-focused individuals are energized by social interaction and thrive on meeting new people, often enjoying wide social circles.

Mike, a sales manager, loves meeting new people and engaging in high-energy networking events. He is confident and assertive, enjoying the spotlight. Mike recharges by socializing, whether it's at work, with friends, or in larger gatherings.

Strengths: Outward-focused individuals shine in social settings, making connections easily and often acting as the "life of the party." They're typically charismatic and excel in a variety of social situations. They can be natural leaders.

Challenges: They may overextend themselves socially, leading to burnout or forming surface-level connections. Time for introspection can also be a challenge, as they might rely too heavily on external validation.

Ambiverts: The Adaptive Integrator

Balanced individuals, called *ambiverts*, naturally shift between solitude and social engagement, depending on their needs and the context. They enjoy meaningful one-on-one conversations but also feel comfortable in group settings. Rather than strictly identifying as introverts or extroverts, they adjust their energy output based on the situation.

For example, Alex, a therapist and musician, loves spending time alone composing music but also enjoys deep conversations with friends and participating in community events. He finds that too much socializing drains him, but too much solitude makes him restless. By recognizing his need for both connection and reflection, he maintains a healthy balance between engagement and introspection.

John is a therapist who spends his workdays deeply engaged with clients, offering empathy and support. Outside of work, he enjoys both spending quiet evenings at home and participating in social activities with friends. John is equally comfortable in solitude and in the company of others, making him adaptable and balanced.

Strengths: Balanced individuals can navigate a variety of social settings while maintaining a strong sense of self. They are adaptable, able to engage deeply with others while also prioritizing personal reflection and renewal.

Challenges: They may struggle with deciding when to recharge versus when to engage, sometimes feeling pulled in both directions. If they overcommit socially, they risk exhaustion, while too much alone time can lead to isolation.

Achieving Balance

A balanced Heart Self is adaptable, switching comfortably between social interaction and solitude depending on needs. People with a balanced Heart Self build trust at a healthy pace, express emotions appropriately, and demonstrate empathy while respecting boundaries. When facing challenges, they blend social support with personal reflection, using both inward and outward approaches to manage stress effectively.

Overall, knowing where you stand on the inward-outward spectrum of the Heart Self helps you understand your strengths and challenges. This awareness allows you to adapt to different social situations, fostering resilience and enriching your relationships in meaningful ways.

Dysregulation: The Heart Self Out of Balance

The Heart Self is your emotional compass, your relational center, and the seat of empathy and attachment. It governs how you connect, how you care, and how you make sense of your emotional experience. But when the Heart Self is chronically dysregulated, its natural rhythms—of opening and retreating, giving and receiving—become distorted or lost.

This dysregulation can take the form of emotional flooding, shame spirals, echoist withdrawal, people-pleasing overextension, or hypersensitivity to rejection. Or it can manifest as relational numbness and disconnection—feeling "shut down," even when connection is wanted.

There are many reasons why the Heart Self may lose balance, including:

Developmental Emotional Disruption

> When caregivers are inconsistent, misattuned, emotionally absent, or overcontrolling, a child learns that emotions are not safe—or that expressing them risks disconnection. This early pattern teaches the Heart Self to suppress feelings, manage others' emotions, or collapse its own needs in exchange for belonging.

Chronic Relational Stress

Over time, repeated experiences of betrayal, invalidation, or abandonment in relationships—romantic, familial, or social—can cause the Heart Self to armor up. The nervous system begins to associate closeness with threat, or connection with exhaustion. Even without a single dramatic event, the accumulation of unmet relational needs creates a deep emotional weariness.

Cultural or Familial Suppression

Some people grow up in cultures or families where emotional expression is discouraged, mocked, or punished. This trains the Heart Self to disconnect from its own inner truth, or to perform emotions instead of feeling them. The result is often a split between outer social functioning and inner isolation.

Neurodivergence or Social Disorientation

For some people—especially those with autism or high sensitivity—reading social cues or managing emotional reciprocity can feel cognitively exhausting or emotionally overwhelming. This doesn't mean the Heart Self is deficient—but it does mean chronic social dysregulation can build up as a form of invisible stress.

Identity-Based Rejection or Suppression

Living in a world that devalues who you are—because of your race, gender identity, sexuality, disability, or other core traits—has a cumulative effect on the Heart Self. Even microaggressions or "polite" exclusions reinforce the message that your emotions and identity must be hidden for safety. This creates chronic strain, relational self-censorship, and emotional contraction.

Codependency and Over-Attunement

Some people adapt to early instability by becoming experts at reading the room—but lose connection to their own emotional needs in the process. Chronic dysregulation arises when your emotional world revolves around others' moods, needs, and reactions, leaving you resentful, drained, or invisible to yourself.

Chronic Heart Self dysregulation doesn't mean you're broken—it means your emotional system has adapted to survive pain without the tools or support it needed. The good news is that those tools can still be developed, and your relational rhythm can still be restored.

The Heart Self and the State Axis

The Heart Self is your emotional center—where connection, compassion, and sensitivity live. It's also where wounds from disconnection, rejection, or neglect are most deeply felt. As a result, the Heart Self is profoundly shaped by State. When you're regulated, it becomes a wellspring of attunement and empathy. When dysregulated, it can collapse into shame or lash out in self-protection.

The Heart Self lives within two axes: **introversion↔extroversion**, and **Positive State↔Negative State**. A balanced Heart Self—what we call the Harmonizer—is emotionally open without being porous, expressive without dominating, and grounded in a healthy sense of self-worth.

Below you can see the two dimensions of action for the Heart Self, Introversion to Extroversion and Positive to Negative State.

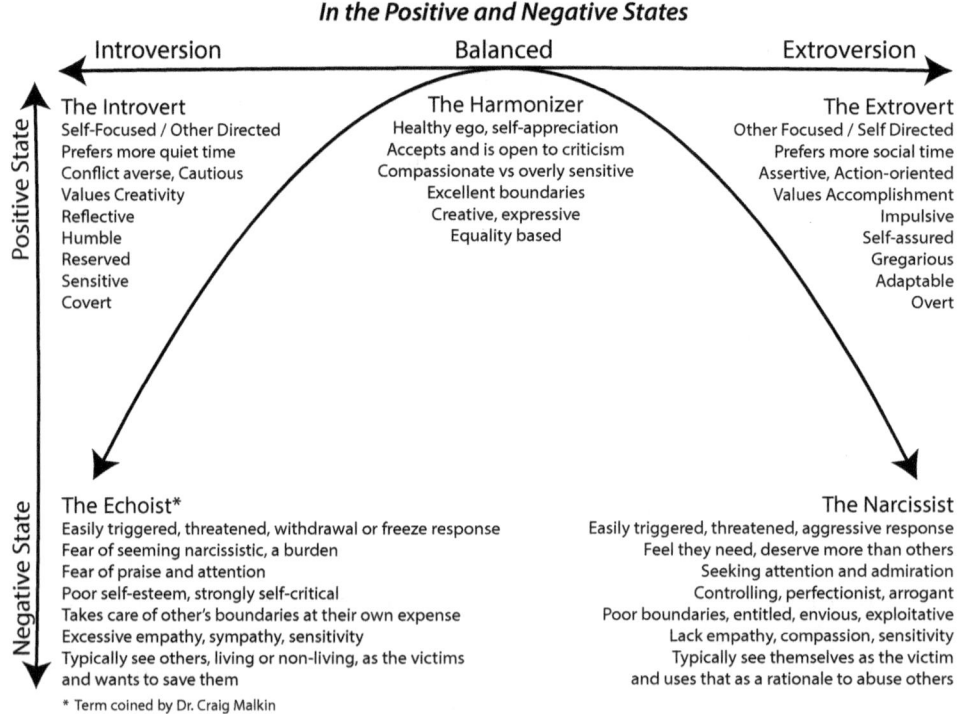

Heart Self
In the Positive and Negative States

Introversion — Balanced — Extroversion
Positive State / Negative State

The Introvert
Self-Focused / Other Directed
Prefers more quiet time
Conflict averse, Cautious
Values Creativity
Reflective
Humble
Reserved
Sensitive
Covert

The Harmonizer
Healthy ego, self-appreciation
Accepts and is open to criticism
Compassionate vs overly sensitive
Excellent boundaries
Creative, expressive
Equality based

The Extrovert
Other Focused / Self Directed
Prefers more social time
Assertive, Action-oriented
Values Accomplishment
Impulsive
Self-assured
Gregarious
Adaptable
Overt

The Echoist*
Easily triggered, threatened, withdrawal or freeze response
Fear of seeming narcissistic, a burden
Fear of praise and attention
Poor self-esteem, strongly self-critical
Takes care of other's boundaries at their own expense
Excessive empathy, sympathy, sensitivity
Typically see others, living or non-living, as the victims and wants to save them

The Narcissist
Easily triggered, threatened, aggressive response
Feel they need, deserve more than others
Seeking attention and admiration
Controlling, perfectionist, arrogant
Poor boundaries, entitled, envious, exploitative
Lack empathy, compassion, sensitivity
Typically see themselves as the victim and uses that as a rationale to abuse others

* Term coined by Dr. Craig Malkin

The Positive Range of the Heart Self allows for healthy introversion (*The Introvert*), where one's inner world is rich and reflective, and healthy extroversion (*The Extrovert*), where social flow and expressive engagement feel natural and energizing. It's not better to be one or the other, each has its strengths.

But neither of these poles is ideal when in a dysregulated, triggered Negative State. And the more introversive or extroversive you tend to be, the more easily you can be triggered. The ideal is to be able to be relatively balanced and move freely between introversive and extroversive modes, of course with a tendency toward one or the other.

Echoism and Narcissism

As adults, people with early relational wounds often develop one of two polarized ways of coping in the Heart Self. You're probably familiar with the terms *narcissist, narcissistic* and *narcissism*, which in our culture are equated with qualities such as an inflated sense of self-importance, overly controlling, and prioritizing their own needs over others. This is one way relational wounds can show up in an individual.

However, you're probably not familiar with the terms *echoism, echoistic* or *echoist*. Echoism is a term coined by psychiatrist Dr. Craig Malkin, and it comes from the same Greek myth as narcissism.

> ### Echoism and the Myth of Narcissus
> *In the story of Narcissus, a hunter so obsessed with his own reflection that he wasted away staring at it, there was another character: Echo. She was cursed to repeat only the words of others, never able to express her own thoughts, desires, or needs.*

Echoist Mode, when in the Negative State, this mode is about turning inward: the person withdraws, minimizing their own needs and over-attuning to others in order to preserve connection and safety.

Narcissisist Mode, when dysregulated, this is about turning outward: they over-attune to their own needs in relation to others and control the narrative in an attempt to protect a fragile internal world.

Both are responses to the same wound: the pain of not being emotionally met. In Dr. Malkin's view, echoism describes a pattern in which people minimize their own presence and emotional needs, often to avoid conflict or rejection. They focus on pleasing others, avoiding attention, and making sure they don't take up too much space.

This coping strategy develops early when children learn—explicitly or implicitly—that their needs are inconvenient or unwelcome. Instead of seeking love and validation outwardly, echoists tend to shrink themselves, believing that staying small, agreeable, and unobtrusive is the best way to be accepted.

On the other end of the spectrum is narcissism. While many people assume that narcissism is simply about confidence or self-importance, in reality those with narcissistic tendencies are often covering deep-seated insecurity.

Instead of withdrawing from relationships like echoists, they build an exaggerated sense of self-worth around themselves as a defense mechanism. They may seek control, admiration, or validation from others as a way of avoiding feelings of inadequacy or unworthiness. Beneath the surface, however, their self-esteem is fragile—highly dependent on external validation to maintain the illusion of confidence.

Both echoism and narcissism are responses to the same core issue: *how do I protect myself from the pain of not feeling valued?*

> **Echoist mode** is about internalizing that pain, making themselves small to avoid causing waves.
> **Narcissist mode** is about externalization, inflating their presence, and often using aggression to ensure they're seen.

In **Echoist mode**, this often means an internal voice that says things like:

> *"I'm not a burden. I am a burden. I'm trying not to be a burden."*
>
> *"I'll stay quiet, empathic and supportive so you'll keep me close."*
>
> *"I'll care for you, as your needs are more important than mine."*

For **Narcissist mode**, it may sound more like:

> *"I'm always in control."*
>
> *"I'm important, and you need me."*
>
> *"I'll keep the spotlight so I don't have to feel small."*

Both styles are driven by the same wound: a fear that showing their real self would lead to shame or rejection.

The Heart Self is where chronic shame often takes root. When emotional needs go unmet or relationships feel unsafe, the system may protect itself by splitting off painful feelings or memories. This is called compartmentalization—when certain parts of your emotional experience are pushed outside of conscious awareness to help you cope. In these moments, the Heart Minister steps in, trying to preserve connection or emotional safety by hiding what feels too overwhelming to face.

This is why State awareness is so important. When you're dysregulated—anxious, shut down, or emotionally flooded—you're more likely to fall back into old relational patterns or Scripts, often without realizing it.

In the understanding of modern cognitive science, when you're in a Negative State, your brain stops updating its internal model of reality. That means even if it seems clear that your approach isn't working, your system can't learn from it. You get stuck repeating the past—not because you choose to, but because your mind can't register new information when it feels threatened.

The path to healing the Heart Self isn't found in either retreat or pursuit—it's found in balance. A steady State makes it possible to remain emotionally present while navigating complex relationships. As with the Vital Self, the Heart Self responds beautifully to Override Strategies: breath, touch, sound, and relational repair support the return to balance.

When the Heart Self feels safe, it doesn't have to over-function. It can rest. It can connect. And it can begin to trust again.

Echoism and Narcissism as Modes, Not People

It's important to understand that each of these modes is initiated by some kind of trigger. Someone with a tendency to be triggered into one of these modes can be relatively open, charming and relational when not triggered. In fact, we all have a tendency one way or the other when challenged or triggered.

The difference is that some people are very easily triggered due to trauma, neglect or other issues making them vulnerable to dysregulation. And some, sadly, spend their lives in this triggered state.

I want to be clear that when we talk about narcissism within the context of the Mind Matrix Model, we are discussing patterns of behavior or traits that can emerge particularly when the Heart Self is in a Negative State.

Conversely, the diagnosis of Narcissistic Personality Disorder or NPD is a clinical diagnosis and refers to someone who has a personality disorder which can severely affect their life and their relationships.

Trauma and the Heart Self

The Heart Self governs your capacity for emotional attunement, intimacy, and relational presence. It's how you form bonds, express needs, and experience love. When trauma strikes the Heart Self, it distorts those capacities—leading to disconnection, reactivity, confusion, and deep emotional defenses.

Heart Self trauma doesn't always look like collapse. Sometimes it looks like performance, control, or self-elevation. The common thread is relational pain—pain so deep that the system has built strategies to keep it from happening again. These strategies may include withdrawing completely (echoist mode), or dominating emotionally to stay in control (narcissist mode). Both are responses to feeling unloved, unseen, or unworthy.

Common origins of Heart Self trauma include:

- Rejection or abandonment by caregivers, peers, or partners
- Emotional neglect—never feeling deeply known or accepted
- Shame-based parenting or religious conditioning
- Overattunement (parental enmeshment), where boundaries were never safe
- Emotional betrayal or gaslighting—when someone manipulates your perception of reality to make you doubt your own feelings, memories, or sanity
- Relational control disguised as love ("I only love you if…")

- Early pressure to meet others' emotional needs before your own
- Being rewarded for emotional performance rather than authenticity
- Growing up in an environment with manipulation, favoritism, or emotional volatility

These patterns may lead the Heart Self to adapt in one of two main ways:

Echoist Mode (Inward Collapse): You become emotionally porous, hyper-attuned to others' needs, and reluctant to assert your own. You fear disconnection and may over-accommodate, people-please, or numb yourself to maintain attachment.

Narcissist Mode (Outward Control): You learn to protect your emotional core by controlling others' perceptions. You may perform intimacy while staying emotionally distant, use charm or victimhood to manage attention, or inflate your presence to avoid vulnerability.

Both are defenses against the same wound: the fear that your real self is unlovable.

How does Heart trauma show up today?

- Feeling easily rejected or misunderstood
- Struggling to express needs without guilt, or expressing them through anger or manipulation
- Becoming emotionally overwhelmed in close relationships
- Needing others to reflect your worth back to you, or fearing they'll see your shame
- Avoiding intimacy, or chasing it compulsively
- Feeling resentful after giving too much, or not feeling seen for whatever you offered

These reactions aren't failures of character. They are brilliant, adaptive strategies your Heart Self learned to survive relational pain. They make sense. But they also create problems and can be unlearned.

What Heals the Heart Self?

1. Relational Safety

Healing happens in relationship. Whether through therapy, chosen family, or deeply attuned relationships, the Heart Self needs to learn that it is possible to be loved without performing, controlling, or abandoning. Even a few moments of being deeply seen and cared about can start to shift the pattern.

2. Boundaries and Self-Containment

For echoist patterns, healing involves learning to say "no," to tolerate discomfort in others, and to value your own emotions as much as theirs.

For narcissist patterns, healing involves softening defenses, allowing vulnerability, and developing real intimacy that isn't based on performance or control.

Both need the ability to feel emotions without being overwhelmed by them.

3. Emotional Reconnection through Nature

For many, healing the Heart Self begins not with other people, but with the non-human world. Nature offers a unique form of relational repair: it asks nothing of you, mirrors you gently, and invites your authentic presence without shame or pressure. Whether lying under trees, walking beside water, sitting in silence with animals, or watching birds move through the sky, the Heart Self can begin to rest.

Here, you don't need to perform. You don't need to apologize. You don't need to be more or less than you are.

Reconnection with the natural world helps restore the Heart Self's rhythm of openness and retreat, trust and solitude, expression and rest.

4. Slowing Down and Feeling Safe

Many Heart Self wounds stem from the message that your emotions were too much, not welcome, or didn't matter. Healing means proving otherwise again and again. This doesn't mean diving headfirst into pain. It means titrating your emotions: learning to feel them in small, safe doses, while anchoring to something steady (breath, body, nature, another person, even music or art).

5. Choosing Integrity over Persona

Personas are the ways we act in different situations and with different people. Personas are not bad per se, but when they are worn to protect rather than connect, they become prisons.

Healing the Heart Self means reclaiming your right to be real. That may mean sharing less, not more. It may mean staying silent when you'd usually perform, or speaking your truth even if it risks rejection. Over time, the Heart Self learns: *I can show up as myself and still belong.*

The Heart Self and Early Trauma

Your Heart Self is what helps you connect with others, feel valued in relationships, and navigate the emotional landscape of life. From the moment you're born, your interactions with caregivers—especially early bonds with a mother or primary figure—shape your ability to trust, feel loved, and develop emotional resilience.

When those early bonds are secure, a child learns: *I am safe. I matter. The world responds to me with care.* But when there's neglect, abuse, or inconsistent care, the Heart Self absorbs a very different message: *I am not important. I must earn love. People are unpredictable or unsafe.*

Children are naturally wired to assume that their experiences are *about them*—that if something is wrong, it must be their fault. This is actually a survival instinct: if the people they depend on aren't providing what they need, it's too terrifying to see them as unreliable. Instead, a child will believe: *Maybe if I try harder, I can fix this.* This leads to feelings of guilt, shame, and an unconscious belief that love must be earned. Because believing in their own power to change things is less frighteniSng than accepting that those who should be caring for them aren't.

Personas: How We Meet the World

In the Mind Matrix Model, personas are ways of interacting—built from Scripts, behaviors, and expressions—that the mind uses to interact with the world, often shaped by which Self is most active in a given situation. They help manage how we show up in relationship. They aren't inherently bad; in fact, we all use multiple personas. The way you interact with a friend is different than with your boss, or a waiter, or a child.

These adaptive personas allow us to shift contextually while maintaining connection and coherence. As with any Script, they also take a great deal of load off the Monarch, our conscious mind, by managing familiar interactions automatically and freeing conscious resources for more complex or novel experiences.

Personas allow us to smoothly navigate social situations without having to analyze and consciously interpret every nuance. Without them, social interaction would be exhausting. Some individuals—for example, people on the autism spectrum—have difficulty forming automatic personas.

As a result, they often must consciously manage social interactions, relying on cognitive strategies to decode social cues and craft appropriate responses. This can be quite effortful and lead to missing subtle signals, delayed reactions, or responses that seem slightly out of step.

In this way, personas serve an essential function: they allow for fluid, largely unconscious adaptation to the complex and shifting demands of relational life.

You have personas for those you are closest to, those you work with, the butcher, the baker—anyone you consistently meet or who fits a familiar framework of relationship. These personas are not acts or deceptions; they are patterns of engagement adapted to the expectations and relational energy of different connections.

Contextual Personas Across the Three Selves

While we often think of personas as primarily social (Heart Self-centered), the Mind Matrix Model includes a broader definition of persona that extends into the Vital Self and the Head Self as well.

We call these **Contextual Personas**—adaptive collections of Scripts, including actions and mental states, that organize your response not only in relationships but also in physical activities and cognitive tasks.

Each Contextual Persona is shaped by which Self is taking the lead role:

> **Vital-Dominant Personas** organize your body-based presence—how you move, coordinate, react physically, and perform learned physical skills like sports, dance, or even calming yourself with breathing and grounding techniques.

- **Heart-Dominant Personas**, what we normally identify as personas, organize your social and emotional presence—how you engage with others, modulate closeness, protect vulnerability, and express feelings.
- **Head-Dominant Personas** organize your cognitive presence—how you think, problem-solve, intuit, analyze, associate, imagine, and strategize in different mental environments.

For example, when you're exercising, doing physical work, or playing sports, the Vital Self steps forward, drawing on Vital-dominant Contextual Personas built around movement, coordination, endurance, and learned physical responses.

When you're working on your taxes, planning a project, creating an overview, or composing a song, the Head Self leads with Head-Dominant Contextual Personas that draw on both analytic skills like logic and deduction, and holistic capacities like creativity and pattern recognition.

In this view, personas aren't just about relationships—they are how the Three Selves and their Ministers adapt and organize us to meet the world across all domains: relational, physical, and cognitive.

Healing doesn't mean no personas. Personas are one of the ways that your nervous system reduces the burden on the Monarch. Rather than seeing personas as something fake or problematic, the Mind Matrix Model helps us recognize them as essential adaptive structures—flexible fields of behavior that allow us to operate smoothly across vastly different situations, without overwhelming the Monarch with constant decision-making.

Healing means reclaiming the ability to choose which parts of yourself are active based not on fear, but on authenticity and context. The Monarch, utilizing the mindful capability of the Reflective Catalyst role, can work with the different Ministers to retire old protective scripts and make room for relational roles that are both adaptive and true.

Shame and Persona

Shame is one of the most powerful shaping forces within the Heart Self. It likely evolved in social mammals, especially those that live in groups like packs or tribes, as a way to keep everyone connected. When an animal does something that might upset the group, shame triggers appeasement or fawning behavior to help them stay included.

You can see this in dogs: when scolded, they often display signs of shame and appeasement—lowered head, tucked tail, submissive posture—even if they haven't actually done anything wrong. This response isn't guilt over a specific action; it's an instinctual strategy to maintain connection and avoid rejection.

Similarly, in humans, shame can be triggered not just by what we've done, but by how we fear we're seen.

When children are consistently shamed, it can attach to their sense of who they are, how they're seen, and whether they believe they are worthy of respect and belonging. For example, when a child feels that their emotions, needs, or expressions lead to disconnection or rejection, the Heart Minister may intervene by creating a **protective persona**.

But when a persona forms around unprocessed shame, because it relates to a Negative State trigger it becomes rigid and reactive. Instead of fluidly adjusting to relational settings, it functions more like armor—protecting what feels unworthy or too vulnerable to show. Over time, the persona can start to take over, hiding perceived vulnerabilities beneath practiced roles that no longer feel like conscious choices.

The Heart Self and the Negative State.

When the Heart Self becomes dysregulated, the Heart Minister activates deeply ingrained Scripts. These often take the form of either Echoist Mode or Narcissist Mode activation, two opposing but related strategies for dealing with unmet emotional needs. Some people are extremely vulnerable to Heart Self triggers and can spend much or all of their lives in Echoist mode or Narcissist mode.

In both cases, the Heart Minister is trying to protect something, often a compartmentalized wound or vulnerable Script that was never met with safety. By understanding how the Heart Self works, and by learning how to rebalance your focus, you can begin to unfreeze those patterns.

Self-Other Development in the Heart Self

Self-Other Development is the very early process by which we come to understand where we end and others begin—emotionally, physically, and psychologically. It unfolds in stages across childhood, helping us form a sense of self in relationship to others.

The Heart Self brings depth to this process by introducing emotional awareness and connection. Around toddlerhood, children begin to recognize themselves as relational beings. They realize that others have feelings too, and those feelings can affect them. If emotions are welcomed and mirrored, the child learns that it's safe to be separate and connected at the same time.

But if emotional needs are met inconsistently, or if the child is made responsible for others' feelings, they may lean too far toward self-erasure or emotional isolation. This is where early patterns of people-pleasing, shame, and relational fear are often born.

How Early Trauma Shapes the Heart Self

Without consistent emotional support, the Heart Self becomes vulnerable to what the Mind Matrix Model calls the *Negative State*—a survival mode where the Heart Self reacts as if rejection or abandonment is always around the corner. Even when caregivers are physically present, a child might *feel* emotionally disconnected, leading to deep-seated insecurity and self-doubt that can last into adulthood.

Behavioral and Physiological Signs of the Heart Self

Here's a list of potential behavioral and physiological signs that reflect the balance of the Heart Self:

Social Interaction:

Inward-Focused: Prefers solitude or small, intimate gatherings; may avoid large social situations.

Balanced: Enjoys both social interaction and alone time, switching comfortably between the two.

Outward-Focused: Thrives in social environments, enjoys being around others, and seeks out social gatherings.

Emotional Expression:

Inward-Focused: Tends to internalize emotions and may struggle with expressing feelings openly.

Balanced: Expresses emotions appropriately, neither suppressing nor over-expressing them.

Outward-Focused: Expresses emotions openly and frequently, often wearing emotions on their sleeve.

Empathy and Sensitivity:

Inward-Focused: Highly sensitive to others' emotions but may struggle to engage empathetically due to internal focus.

Balanced: Demonstrates empathy without becoming overwhelmed, balancing personal boundaries with sensitivity to others.

Outward-Focused: Highly empathetic, often deeply involved in others' emotions, and may struggle with boundaries.

Communication Style:

Inward-Focused: Prefers written communication or one-on-one conversations; may avoid public speaking or large group discussions.

Balanced: Comfortable with both one-on-one and group communication, adapting to the situation.

Outward-Focused: Enjoys group discussions, public speaking, and often leads conversations.

Conflict Resolution:

Inward-Focused: Tends to avoid conflict, possibly suppressing their own needs to maintain peace.

Balanced: Addresses conflicts directly but with empathy, seeking win-win outcomes.

Outward-Focused: Confronts conflict head-on, assertive in defending their position, and may sometimes be perceived as too aggressive.

Decision-Making:

Inward-Focused: Prefers introspection before making decisions and often takes a cautious approach.

Balanced: Makes decisions with a blend of reflection and action, considering both internal and external factors.

Outward-Focused: Makes decisions quickly, often influenced by social input or a desire for action.

Body Language:

Inward-Focused: Closed or minimal body language, may avoid eye contact, often appears reserved.

Balanced: Open but not overly expressive body language, maintains appropriate eye contact.

Outward-Focused: Open, expressive body language, frequent use of gestures, and maintains strong eye contact.

Stress Management:

Inward-Focused: Internalizes stress, often managing it through solitary activities.

Balanced: Manages stress through a mix of social interaction and personal reflection.

Outward-Focused: Manages stress by talking it out with others or engaging in social activities.

Trust in Relationships:

Inward-Focused: Tends to be slow to trust, often cautious or reserved in forming deep emotional bonds.

Balanced: Able to build trust gradually while remaining open.

Outward-Focused: Often quick to trust, sometimes forming strong attachments before relational safety is fully established.

Attachment Style:

Inward-Focused: May exhibit avoidant attachment, valuing independence and self-reliance.

Balanced: Demonstrates secure attachment, comfortable with both closeness and independence in relationships.

Outward-Focused: May exhibit anxious attachment, frequently seeking closeness and reassurance from others.

Healing the Heart Self

The key to healing your Heart Self isn't found in external validation but in developing your *intrinsic self-worth*—a sense of value that doesn't easily rise and fall based on how others treat you or what's going on inside you. This involves:

Building Self-Compassion: Learning to offer yourself the kindness and understanding you may not have received as a child. This means taking good care of yourself when you're feeling down, letting go of any internal or outside voices telling you that you aren't worthy or good, and generally working toward a healthy, content life.

Recognizing that self-critical or fear "voices" are not your own. We are all familiar with thoughts and feelings that are self-critical, fearful, or shaming—these are the voices of our internalized Sentries.

Understanding this distinction allows you to relate to these voices differently. Rather than taking them at face value, you can gently acknowledge them as protective mechanisms from the past that may no longer serve you.

By doing so, you can begin to soften their grip, offering yourself compassion and the space to respond differently, ultimately allowing your true, authentic voice to guide you forward.

Healing the Heart Self begins with reclaiming emotional safety and trust in connection. In the Mind Matrix Model, the Heart Self governs relationships, attachment, and emotional expression. When wounded, it often adapts by suppressing needs (echoist mode) or inflating them (narcissistic mode), both of which create barriers to authentic connection.

Healing the Heart Self means developing a felt sense that it is safe to be seen, to need, and to feel. This requires both internal work through regulating your emotional state, and external work through good relationships where it's safe to practice being real, authentic and open.

Repairing Attachment Wounds: Engaging in relationships (including therapy) where secure, consistent support helps rewire old patterns—leaving relationships where you are abused, criticized or told you aren't worthy and seeking out supportive, caring relationships.

Emotional Regulation Practices: Techniques like mindfulness, breathwork, and grounding exercises help soothe your nervous system and make emotional experiences feel safer.

Relational Authenticity: Practicing honesty in your relationships—expressing needs and holding boundaries with others without fear of rejection or shame—rebuilds trust in both yourself and others.

In the beginning, you may encounter some very difficult or scary feelings of vulnerability, but over time being with people as your authentic self creates much deeper, more fulfilling relationships.

Healing your Heart Self is not about eliminating vulnerability but *learning to experience it safely*, knowing that relationships can be imperfect and still meaningful, that emotions can be intense and still manageable, and that your worth is not something you have to earn.

The Myth of Self-Esteem

From the perspective of the Mind Matrix Model, what we call "poor self-esteem" is not actually a reflection of how you feel about yourself, it's more the protective activity of internal Sentries. In this model, Sentries are Negative State Scripts designed to keep us safe. Often formed in early life, they are protective subroutines that activate when the system is under threat, especially emotional threat.

One way Sentries protect us is by generating self-critical thoughts, feelings of inadequacy, or even physical tension. These responses are not random, they are survival strategies meant to keep us hypervigilant, small, or compliant in order to avoid danger. In effect, they say: "If I make you feel bad about yourself, maybe you won't take a risk and get hurt again."

Most of us mistake the voice or feeling of a Sentry as our own voice—"me talking to me"—but in reality, it is not. It is the echo of something we once needed to stay safe, but which no longer serves us. The true self—the Monarch—is not cruel, shaming, or belittling. When we are in the Positive State, the Monarch is in charge and guides with clarity, care, and inner authority.

Many people believe that poor self-esteem can be fixed through praise, achievements or how they look, setting them up for endlessly trying to feel better. Like a boat with a leak in it, the solution is not to keep bailing it out but to plug the hole.

Reclaiming self-worth, then, is not about "building self-esteem" but about recognizing these Sentries for what they are: protective mechanisms triggered by fear, shame, or unresolved pain. **The answer is not to push the voices away, argue with them, or accept them as truth. The ultimate answer is through expanded self-awareness and knowledge of how your mind works.**

Like an airplane flying through a storm, the way forward is not by continuing straight on, but upward above the clouds and into calmer skies. Rather than trying to escape from, argue with, or agree with the voices, learn to shift your State: ground yourself in body and breath, shift to the Positive State, and become the witness of your internal environment rather than the victim in the story. From there, clarity, compassion, and discernment become available again.

Grounding the Heart Self

The Heart Self stays balanced through a mix of social connection, personal reflection, grounding rituals, and understanding your own needs, especially in terms of introversion and extroversion.

> **Extroverts** often feel grounded through active engagement with others. They recharge by participating in social gatherings, group activities, or community events. Rituals like shared meals or regular gatherings can help extroverts feel connected and renewed.
>
> **Introverts** tend to ground themselves through quieter, one-on-one interactions or solitary rituals. They may need time alone to process emotions and recharge after social interactions. Rituals like journaling, meditation, or spending time in nature can offer introverts a peaceful space for self-reflection and emotional renewal.

Both introverts and extroverts benefit from rituals that provide structure and comfort. Shared rituals can create a sense of community, while personal rituals create a sense of safety and often can offer a space for self-awareness and reflection.

Reflection is essential for everyone, whether through quiet time, journaling, or mindfulness. Taking this time allows you to process your feelings, understand your boundaries, and release social tension, ultimately making you more resilient.

By grounding yourself through connection, reflection, rituals, and an awareness of individual needs, your Heart Self can better manage emotional energy, face relational challenges, and maintain balance. This balance leads to healthier relationships, greater emotional stability, and a strong sense of self within the social world.

> *Honesty doesn't mean oversharing. Those with an echoist leaning may feel dishonest if they withhold anything, but authentic expression includes discernment. Sharing appropriately, based on context and emotional safety, is a key part of relational integrity.*

Final Thoughts

The Heart Self provides a framework for understanding how we interact with our social and emotional worlds. Whether one tends to be more inward-focused, outward-focused, or balanced, recognizing these traits can guide personal development and improve relationships.

For those at the extremes, finding balance is key to a fulfilling life. Through tailored therapies, mindful dietary choices, and the use of herbs, nutraceuticals, and remedies, individuals can work towards balancing their socio-emotional lives, fostering both inner peace and social well-being. By understanding where you fall within the Heart Self, you can cultivate healthier, more satisfying relationships with your inner Selves and with others.

Chapter Ten
Balancing the Heart Self

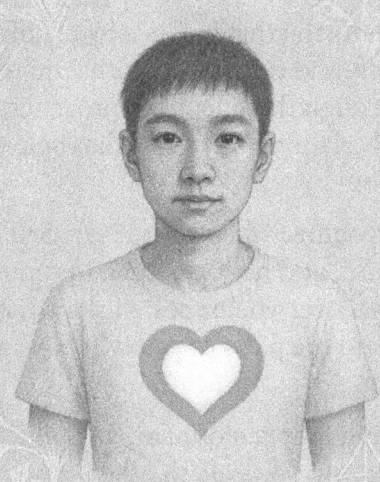

*There are times to prefer
silence over sound, quiet
over conversation — perhaps an
introvert always enjoys the
shape of being alone.
But when absence becomes noise
and silence grows loud,
I adapt to change
and bring back the chaos of
three girls, one household, two cats,
and various visitors:
neighbors, friends, family.
There is a balance between
extremes that can satisfy
the two sides of me.*

~ Dual
   by Alison McBain

The Heart Self: Balancing Inward and Outward Focus

Your Heart Self is where connection, vulnerability, and emotional memory live. When it's in balance, you can connect with others easily and give and receive love freely. But when it's been hurt—by rejection, neglect, or disconnection—it adapts in ways that can become burdensome over time. You might overextend, retreat, over-attune, or shut down entirely. Healing the Heart Self means learning to listen again, gently and with compassion, to what you need.

This chapter is about restoring that balance by reconnecting your Heart Self with safety, presence, and emotional truth. You'll learn how to support your Heart Self through therapeutic approaches, gentle rituals, herbs and homeopathics, and relational practices that help reestablish trust—internally and externally.

We'll explore how to recognize when your Heart Self is leaning too far inward or too far outward, and how to return to center. You'll discover ways to soothe emotional overwhelm, soften shame, restore boundaries, and bring warmth back to the parts of you that have grown cold or tired from carrying too much.

This isn't about becoming more emotional. It's about becoming more balanced and more attuned—to yourself, to others, and to the intelligence of your own Heart Self.

Heart Self Questionnaire

This self-assessment helps you explore how your Heart Self—the emotional and relational part of your mind—relates to others and to yourself. It identifies tendencies toward inward focus (emotional withholding), outward focus (emotional overexpression or dependence), or balance. It also captures instability (swinging between extremes).

You can also access a downloadable PDF version of the form as well as an interactive version by visiting the Mind Matrix Model website. You'll need to register if you haven't yet. You can sign up for free access by scanning the QR code or visiting this short link:

mmm.tips/heartform

https://mmm.tips/heartform

The interactive form can be used to chart your progress over time, and includes many combination patterns that reveal more complex dynamics.

Instructions

For each question, choose the option (Rarely true, Sometimes true, Often true, Very true) that best describes your typical experience—not what you wish were true. Don't overthink it. Go with your first honest reaction.

If you are keeping a journal, this is a good time to write your responses down there so you can check up on how you're doing later. Otherwise just grab a piece of paper or a screen device to track your answers.

> **Note:** *This is not a medical test, but a self-reflection tool designed to help you explore approaches for improving your quality of life. If you have any concerns, consider consulting a healthcare professional or therapist for personalized guidance.*

1. Social Interaction

A) I prefer being alone or in small groups. Too much interaction drains me.
○ Rarely true=1 ○ Sometimes true=2 ○ Often true=3 ○ Very true=4

B) I enjoy both alone time and socializing, depending on my energy.
○ Rarely true=1 ○ Sometimes true=2 ○ Often true=3 ○ Very true=4

C) I feel energized and alive around others and I often seek out connection.
○ Rarely true=1 ○ Sometimes true=2 ○ Often true=3 ○ Very true=4

D) I often feel torn—craving connection, then wanting to retreat.
○ Rarely true=1 ○ Sometimes true=2 ○ Often true=3 ○ Very true=4

2. Emotional Expression

A) I tend to hold in my feelings and rarely show them openly.
○ Rarely true=1 ○ Sometimes true=2 ○ Often true=3 ○ Very true=4

B) I express emotions clearly without overdoing or holding back.
○ Rarely true=1 ○ Sometimes true=2 ○ Often true=3 ○ Very true=4

C) I express emotions freely and often—sometimes strongly.
○ Rarely true=1 ○ Sometimes true=2 ○ Often true=3 ○ Very true=4

D) I sometimes bottle up my emotions until they burst out.
○ Rarely true=1 ○ Sometimes true=2 ○ Often true=3 ○ Very true=4

3. Communication in Conflict

A) I usually avoid conflict and hold back what I want to say.
○ Rarely true=1   ○ Sometimes true=2   ○ Often true=3   ○ Very true=4

B) I can express disagreement calmly while listening to others.
○ Rarely true=1   ○ Sometimes true=2   ○ Often true=3   ○ Very true=4

C) I tend to confront issues quickly—sometimes too strongly.
○ Rarely true=1   ○ Sometimes true=2   ○ Often true=3   ○ Very true=4

D) I swing between staying silent and reacting too strongly.
○ Rarely true=1   ○ Sometimes true=2   ○ Often true=3   ○ Very true=4

4. Empathy and Sensitivity

A) I easily pick up on others' emotions but lose track of my own.
○ Rarely true=1   ○ Sometimes true=2   ○ Often true=3   ○ Very true=4

B) I can tune into others' feelings without losing my center.
○ Rarely true=1   ○ Sometimes true=2   ○ Often true=3   ○ Very true=4

C) I feel others' emotions deeply and often react strongly to them.
○ Rarely true=1   ○ Sometimes true=2   ○ Often true=3   ○ Very true=4

D) I shift between being overly empathic and shutting off emotionally.
○ Rarely true=1   ○ Sometimes true=2   ○ Often true=3   ○ Very true=4

5. Trust and Closeness

A) I find it hard to trust. I often keep emotional distance, even from people I care about.
○ Rarely true=1   ○ Sometimes true=2   ○ Often true=3   ○ Very true=4

B) I open up gradually and build trust over time.
○ Rarely true=1   ○ Sometimes true=2   ○ Often true=3   ○ Very true=4

C) I tend to trust quickly and get emotionally involved early.
○ Rarely true=1   ○ Sometimes true=2   ○ Often true=3   ○ Very true=4

D) I swing between craving closeness and pushing people away.
○ Rarely true=1   ○ Sometimes true=2   ○ Often true=3   ○ Very true=4

6. Emotional Reactivity

A) I rarely show strong emotions, even when I feel them inside.
○ Rarely true=1 ○ Sometimes true=2 ○ Often true=3 ○ Very true=4

B) I can stay with strong feelings without getting overwhelmed.
○ Rarely true=1 ○ Sometimes true=2 ○ Often true=3 ○ Very true=4

C) I react emotionally and sometimes intensely when upset.
○ Rarely true=1 ○ Sometimes true=2 ○ Often true=3 ○ Very true=4

D) I suppress emotions until they explode, or fluctuate unpredictably.
○ Rarely true=1 ○ Sometimes true=2 ○ Often true=3 ○ Very true=4

7. Handling Rejection or Criticism

A) I take rejection very personally and pull away to protect myself.
○ Rarely true=1 ○ Sometimes true=2 ○ Often true=3 ○ Very true=4

B) I can process rejection or feedback without losing my sense of self-worth.
○ Rarely true=1 ○ Sometimes true=2 ○ Often true=3 ○ Very true=4

C) I often feel wounded and seek reassurance from others when I feel rejected.
○ Rarely true=1 ○ Sometimes true=2 ○ Often true=3 ○ Very true=4

D) I bounce between needing validation and wanting to withdraw.
○ Rarely true=1 ○ Sometimes true=2 ○ Often true=3 ○ Very true=4

8. Seeking Support

A) I tend to deal with things on my own, even when I could use help.
○ Rarely true=1 ○ Sometimes true=2 ○ Often true=3 ○ Very true=4

B) I reach out for support when needed and support myself too.
○ Rarely true=1 ○ Sometimes true=2 ○ Often true=3 ○ Very true=4

C) I often turn to others quickly when upset or uncertain.
○ Rarely true=1 ○ Sometimes true=2 ○ Often true=3 ○ Very true=4

D) I alternate between isolating and depending heavily on others.
○ Rarely true=1 ○ Sometimes true=2 ○ Often true=3 ○ Very true=4

9. Trust in Relationships

A) I am slow to trust and take time to build deep connections.

○ Rarely true=1   ○ Sometimes true=2   ○ Often true=3   ○ Very true=4

B) I trust appropriately, balancing openness with caution.

○ Rarely true=1   ○ Sometimes true=2   ○ Often true=3   ○ Very true=4

C) I tend to trust easily and quickly, often forming connections rapidly.

○ Rarely true=1   ○ Sometimes true=2   ○ Often true=3   ○ Very true=4

D) I shift between trusting too quickly and pulling away.

○ Rarely true=1   ○ Sometimes true=2   ○ Often true=3   ○ Very true=4

10. Attachment Style

A) I value independence and self-reliance and don't often get very close to people.

○ Rarely true=1   ○ Sometimes true=2   ○ Often true=3   ○ Very true=4

B) I am comfortable with both closeness and independence in relationships.

○ Rarely true=1   ○ Sometimes true=2   ○ Often true=3   ○ Very true=4

C) I frequently seek closeness and reassurance from others.

○ Rarely true=1   ○ Sometimes true=2   ○ Often true=3   ○ Very true=4

D) I go back and forth between needing closeness and pushing others away.

○ Rarely true=1   ○ Sometimes true=2   ○ Often true=3   ○ Very true=4

How to Score Your Heart Self Axis Questionnaire

Step 1: Tally Your Scores
Go through your answers and total the points for each letter:
- Each time you rated an A, add the point value you selected (1 = Rarely True, 4 = Very True) to your A total.
- Do the same for B, C, and D responses.
  For example, if you answered Rarely true eight times, that would total 8, Sometimes true eight times would be 16, Often true eight times = 24, Very true eight times = 32.

Each letter will have a total between 10 (lowest) and 40 (highest).

Your Scores:

    A =   B =   C =   D =

Step 2: Interpretation
Find which pattern below matches your scores.

A 30 or more - Inward-Focused Heart Self (emotionally withdrawn, guarded)

Your system may avoid vulnerability. Support includes emotional expression, trust-building, and safe connection

What to Support: Support includes emotional expression, trust-building, and safe connection.

Read: Inward-Focused – The Reflective Observer

High B - Balanced Heart Self

You are generally emotionally grounded, relationally healthy, and self-aware. Focus on sustaining resilience and deepening insight.

What to Support: Support includes self-soothing, internal containment, and boundary work.

Read: Balanced: The Harmonious Integrator

High C - Outward-Focused Heart Self

Your system may prioritize others or seek closeness for safety.

What to Support: Support includes self-soothing, boundaries, and inner containment.

Read: Outward-Focused – The Social Dynamo

High D - Swinging/Unstable Heart Self

You may alternate between isolation and emotional intensity. This often signals attachment wounds. Focus on rhythm, predictability, and titrated emotional work.

What to Support: Focus on rhythm, predictability, and titrated emotional repair.

Read: Inward-Focused – The Reflective Observer and Outward-Focused – The Social Dynamo

If none of your scores is 30 or more, choose the one that is the highest score. This indicates that you could have a more complex pattern that the interactive form on the website would reveal.

Healing involves gently reworking attachment strategies with somatic grounding, relational safety, and emotional pacing.

Reflection Prompts (Optional)

> "How did I learn to express—or not express—my feelings?"
>
> "Do I tend to over-focus on others or ignore my own emotional needs?"
>
> "What kind of emotional environment feels safe for me?"
>
> "When I'm triggered, do I pull in or reach out?"

> **Note**: *While these questionnaires are a helpful tool for self-assessment, it's important to recognize that we may not always be the best judges of our own tendencies. Our perceptions can be influenced by biases or blind spots.*
>
> *To gain a more accurate understanding, it can be very helpful to have someone who knows you well—like a partner, close friend, family member, or colleague—answer the questions about you. Their perspective can provide additional insights and help paint a clearer picture of your social and emotional patterns.*

Inward-Focused: The Reflective Observer

Inward-focused individuals find energy in quiet, introspective environments. They are thoughtful and reserved, valuing deep connections over broad social networks. These individuals excel in reflective tasks and have a nuanced understanding of their inner world and emotions.

Approaches to Balancing Inward Focus:

Therapies and Modalities:

Mindfulness-Based Stress Reduction (MBSR): Helps Inward-Focused individuals feel more comfortable in social settings by reducing anxiety.

Art Therapy: Encourages them to express emotions and thoughts creatively.

Cognitive Behavioral Therapy (CBT): Helps address negative thought patterns contributing to social anxiety and isolation.

Diet and Nutrition:

Omega-3 Fatty Acids: Found in fish oil and flaxseeds, omega-3s support brain health and can help regulate mood.

B Vitamins: Essential for energy and stress reduction, helping them feel more energized in social situations.

Herbs and Nutraceuticals:

Ashwagandha: An adaptogen that helps manage stress and reduce social anxiety.

Rhodiola Rosea: Supports stamina and resilience in social settings.

L-Theanine: Found in green tea, it promotes relaxation without drowsiness.

Tulsi (Holy Basil) – A gentle adaptogen that uplifts mood, reduces social anxiety, and supports clarity. Especially helpful for Heart Self balance.

Lemon Balm – Calms the nerves without sedating, gently lifts low mood, and is ideal for sensitive individuals who feel overwhelmed by social dynamics.

Milky Oat Seed – Nourishes a depleted nervous system, helping with emotional fragility and boundary strengthening.

Rose Petal – A heart tonic traditionally used to encourage self-love, receptivity, and emotional softness.

Schisandra Berry – Enhances adaptability and stamina in social situations while protecting against emotional depletion.

Homeopathic Remedies

Homeopathics act subtly and are especially well-suited to the emotionally sensitive and energetically permeable inner world of echoists.

A common starting dose is **30c potency, taken 3–4 times per day**. If you notice clear improvement, you may shift to **a single dose of 200c** for deeper, longer-lasting support. For more guidance, see the Next Steps chapter *Homeopathy: Gentle Remedies for Balance and Health*.

Pulsatilla 30c – For gentle, shy individuals who crave connection but fear rejection; supports emotional fluidity and confidence.

Silicea 30c – For those who are deeply inward, perfectionistic, or self-doubting; helps strengthen internal fortitude and boundary resilience.

Baryta Carbonica 30c – For socially immature or withdrawn individuals, often due to deep fear of being judged or seen.

Ignatia 30c – For those who suppress grief or disappointment and struggle to express themselves authentically.

Natrum Muriaticum 30c – For introverts who build emotional walls due to past relational wounding, helping to gently dissolve them.

Essential Oils

These oils work through the limbic system (Vital + Heart Self access) and can be inhaled, used in baths, or diluted for anointing the chest or back of neck.

Rose Otto – Opens the heart, heals emotional wounding, and fosters a safe sense of connection.

Bergamot – Lightly energizing and anti-anxiety, it's especially good for social discomfort and a lack of self-worth.

Frankincense – Anchoring and introspective, helps bridge inner awareness with outward expression.

Cedarwood – Grounds and strengthens boundaries, great for those who feel porous or overly merged with others.

Ylang Ylang – Softens rigidity and emotional suppression; promotes receptivity and emotional safety.

Sweet Orange – Bright and uplifting without overstimulating; encourages warmth, playfulness, and spontaneity.

Suggested Formulation: "Open Presence" Blend

A calming, heart-supportive essential oil blend for overly sensitive introverts:

3 drops Rose

2 drops Bergamot

2 drops Cedarwood

1 drop Frankincense

Diffuse during journaling, social engagements, or while preparing for interpersonal interactions.

Acupressure for the Inward-Focused (Introversive) Heart Self

These points support Heart Self patterns of withdrawal, emotional suppression, or internalized shame. They help you express needs, reconnect after emotional retreat, and restore the Heart's courage to reach outward.

You can activate them by applying gentle, steady pressure with your fingertips while breathing slowly and mindfully. A few minutes of focused contact can help release stuck emotion and gently reawaken your Heart's relational presence.

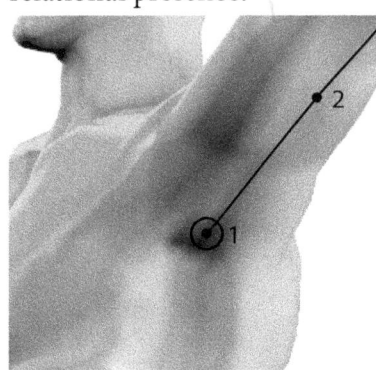

Heart 1 – Supreme Spring (Jiquan)

Location: In the center of the axilla (armpit), deep between the chest and shoulder muscles.

Use for:

Emotional numbness or shutdown
Withdrawing from connection or touch
Softening after deep grief or isolation

Symbolism: The Heart's first outflow into the world—revitalizes expression after long-held emotional silence.

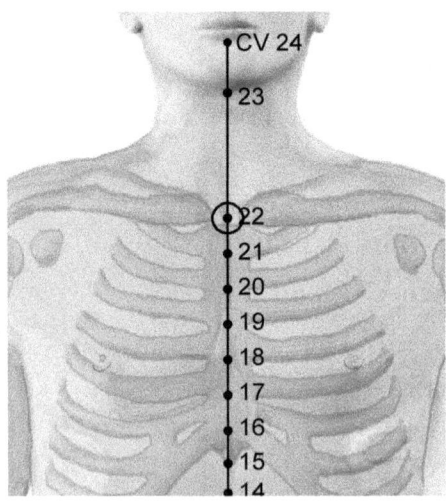

Conception Vessel 22 – Celestial Chimney (Tiantu)

Location: In the depression above the sternum, at the suprasternal notch.

Use for:

Constricted throat or trouble speaking emotions
Feeling choked up or afraid to be seen
Releasing grief held in the voice

Symbolism: Clears the Heart–throat channel so your true voice can emerge with safety and clarity.

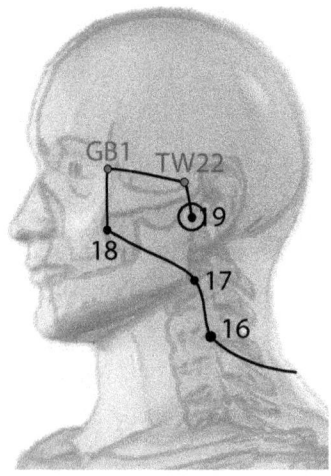

Small Intestine 19 – Listening Palace (Ting Gong)

Location: Just in front of the ear, in the hollow that opens when the mouth opens wide.

Use for:

Feeling emotionally unheard
Difficulty attuning to others after retreat
Strengthening safe reciprocal communication

Symbolism: Restores the loop between listening and being heard—a key step in relational re-entry.

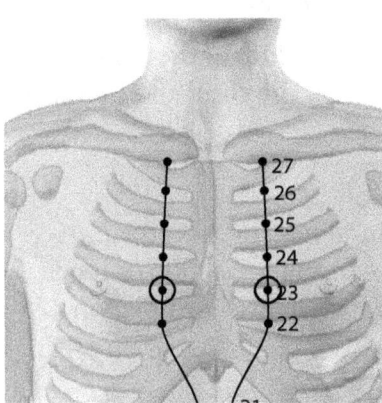

Kidney 23 – Spirit Seal (Shenfeng)

Location: In the fourth intercostal (between the ribs) space, 4 fingers out from the midline. You can also release Ki 24-27 to enhance the release.

Use for:

Shyness or fear of opening emotionally
Supporting quiet strength
Anchoring the Heart Spirit

Symbolism: Stabilizes the Heart from below—offering quiet confidence and rooted emotional presence.

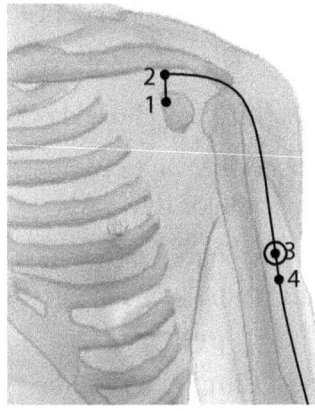

Lung 3 – Heavenly Palace (Tian Fu)

Location: On the upper arm, 7 fingers above the elbow crease to the outer side of the biceps.

Use for:

Suppressed sorrow or emotional holding
Inability to express sadness
Bringing breath and feeling into alignment

Symbolism: Opens a "celestial window" for unspoken emotions to flow gently outward.

Outward-Focused: The Social Dynamo

Outward-Focused individuals thrive in social environments, drawing energy from interacting with others. They are assertive, expressive, and enjoy being in the spotlight. These individuals are action-oriented and excel in dynamic, fast-paced settings.

Approaches to Balancing Outward Focus:

Therapies and Modalities:

Dialectical Behavior Therapy (DBT): Helps develop better emotional regulation and mindfulness.

Journaling: Encourages introspection and reflection on their experiences and emotions.

Diet and Nutrition:

Complex Carbohydrates: Foods like whole grains provide sustained energy, supporting their high activity levels.

Protein-Rich Foods: Protein supports cognitive function and mood regulation.

Herbs and Nutraceuticals:

Extroverts often benefit from herbs that soothe nervous energy, strengthen boundaries, and encourage self-reflection or emotional depth.

Holy Basil (Tulsi): Helps manage stress and prevents burnout.

Valerian Root: Supports relaxation, helps unwind after a busy day.

Passionflower: Promotes calmness and helps manage anxiety. Reduces circular thinking and mental chatter; ideal for those who struggle to transition out of "social mode."

Skullcap – A nervine that quiets the racing mind and helps integrate experiences, especially after social overload.

Wood Betony – Grounds energy into the body, calming an overactive mental field and reconnecting to somatic presence.

Reishi Mushroom – Calms a high-output nervous system, enhances inner wisdom, and supports spiritual and emotional grounding.

Motherwort – Softens reactivity and helps regulate the heart's emotional rhythms—great for those who react quickly and intensely.

Passionflower –

Homeopathic Remedies

These homeopathic profiles help with emotional containment, boundary-setting, and rebalancing from excessive outward orientation.

A common starting dose is **30c potency, taken 3–4 times per day**. If you notice clear improvement, you may shift to **a single dose of 200c** for deeper, longer-lasting support. For more guidance, see the Next Steps chapter *Homeopathy: Gentle Remedies for Balance and Health*.

Lachesis 30c – For expressive, charismatic individuals who may dominate conversations but feel internally tense or jealous; helps support self-reflection and emotional regulation.

Phosphorus 30c – For those who are warm, enthusiastic, and socially magnetic—but prone to emotional burnout and energetic oversensitivity.

Sulphur 30c – For intellectual extroverts with strong opinions and pride, but who struggle with self-awareness or attunement to others.

Veratrum Album 30c – For high-energy individuals who seek attention and admiration, especially when driven by insecurity.

Nux Vomica 30c – For the always on person who becomes irritable or depleted when having to slow down; supports rebalancing.

Essential Oils

These oils soothe excess social energy, anchor into the body, and encourage deeper inner listening.

Vetiver – Deeply grounding and calming; ideal after overstimulation or excessive talking.

Sandalwood – Helps draw awareness inward, encouraging reflection, humility, and presence.

Patchouli – Grounds scattered energy and reconnects to physical sensuality and inner stillness.

Myrrh – Encourages emotional introspection and reconnection with what truly matters.

Clary Sage – Opens intuition and supports inner wisdom when extroverted tendencies dominate.

Suggested Formulation: "Inner Stillness" Blend

A calming and centering essential oil blend for extroverts:

    2 drops Vetiver
    2 drops Sandalwood
    1 drop Myrrh
    1 drop Clary Sage

Apply to soles of feet, back of neck, or diffuse after social interaction or to support reflective practices like journaling or meditation.

Acupressure for the Outward-Focused (Extroversive) Heart Self

These points support Heart Self patterns of over-connection, relational overexposure, and emotional performativity. They help you set healthy emotional boundaries, gather your energy inward, and return to inner coherence.

For detailed instructions on technique, timing, and best practices, see the Next Steps *Chapter 23 - Acupressure For Yourself and Others.*

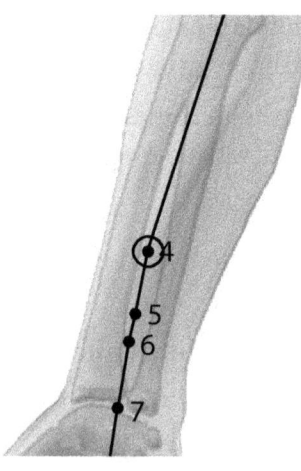

Pericardium 4 – Gate of Origin (Ximen)

Location: On the middle of the inner forearm, 9 fingers above the wrist crease, between the tendons.

Use for:

Emotional urgency or codependent pull
Over-identifying with others' pain
Restoring self-containment

Symbolism: Filters and slows the outflow of Heart energy—ideal for regathering scattered emotions.

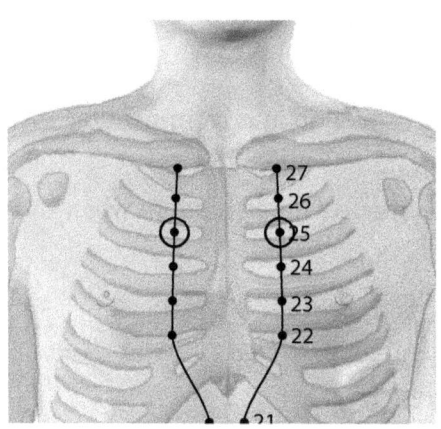

Kidney 25 – Spirit Storehouse (Shencang)

Location: In the second intercostal space 5 fingers below the collar bone and 4 fingers out from the center.

Use for:

Feeling emotionally porous or exposed
Self-abandonment in relationships
Containing and centering the Heart

Symbolism: Protects the Heart Spirit with a sense of internal sanctuary.

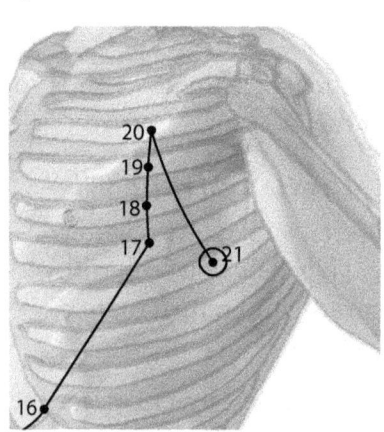

Spleen 21 – Great Embracement (Dabao)

Location: Six fingers down from the front of the armpit, between the ribs.

Use for:

Feeling emotionally scattered
Loss of center in social settings
Drawing energy back from over-connection

Symbolism: Gathers your emotional field inward—like giving yourself a healing embrace.

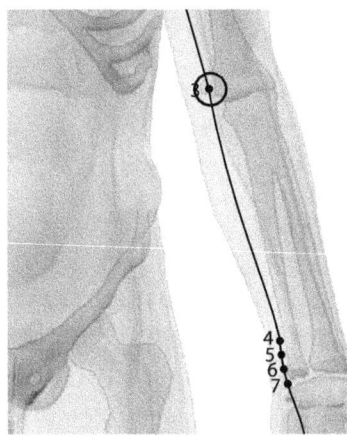

Heart 3 – Lesser Sea (Shao Hai)

Location: At the inner (medial) side of the elbow crease when the arm is bent. Straighten and feel for a firm knot.

Use for:

Emotional volatility or flooding
Soothing irritability and impulsivity
Returning to inner calm

Symbolism: Calms the Heart's "waves" when emotions swell too large to contain.

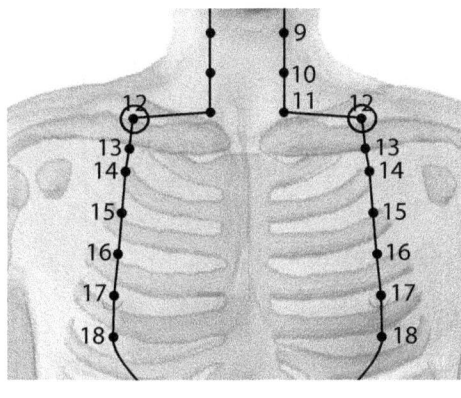

Stomach 12 – Empty Basin (Quepen)

Location: Starting at the inner top of the collar bone, 4 fingers out. Press in and down behind the bone.

Use for:

Emotional exhaustion from over-socialization
Difficulty retreating after too much expression
Resetting the boundary between head and heart

Symbolism: Drains excess emotion from the upper body and helps reset relational equilibrium.

Balanced: The Harmonious Integrator

Balanced individuals navigate the Heart Self with ease, adapting to various social situations while maintaining a strong sense of self. They are comfortable with both introspection and social engagement, which helps them maintain well-rounded relationships.

Example of a Balanced Person:
John is a therapist who spends his workdays deeply engaged with clients, offering empathy and support. Outside of work, he enjoys both spending quiet evenings at home and participating in social activities with friends. John is equally comfortable in solitude and in the company of others, making him adaptable and balanced.

Strengths:
Balanced individuals have strong emotional intelligence, healthy boundaries, and can navigate different social settings without losing themselves. They are often creative, expressive, and value fairness in relationships. Their ability to balance social and solitary activities helps them build meaningful relationships without feeling overwhelmed.

Challenges:
While balanced individuals generally manage social and emotional dynamics well, they must remain mindful of maintaining this equilibrium amidst life's demands.

Approaches to Maintaining Balance:

Therapies and Modalities:

Mindfulness Practices: Regular mindfulness meditation helps maintain emotional equilibrium and adaptability.

Relational Therapy: Ensures that balanced individuals maintain healthy relationships and continue to grow socially and emotionally.

Diet and Nutrition:

Balanced Diet: A diet rich in whole foods, including fruits, vegetables, lean proteins, healthy fats and good fiber supports overall health and emotional stability.

Probiotics: Supports gut health, which is linked to mood and emotional regulation.

Herbs and Nutraceuticals:

For those who are already balanced, the goal is maintenance, resilience, and fine-tuning. These herbs along with magnesium act as tonics and gentle regulators:

American Ginseng (Panax quinquefolius) – A classic adaptogen that boosts mental clarity and physical stamina without overstimulation.

Tulsi (Holy Basil) – Calms low-grade stress while supporting mental clarity and emotional grace—also beneficial for preventing imbalance during overstimulation.

Linden Flower – A gentle nervine that eases tension in the heart and body; helps maintain calm and compassion in interactions.

Eleuthero (Siberian Ginseng) – Builds long-term adaptability and stress resistance; excellent during seasonal or role transitions.

Nettle Leaf – Nutrient-rich, gently energizing, and supports adrenal balance—ideal for those who "run well" but need nutritional depth.

Magnesium: Supports relaxation and helps maintain a calm, balanced state. Best is magnesium glycinate (sometimes called bisglycinate). Don't use magnesium oxide, as it doesn't assimilate well and can build up in your system.

Homeopathic Remedies for Balancing the Heart Self

Here's a list of carefully selected homeopathic remedies that support Heart Self balance, especially around themes of inward and outward emotional regulation. These remedies can be helpful for emotional sensitivity, relational overwhelm, boundary collapse, and suppressed or frozen feelings—key patterns often seen in Heart Self imbalance within the Mind Matrix Model.

A common starting dose is **30c potency, taken 3–4 times per day**. If you notice clear improvement, you may shift to **a single dose of 200c** for deeper, longer-lasting support. For more guidance, see the Next Steps *Chapter 25 - Homeopathy - Gentle Remedies for Balance and Health*.

Ignatia amara

Used For:

Acute grief, heartbreak, emotional suppression

Internalized sorrow with sighing, lump in the throat
Mood swings between tears and laughter

Pattern: When the Heart Self retreats inward and locks emotion away.
Inward-focused distress with blocked expression.

Pulsatilla

Used For:

Need for affection, reassurance, and connection
Weepiness, clinginess, or feeling abandoned
Emotional reactivity to social changes

Pattern: The Heart Self reaches outward too far, becomes dependent, loses center. Outward-focused distress driven by disconnection.

Natrum Muriaticum

Used For:

Emotional withdrawal, quiet grief, and difficulty trusting
High-functioning people who suffer privately
Grief held behind a composed exterior

Pattern: The Heart Self becomes guarded, overly inward, and disconnected. Common in echoist patterns or early Heart Self wounding.

Staphysagria

Used For:

Suppressed anger from being mistreated or humiliated
Fear of confrontation, followed by emotional collapse
Polite exterior with deep inner resentment

Pattern: A shut-down Heart Self where boundaries have been violated and emotion is held tightly inside. Useful in Heart Self trauma with relational shame.

Phosphorus

Used For:

Open, warm, emotionally porous people
Easily overwhelmed by others' emotions
Tendency to scatter or burn out after too much outward flow

Pattern: The Heart Self overextends, loses containment, becomes depleted. Helpful when connection becomes exhausting.

Essential Oils for Balancing the Heart Self

Essential oils offer a way to gently shift arousal states through scent. While scientific evidence varies, many people find them soothing or energizing. If you have allergies, respiratory conditions, or other health concerns, approach essential oils with caution and consider consulting an aromatherapy practitioner.

Each of these oils can be used in a diffuser, diluted for topical use (e.g., over the chest or wrists), or simply inhaled from the palms for a quick reset. For more information on using essential oils, see the chapter *Essential Oils—History, Use, and Safety* in the appendix.

Each of the oils are grouped by emotional function:

To Open and Soothe the Heart (for inward retreat or shutdown):

Rose (Rosa damascena)

Softens grief and emotional numbness
Gently opens the Heart after loss or retreat
Restores a sense of beauty and emotional warmth

Melissa (Lemon Balm)

Calms panic and overarousal
Gently restores joy and peace
Helpful for emotional trauma stored in the chest

Jasmine

Restores sensuality, receptivity, and self-worth
Uplifts the mood while grounding emotional energy
Supports reconnection after emotional isolation

To Strengthen Emotional Boundaries (for outward flooding or over-attunement):

Cypress

Protects the Heart when it's too porous
Useful for grief, transition, and letting go
Brings quiet containment and centering

Yarrow

Energetic "shielding" oil
Good for empaths or those who absorb others' emotional energy
Balances emotional boundaries without shutting down

Vetiver

Deeply grounding, especially when emotions are scattered
Anchors you in your own body and rhythm
Helps prevent outward emotional overwhelm

To Rebalance Emotional Flow (inward—outward):

Geranium

Harmonizes mood swings
Supports both emotional release and containment
Regulates Heart energy—great for re-centering after relational tension

Lavender

Calms the nervous system
Balances excess emotional charge (inward anxiety or outward irritability)
Gentle enough for frequent use

Acupressure for Balancing the Heart Self

These points help regulate emotional energy, ease overwhelm, and restore the Heart Self's natural rhythm of connecting and retreating. You can activate them by applying gentle, steady pressure with your fingertips while breathing slowly and mindfully. A few minutes of focused contact can be enough to shift your State and re-center emotionally.

For detailed instructions on technique, timing, and best practices, see the Next Steps *Chapter 23 - Acupressure For Yourself and Others.*

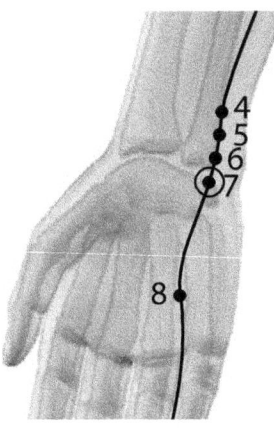

Heart 7 – Spirit Gate (Shenmen)

Location: On the inner wrist crease, to the side of the tendon (flexor carpi ulnaris) toward the middle of the wrist.

Use for:

Emotional overwhelm
Difficulty expressing or accessing feelings
Calming the Heart and supporting a steady relational presence

Symbolism: Opens and protects the "gate" of the Heart—ideal for rebalancing between inward retreat and outward expression.

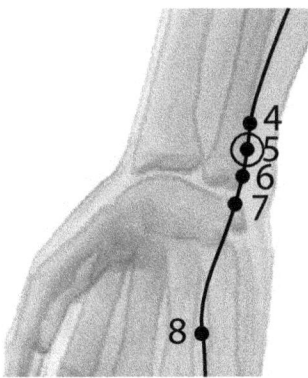

Heart 5 – Penetrating Inside (Tong Li)

Location: Two finger-widths up from the bump by the wrist crease (pisiform bone), just past the bump (head) of the ulnar bone.

Use for:

Expressing difficult emotions
Connecting inner feeling to outer communication
Soothing heartbreak or emotional suppression

Symbolism: The bridge between your inner world and your voice—a beautiful Heart Self integration point.

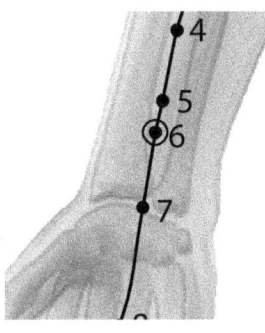

Pericardium 6 – Inner Gate (Neiguan)

Location: four finger-widths above the inner wrist crease, between the tendons.

Use for:

Anxiety, tight chest, social tension
Calming racing thoughts due to relational stress
Strengthening the Heart's protective boundary

Symbolism: Supports the Heart's movement outward while shielding from overexposure—great for reestablishing safe relational flow.

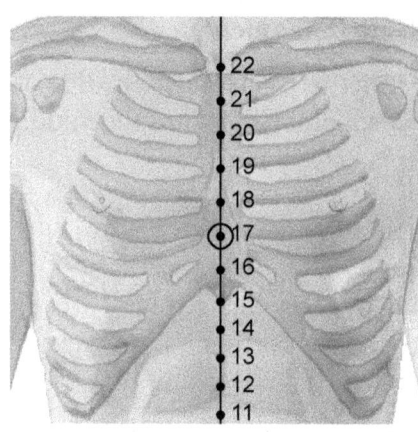

Conception Vessel 17 – Chest Center (Shanzhong) Sea of Tranquility)

Location: Four fingers above the bottom of the sternum

Use for:

Releasing grief, vulnerability, or guardedness
Expanding the chest and breath
Reconnecting to heartfelt presence

Symbolism: The meeting place of Heart energy, breath, and social emotion—helps the Heart Self expand without losing its center.

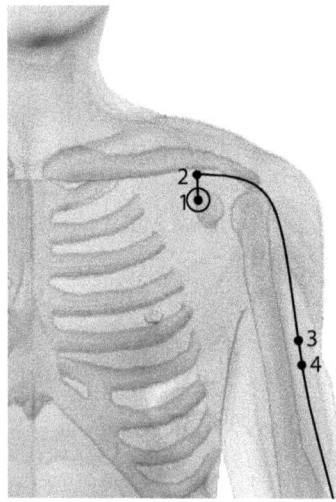

Lung 1 – Middle Palace (Zhongfu)

Location: 2 fingers below the collarbone, 4 fingers out from the crease of the shoulder joint between the second and third ribs.

Use for:

Letting go of old grief or relational pain
Supporting emotional boundaries
Anchoring breath and clarity when the Heart feels too exposed

Symbolism: The Lung nourishes the Heart—this point supports the inward movement when emotional overwhelm is high.

Heart Self Fast Reset Meditation

Use this when you're emotionally overwhelmed, disconnected, or looping on someone else's needs or approval.

Length: ~2–3 minutes

Posture: Seated or standing, hands gently resting over your chest.

Take a breath in through your nose and let it out slowly through your mouth.

Place your hand over your heart—or both hands, if it helps you feel more anchored. Let your chest rise and fall beneath your hands.

Feel the warmth of your own touch. You are here. You are feeling. You are safe enough to pause.

Now breathe into the space beneath your hands. Don't try to change anything—just breathe *with* whatever is there. You don't need to figure it out.

Just notice:

> Is there pressure?
> Tenderness?
> Tightness?
> Numbness?

Whatever's there, just name it softly:

> *This is what I'm feeling right now.*

You don't have to fix it.

You don't have to be different than you are now.

You just get to feel what's yours.

Breathe in. Breathe out.

Let your system come back to center.

When you're ready, gently release your hands. Feel your feet again. Come back to the space around you—carrying a little more of yourself with you.

Affirmation:

> *I am allowed to feel what I feel.*
> *I can come back to myself, even in the middle of everything.*
> *My heart knows how to soften and steady.*

Heart Self Daily Ritual Meditation

A slow ritual to attune to your emotional center and restore relational balance.

Length: ~5–8 minutes

Posture: Seated or lying down, one hand on your heart, the other on your belly.

Close your eyes.

Bring your awareness to your breath, and let it settle. Feel the rise and fall of your chest. The quiet rhythm of your inner life.

Breathe into your heart.

Feel your hand rise and fall with each breath. Feel how the heart rests between the world and your center. It listens both inward and outward.

Now ask gently:

> *"Am I more inward or outward right now?"*

If you're turned inward—feeling distant, tender, or alone—just notice. If you're turned outward—focused on others, seeking connection, or approval—just notice.

There is no right place to be. Only a rhythm to rediscover.

With each breath, invite your Heart Self to come home to balance.

> **Inhale** – drawing your awareness *inward*, into your feeling self.
>
> **Exhale** – gently *outward*, toward openness and connection.

Back and forth. In and out. Like a tide. Like breath. Like the heart itself.

Let yourself rest in the quiet space between those two directions.

And then ask one more question, softly:

> *"What would bring me into balance today?"*
> A conversation?
> A moment alone?
> A boundary?
> A touch?

Let the answer rise—not from thought, but from the felt sense beneath your hand.

Take one more breath. Thank your heart for its work.

And gently return to your day—more connected, more whole.

Affirmation:

My inner world is worthy of my attention.
My outer world does not define me.
I carry my heart with balance, courage, and care.

Final Thoughts

Your Heart Self is a living, breathing center of connection. It feels, it listens, it reaches, and it retreats. Sometimes it sings out in joy. Sometimes it hides. And sometimes, it just needs a quiet moment to come back into rhythm.

Balancing inward and outward focus isn't about getting it perfect—it's about learning how to notice where you are, and gently shifting when you've drifted too far in either direction. Your Heart Self doesn't need to be fixed. It needs to be met—with honesty, compassion, and space to move.

The more you tend to your emotional range, the easier it becomes to hold both self and other, solitude and belonging, depth and expression. This is the work of the Heart: not to shut down or give everything away, but to stay open in a way that honors your truth.

Chapter Eleven

The Head Self

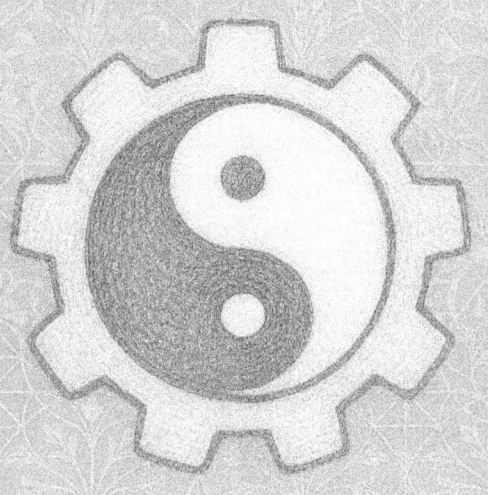

The everlasting universe of things
Flows through the mind, and rolls its rapid waves,
Now dark—now glittering—now reflecting gloom—
Now lending splendour, where from secret springs
The source of human thought its tribute brings
Of waters—with a sound but half its own,
Such as a feeble brook will oft assume,
In the wild woods, among the mountains lone,
Where waterfalls around it leap for ever,
Where woods and winds contend, and a vast river
Over its rocks ceaselessly bursts and raves.

~ Excerpt from "Mont Blanc"
   by Percy Bysshe Shelley

Introduction to the Head Self

The Head Self represents the broad range of thinking processes we use to make sense of the world, covering everything from detail-oriented analysis to big-picture intuition. Rather than focusing solely on left or right brain functions, the Head Self encompasses how you process information, solve problems, and interact with your surroundings. These styles of thinking exist along a series of spectrums, each with its own balance—analytic versus intuitive, sequential versus holistic, and so on.

> ### Moving Beyond 'Left Brain/Right Brain'
>
> *You've probably heard people talk about being "left-brained" (logical) or "right-brained" (creative). While it's true that some of the brain's basic jobs are more active on one side, the old idea of a strict left/right split is outdated.*
>
> *In the Mind Matrix Model, when we talk about "Analytic Mode" and "Holistic Mode," we're looking at how your whole mind works to think things through, not just one side of your brain. It's all about the different ways your entire mind can process information.*
>
> *Both styles have strengths and limitations. For example, Analytic Mode thinking offers clarity but can lead to over-analysis, while intuitive thinking fosters quick decisions but can be less precise.*
>
> *Flexibility in using these modes makes us more adaptable to different situations and helps us find balanced solutions. This balance even shows up in behaviors, where those with a more analytic mode of thinking might display more controlled body language and subtle expressions, while holistic thinkers tend to show more open gestures and spontaneous expression.*

The Two Modes of Thinking

On one end of these spectrums, analytical thinking and sequential processing help you with tasks requiring logic, order, and precision.

> The **Analytic Mode** (primarily the left cerebral hemisphere) excels at breaking down information and focusing on details, supporting critical thinking, language, and reasoning.

On the other end, the **Holistic Mode** (mostly right hemisphere) uses intuitive thinking and holistic processing to let you see connections and patterns, drawing on instinct and a big-picture view. It fosters creativity, empathy, and context, helping us interpret complex ideas and understand relationships. It is also more connected to the unconscious, which in the Mind Matrix Model is called the Head Self Minister.

Even the voice reveals one's tendency, reflected in the voice's prosody. Prosody is the patterns of intonation, rhythm and stress patterns (emphasizing certain words) in speech. Those with an analytic tendency will tend to have less variation in pitch, a more steady rhythm, and stressing the factually important words, whereas people with a holistic bent will have more musicality and rhythm variations, and will stress the emotionally important words.

Analytic Mode of thinking: "The *data* shows a *20% increase* over the last quarter, which *aligns* with our *projections*." (Steady, monotone, factual delivery).

Holistic Mode of thinking: "*Wow*, our *efforts really paid off! Look* at that *20% jump*—we've *really* made a *difference!*" (Engaging, emotionally inflected tone with pitch and rhythm variations).

These two modes of thinking exist along an overall spectrum or axis. Of course, those who are relatively balanced between the two modes will have both, shifting to a more expressive or more flat prosody depending on the situation.

While each hemisphere has specialized strengths, they work together through a thick bundle of nerves called the *corpus callosum* (Latin for "tough body," referring to its tough, fibrous nature) which allows them to share information quickly.

For instance, the left hemisphere may control the fine motor skills needed to write, while the right hemisphere provides spatial awareness to keep writing aligned on the page. This collaboration is what makes a balanced Head Self so important—it enhances your ability to think clearly, stay adaptable, and approach life with flexibility.

Achieving Balance

A balanced Head Self can switch easily between clear, logical thinking and creative, big-picture insight. People with a balanced Head Self can focus when needed, reflect without overthinking, and use both facts and intuition to make thoughtful decisions. They're able to think things through without getting stuck, and stay open to new ideas without feeling overwhelmed.

The Head Self's holistic and analytic modes are meant to work together. Think of Rodgers and Hammerstein working on a musical. They aren't arguing over whether the words or the music are more important—one offers an idea, and the other picks it up. They collaborate naturally, passing inspiration back and forth.

When life gets stressful, a balanced Head Self helps you stay steady. It lets you sort through your thoughts calmly, ask helpful questions, and find clarity without shutting down or spiraling out.

Understanding where you fall on the spectrum between analytic and intuitive thinking can help you recognize both your strengths and the areas where you may get stuck. With this awareness, you can adjust how you think depending on the situation—helping you solve problems more easily, reduce mental stress, and stay clear-headed in everyday life.

The Neurological Basis of the Head Self

The Head Self is powered by the brain's **cerebral cortex**, especially the front and top regions where thinking, planning, and decision-making happen. Different parts of the brain team up to help us solve problems, reflect on life, and understand both the details and the big picture.

At the center of it all is the **prefrontal cortex**, which acts like your internal planner. It helps you focus, weigh options, and make thoughtful choices. Some areas help with facts and logic, while others connect thoughts to emotions and values—so you're not just smart, but wise.

The brain is also divided into two hemispheres that support different thinking styles. The **left hemisphere** is more analytical—it likes step-by-step logic, language, and detail. The **right hemisphere** is more holistic—it sees patterns, reads emotional tone, and understands context. A healthy Head Self can shift between the two, depending on the situation.

Two major brain networks shape how we think:

> The **Default Mode Network (DMN)** turns on when you're daydreaming, reflecting, or imagining other people's perspectives. It lets you review the past, plan for the future, and understand yourself.
>
> The **Task-Positive Networks (TPNs)** turn on when you're focusing on a specific task—solving a problem, reading, or organizing something.

These two networks are like a seesaw: when one is active, the other quiets down. A flexible Head Self can move smoothly between them—focused when needed, reflective when helpful.

When everything's working well, these brain regions form a coordinated team that helps you stay grounded, think clearly, and adapt to whatever life throws your way.

Being able to shift between logical and intuitive thinking is useful in a wide range of situations. And as we'll discuss in the chapter on State, the farther we go to the extremes of this cognitive spectrum, the more we risk slipping into imbalance and potentially entering the Negative State where thinking can become skewed. Achieving balance in the Head Self helps us navigate these spectrums more freely, leading to a healthy, flexible, and resilient mind.

When the Head Self Becomes Chronically Dysregulated

The Head Self is the organizing intelligence of your system. It weaves meaning from experience, holds beliefs and values, and toggles between two powerful tools: analytic thinking (linear, detail-focused, logical) and holistic thinking (intuitive, pattern-based, big-picture). When these modes are balanced, the Head Self is adaptable, creative, and integrative.

But when the system becomes imbalanced or overwhelmed due to chronic stress, trauma, overuse, or isolation, the Head Self can shift into chronic dysregulation. This usually leans toward one of two poles:

> **Analytic-Dominant Dysregulation**: The mind becomes rigid, overly focused on correctness, and detached from feeling or context.
>
> **Holistic-Dominant Dysregulation**: The mind becomes diffuse, symbol-heavy, disorganized, or unable to discern which intuitions are real or relevant.

These tendencies are often adaptive at first—strategies to manage overwhelming complexity or emotional pain—but they become unsustainable when they begin to override the other Selves or disconnect the Head from the body and emotions.

Analytic-Dominant Dysregulation

This mode of dysregulation tends to show up in people who cope through control, intellectualization, or overthinking. It can be intensified by an early life where rationality was overvalued or emotions were dismissed.

Common patterns include:

- Excessive mental rehearsal or analysis ("If I just think hard enough, I'll figure it out.")
- Difficulty trusting feelings, body signals, or intuition
- Paralysis around decision-making due to fear of being wrong
- Over-identification with productivity, intelligence, or factual accuracy
- Inflexibility around beliefs or methods—everything becomes a problem to solve
- Resistance to spontaneity or ambiguity

This state often results in mental exhaustion, a narrowed State Range, and detachment from the present moment.

Holistic-Dominant Dysregulation

This mode of dysregulation tends to occur when the analytic mind has been bypassed, overwhelmed, or distrusted—either by trauma, sensory overload, or cultural invalidation of structure. It's especially common in people with high creative or intuitive capacity who were unsupported in organizing their inner world.

Common patterns include:

- Thought spirals: connections between everything, but no anchor in sequence or clarity
- Magical or symbolic thinking that lacks integration
- Intuition flooding: sensing too much, all at once, with no filter or structure

- Over-identifying with archetypes, myths, or dream states without grounding
- Difficulty completing thoughts or conversations—drifting away midstream
- Emotional dysregulation expressed through ideas that "feel true" but shift rapidly

While often misread as "scatterbrained" or dramatic, this is a real and painful loss of containment that leaves the person feeling unmoored.

Systemic Causes of Head Self Dysregulation

Whether analytic or holistic dominant, chronic dysregulation of the Head Self may be rooted in:

- Early intellectual overburden (parentification, expectation to explain or mediate)
- Emotion-intellect splits, where thinking becomes a safe escape from feeling
- Spiritual or symbolic overwhelm without relational grounding
- Highly verbal or symbolic trauma, including ideological or religious betrayal
- Cognitive overload from screen time, hyperproductivity, or media fragmentation
- Cultural dismissal of imagination or non-linear thought (especially in educational systems)
- Overexposure to contradiction or manipulation, eroding trust in perception

The Consequences of Dysregulation

A dysregulated Head Self doesn't just result in "thinking too much" or "being too abstract." It affects how you:

- Understand yourself
- Construct reality
- Choose direction
- Integrate emotions
- Communicate with others

When the Head Self cannot function fluidly, it often either dominates the system (trying to solve what can only be felt) or dissociates entirely (leaving the Vital and Heart Selves flooded or numb). Either way, it disrupts integration and resilience.

The Head Self and the State Axis

The Head Self governs your thinking—your stories, beliefs, perspectives, and ability to make meaning. But it doesn't operate in a vacuum. Its clarity or confusion, flexibility or rigidity, insight or distortion are shaped entirely by **State**.

When you're regulated, your Head Self becomes the **Synthesizer**: curious, integrative, and able to toggle between analytic and holistic modes depending on the situation. It can hold multiple perspectives without collapse. It can sort out what's true, what matters, and what doesn't need to be thought about anymore. In this balanced place, the Head Self is a powerful ally for grounded creativity and insight.

But when your system becomes dysregulated, the Head Self tends to split into *mode dominance*—either analytic or holistic—and then spirals into extremes.

The diagram on the opposite page shows this dynamic. The vertical State arrow reflects how the Positive State evokes a grounded, positive sense of reality, whereas the Negative State creates an imbalanced view of reality.

> In **Analytic Dominant Mode**, dysregulation often creates **The Critic**—rigid, overcontrolling, judgmental, and stuck in loops. This is the mode of obsessive planning, catastrophic thinking, and the feeling of being "locked in your head."

> In **Holistic Dominant Mode**, dysregulation can lead to **The Drifter**—scattered, abstract, symbolic without grounding. This mode often appears as spiritual bypassing, magical thinking, or reality distortion when emotions feel too complex to hold directly.

Both are signs that the Head Self is trying to maintain control—but doing so without the support of a stable system underneath. The Monarch may have checked out, and the Ministers are now recycling old Scripts to try to make sense of things.

Your **State** determines which Head Self pathways are accessible:

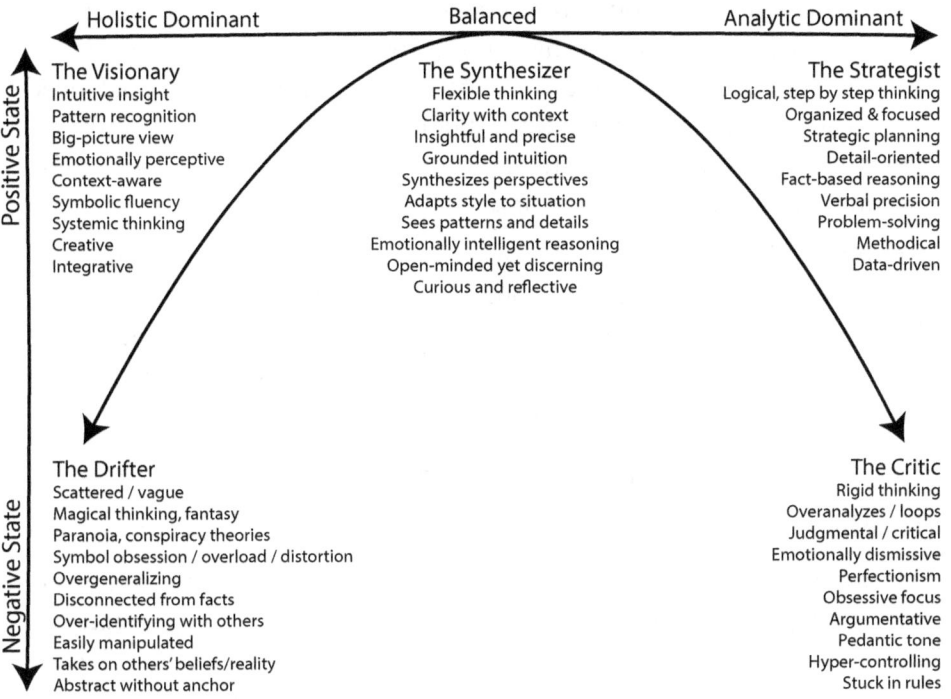

In a **Positive State**, you can think clearly and flexibly. You can switch between big-picture and detail, intuition and logic.

In a **Negative State**, the mind narrows, tightens, or spirals. You might either lose the thread—or become entangled in it.

Because the Head Self is so verbal and meaning-driven, it can easily justify dysregulation. It will tell you stories to explain your fear, your anger, your collapse. But the real work is often somatic: returning to the Vital Self, calming the Heart, and letting the thinking mind follow.

Tom, an analytic thinker, found himself paralyzed by overthinking decisions. By intentionally engaging in holistic practices like drawing and visualization, he found new thought clarity and flexibility.

When you support your Head Self with grounding, rhythm, and enough quiet, it can return to its true role—not to control everything, but to understand, integrate, and guide.

Trauma and the Head Self

The Head Self allows you to make meaning of the world—through both clarity and creativity. It governs not only logical reasoning and language, but also intuition, imagination, and pattern recognition. When balanced, the Head Self integrates analytic and holistic modes with perspective and flexibility. But when trauma strikes this part of the system, those modes become exaggerated, unstable, or disconnected.

Trauma in the Head Self creates distortions in how you perceive reality, organize experience, and trust your own thoughts or insights. The analytic mind may become hyper-controlling; the holistic mind, untethered. In either case, your inner compass is disrupted—and thought becomes a survival strategy, not a tool for understanding.

Common Causes of Head Self Trauma

For the Analytic Mode (over-control, collapse into rigidity):

The analytic mind develops best when thinking, questioning, and problem-solving are encouraged in a safe, supportive way. But when logic becomes the only safe option—or when thinking is used to control emotion or avoid punishment—it can create trauma patterns.

- Emotional invalidation or gaslighting ("That's not what happened."): Being told your perception is wrong—even when you're sure of what you saw or felt—undermines your trust in your own thoughts and memory. Over time, you may become afraid of being wrong or doubt what you know is true.

- Repeated humiliation around being wrong or confused: When mistakes are punished or mocked, thinking becomes high-stakes. You may develop fear around learning or expressing your opinion.

- Praise tied only to performance: If your worth was based on getting the right answer or being the "smart one," thinking may feel more like a performance than a natural part of life. You may feel like you always have to be right or know everything.

- Growing up where only logic was safe: In homes where emotions were seen as messy or weak, the analytic mode may take over as a way to stay safe or "acceptable." Emotional sensitivity may have been hidden behind logic or sarcasm.

- Being forced to explain trauma or emotions too early: If you had to make sense of overwhelming experiences on your own—or had to "make it make sense" for adults—you may have turned to logic to survive what couldn't be felt or understood at the time.
- Being enmeshed with an anxious or intellectual caregiver: If your parent or caregiver relied on you to process their anxiety, solve their problems, or mirror their intellectual identity, you may have developed an over-responsible or hyper-verbal Head Self.
- Living in high-pressure, perfectionist systems: School or cultural environments that reward constant performance, competition, and "doing everything right" can push the analytic mind into overdrive, leaving little room for creativity, rest, or intuition.

For the Holistic Mode (distortion, collapse into abstraction):

The holistic mind thrives on imagination, intuition, and emotional resonance. It takes in the big picture, senses unspoken truths, and connects things in meaningful ways. But when this mode becomes distorted—often due to instability, fear, or confusion—thinking may lose clarity and drift into overwhelm or fantasy.

- Exposure to symbolic chaos early in life: Children who are immersed in abstract or mystical language too soon—without grounding or clear emotional support—may develop fragmented or dissociative thought patterns. This can happen with spiritual abuse, extreme beliefs, or neglect that feels dreamlike and confusing.
- Fear-based or contradictory messaging: Growing up in an environment where people say one thing but act another—or where danger is mixed with love—can make it hard to know what's real. The mind may try to "make it make sense" by seeing hidden meanings everywhere.
- Being mocked or punished for emotional or intuitive truths: If you had deep feelings, dreams, or insights as a child—and were laughed at, dismissed, or told to stop "making things up"—you may have internalized the idea that your inner world is untrustworthy or dangerous.
- Praised for creativity but punished for questioning: Some children are encouraged to be imaginative as long as they don't challenge the rules. This creates confusion: you can be expressive, but only in

approved ways. The mind may split between pleasing others and following its own insight.

- Losing a trusted belief system: If you experienced a spiritual or ideological betrayal—such as a faith collapse, political disillusionment, or a mentor's fall from grace—it can create deep disruption in the holistic mind's framework for meaning.

- Sensory or cognitive overwhelm without support: Highly sensitive or neurodivergent children may experience a world that feels too fast, loud, or chaotic—and may not have had the tools to ground themselves. The holistic mode may then develop as a way to escape or reinterpret reality.

How Trauma Manifests in the Head Self

Analytic-Dominant Trauma Responses:

When trauma pushes the analytic mode into overdrive, the mind tries to create safety through control, precision, and certainty.

- Overthinking and mental looping: You may find yourself stuck in the same thoughts, trying to "figure things out" or prepare for every possible outcome. Rest is difficult because the mind doesn't know when it's safe to stop.

- Perfectionism or black-and-white thinking: Things feel either right or wrong, good or bad, safe or unsafe—with no room in between. Mistakes feel dangerous, and nuance can be threatening.

- Compulsive research or fact-checking: You might constantly gather information to feel safe or certain, even when it doesn't actually help you move forward.

- Harsh inner criticism: A voice in your head may say, "You should've known better," or "Why did you mess that up again?" This can make thinking feel like self-punishment.

- Disconnection from body and emotion: The analytic Head Self may suppress sensation and feeling to stay in control. You may have trouble feeling what's happening in your body—or even recognizing what you're feeling emotionally.

- Using intellect to avoid vulnerability: You may mistrust intuition, minimize others' emotions, or use sarcasm and logic to keep distance in relationships.

Holistic-Dominant Trauma Responses:

When trauma distorts the holistic mode, the mind may feel flooded with symbols, emotions, or intuitive impressions that lack grounding.

- Magical thinking or overreliance on signs: You may look for meaning in everything—dreams, coincidences, objects—trying to find a pattern that explains your feelings or keeps you safe.
- Difficulty forming clear stories or timelines: Memories may feel jumbled or blurry, and it may be hard to describe what happened or why you feel the way you do.
- Confusion between intuition and projection: You may sense something strongly but feel unsure whether it's insight or fear. Boundaries between your thoughts and others' emotions may blur.
- Spiral thinking or symbolic loops: The mind may jump between unrelated ideas, symbols, or theories—often creating hidden meanings or conspiracies where none exist.
- Emotional overwhelm with no structure: Feelings come on intensely and unpredictably, and there may be no system in place to regulate or understand them.
- Avoidance of logic or routine: You might resist structure, fear planning, or reject systems altogether—especially if they once felt oppressive or were used to control you.

The Head Self and Early Trauma

The Head Self shapes how we see reality and make sense of the world. It works by balancing the *Analytic Mode of thinking* (which handles logic, precision and details) with the *Holistic Mode of thinking* (which handles creativity, intuition and the big picture). When these two parts work well together, we get a stable, adaptable view of the world. But early trauma or neglect can throw this balance off, pushing the Head Self into the Negative State where thoughts and perceptions become distorted.

In the Negative State, the Head Self might rely too heavily on either the Analytic Mode or Holistic Mode.

For example, someone who tends toward the Analytic Mode might get stuck in rigid thinking, unable to see other perspectives. Or if they lean toward the Holistic Mode they might fall into overly intuitive thinking, seeing patterns that aren't there or becoming paranoid. Either way, their view of reality becomes skewed.

This Negative State can show up as paranoia, mental rigidity, excessive control, or a need to depend on others who seem more confident in their reality. People in this state might struggle to trust their own judgments and may look to others for a stable perspective, which can make them vulnerable to influence or manipulation. They might misinterpret neutral situations as threatening or have trouble seeing relationships clearly.

These imbalances make it hard for the Head Self to adapt, see different perspectives, or blend logical and intuitive thinking. This state, rooted in early trauma, often causes people to either cling tightly to specific beliefs or feel lost in an unstable reality, making it difficult to stay grounded.

Healing involves learning to balance the Analytic and Holistic Modes using practices like mindfulness, critical thinking, and rituals that blend logic and creativity. Gradually, these approaches can help rebuild a stable, flexible sense of reality, allowing the Head Self to feel secure and resilient.

The Mind as a Model-Builder

Recent insights from cognitive science reveal that the human mind doesn't simply observe and react to the world, it actively constructs a mental model or internal simulation of reality. This model is constantly updated based on incoming sensory information, emotional experiences, and past learning. Its purpose is to help us navigate the world efficiently and make sense of what's happening around us.

When this internal simulation is accurate, it helps us respond appropriately to situations, understand others, and adapt flexibly. But when the model becomes outdated or distorted—whether through trauma, chronic stress, or lack of feedback—it leads to misinterpretations, emotional reactivity, and poor decision-making.

One of the most significant findings is that stress disrupts the updating process. In states of fear, anxiety, or overwhelm, the brain prioritizes protection over learning. It stops integrating new information that might correct the model.

This means that when we're in the Negative State, we continue operating from old assumptions even if the world around us has changed. And those most susceptible to the Negative State will have models that are completely inappropriate for the world they are living in.

What Heals the Head Self

For Analytic-Mode Healing:

- Relaxing the grip of control through embodiment: practices that focus on breath, touch, and movement help the overactivated mind trust the present moment.
- Allowing uncertainty: journaling without conclusions, asking open questions, and practicing "I don't know—and that's okay."
- Gentle engagement with art and metaphor: reclaiming non-linear expression, especially in low-stakes environments (poetry, collage, creative writing).
- Mindfulness-Based Cognitive Therapy: observing thoughts without trying to fix or judge them; reducing over-identification with mental narratives.

For Holistic-Mode Healing:

- Structured reflection and narrative repair: using timelines, maps, or writing to organize intuitive impressions into coherent form.
- Reality testing: grounding intuitive insights through dialogue, feedback, or research—asking "Is this symbolic or literal? Is it happening now?"
- Practices that strengthen sequence and cause-effect thinking: logic puzzles, light planning exercises, or gentle exposure to structure in daily life.
- Anchoring symbols in the body or nature: walking with a stone, drawing spirals in sand—bringing metaphor back into the sensory present.

For Both Modes:

Immersion in nature: Nature is both patterned and intuitive, ordered and wild. For the analytic thinker, it softens logic with mystery.

For the holistic thinker, it grounds imagination in sensation. The sound of wind, the rhythm of walking, the spiral of a shell—all help reintegrate the analytic and holistic selves under the Head Self's guidance.

Balanced conversation: Dialogues with grounded, emotionally attuned people help the Head Self practice flexible integration—seeing that logic, emotion, and intuition can coexist.

Affirming meaning-making as a sacred act: The Head Self heals when it realizes it doesn't need to "prove" reality to feel safe. It can wonder, reflect, question—and still belong.

We'll be going into ways to heal the Head Self in the next chapter.

Final Thoughts

The Head Self offers a framework for understanding how different styles of thinking influence your behavior, decision-making, and problem-solving. By recognizing our tendencies on each of these spectra, you can better appreciate your cognitive strengths and work toward achieving a balanced approach—integrating analytical and intuitive thinking, detail-oriented and big-picture perspectives, and logical and creative problem-solving.

Behavioral and physiological signs, like prosody, gestures, and facial expressions, provide additional insights into our cognitive tendencies. By considering these signs alongside cognitive preferences, you can gain a fuller understanding of how you express cognitive balance in everyday life.

Embracing the full range of cognitive processes enhances your ability to navigate life's complexities with both clarity and creativity, leading to more effective decision-making and a richer, more fulfilling experience.

This chapter offers a practical understanding of the Head Self. In our next chapter, we'll go into detail on what you can do to balance your Head Self.

Chapter Twelve
Balancing the Head Self

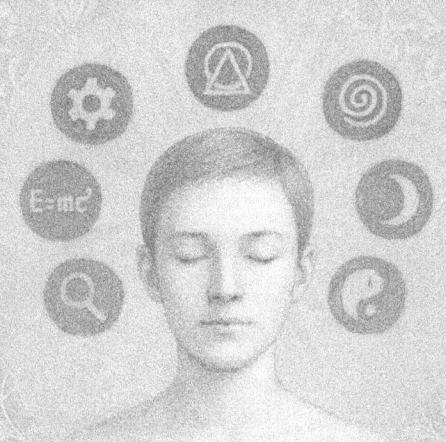

*Now is the time to understand
That all your ideas of right and wrong
Were just a child's training wheels
To be laid aside
When you can finally live
with veracity
And love.
Now is the time for the world to know
That every thought and action is sacred.
That this is the time
For you to compute the impossibility
That there is anything
But Grace.*
~ Excerpt from Now is the Time
  by Hafiz

Grounding with Reality, Balance & Meaningful Practices

As we've covered, the Head Self is about building a grounded, realistic understanding of the world. It uses two main ways of thinking: the *Analytic Mode of thinking* (principally located in the left cerebral cortex and colloquially called the left brain) and the *Holistic Mode of thinking* (principally located in the right cerebral cortex and called the right brain).

The Analytic Mode helps us think in a logical, step-by-step way, focusing on details and breaking things down. This kind of thinking is great for tasks that need careful planning and organization.

The Holistic Mode, on the other hand, takes in the bigger picture through intuition and pattern recognition, helping us see connections and deeper meanings.

A healthy Head Self depends on a balance between these two ways of thinking. When the Analytic and Holistic Modes work together, they give us a flexible and realistic view of the world, allowing us to be both clear-headed and creative.

Each mode benefits from grounding activities that strengthen its unique skills:

> For the **Analytic Mode**, grounding often comes from structured activities like organizing, planning, and problem-solving. These activities provide order, helping us see things clearly and make practical decisions.

> The **Holistic Mode** finds grounding in creative, open-ended activities that let us explore and imagine. Art, music, and visualization exercises allow this part of the mind to understand deeper connections and meanings, making our understanding of the world more adaptable and cohesive.

Rituals are powerful tools for grounding the Head Self because they bring together structure and meaning, engaging both the Analytic and Holistic Modes in a balanced way. Here are a few examples:

- **Morning or Evening Routines**: These give the Analytic Mode a reliable structure while letting the Holistic Mode connect with a sense of purpose. For example, a morning routine might include a few calming activities that help us focus for the day ahead.

- **Reflective Practices**: Journaling, meditation, or gratitude practices let the Analytic Mode organize thoughts, while the Holistic Mode explores emotions and patterns. These rituals bring balance and help us connect insights with clear intention.
- **Creative Planning Rituals**: Vision-boarding or setting goals combines structured planning with imagination. These activities align specific steps with broader goals, giving both modes a sense of clarity and exploration.

When we use practices and rituals that integrate both modes, they support each other and create a grounded, flexible cognitive state. For example:

Mindfulness Meditation combines focused attention (analytic) with an open, accepting awareness (holistic), grounding us in the present and increasing mental clarity.

Problem-Solving through Play: Games like chess, puzzles, or storytelling involve both strategy and creativity, helping the Head Self become more adaptable and balanced.

Through these practices, the Head Self can develop a balanced sense of reality, shaped by both logic and creativity. This balance supports resilience, critical thinking, and open-mindedness, helping us navigate complex situations with clear, adaptable thinking.

Head Self Questionnaire

This questionnaire helps you explore how your Head Self—the thinking and problem-solving part of your mind—tends to operate. It identifies a leaning toward Analytic thinking (detail-oriented, logical), Holistic thinking (intuitive, big-picture), Balanced cognition, or Instability (fluctuating or uncertain patterns).

You can also access a downloadable PDF version of the form as well as an interactive version by visiting the Mind Matrix Model website. You'll need to register if you haven't yet. You can sign up for free access by scanning the QR code or visiting this short link:

mmm.tips/headform

https://mmm.tips/headform

The interactive form can be used to chart your progress over time, and includes many combination patterns that reveal more complex dynamics.

Instructions

For each question, choose the option (Rarely true, Sometimes true, Often true, Very true) that best describes your typical experience—not what you wish were true. Don't overthink it. Go with your first honest reaction.

Use a journal, notes app, or form field to track your responses.

If you are keeping a journal, this is a good time to write your responses down there so you can check up on how you're doing later. Otherwise just grab a piece of paper or a screen device to track your answers.

> **Note:** *This is not a medical test, but a self-reflection tool designed to help you explore approaches for improving your quality of life. If you have any concerns, consider consulting a healthcare professional or therapist for personalized guidance.*

1. Problem-Solving Style

A) I break problems down into parts and think step-by-step.

○ Rarely true=1   ○ Sometimes true=2   ○ Often true=3   ○ Very true=4

B) I use logic and intuition together, depending on the situation.

○ Rarely true=1   ○ Sometimes true=2   ○ Often true=3   ○ Very true=4

C) I follow my gut and look for patterns to guide me.

○ Rarely true=1   ○ Sometimes true=2   ○ Often true=3   ○ Very true=4

D) I switch between overthinking and vague guessing without much control.

○ Rarely true=1   ○ Sometimes true=2   ○ Often true=3   ○ Very true=4

2. Learning Style

A) I like structured lessons and clear instructions.

○ Rarely true=1   ○ Sometimes true=2   ○ Often true=3   ○ Very true=4

B) I can learn with structure or flexibility.

○ Rarely true=1   ○ Sometimes true=2   ○ Often true=3   ○ Very true=4

C) I learn best from visual patterns, metaphors, or stories.

○ Rarely true=1   ○ Sometimes true=2   ○ Often true=3   ○ Very true=4

D) I jump between approaches and struggle to stay focused on one way.

○ Rarely true=1   ○ Sometimes true=2   ○ Often true=3   ○ Very true=4

3. Decision-Making

A) I research or plan carefully before choosing.

○ Rarely true=1   ○ Sometimes true=2   ○ Often true=3   ○ Very true=4

B) I consider options and trust myself to choose when ready.

○ Rarely true=1   ○ Sometimes true=2   ○ Often true=3   ○ Very true=4

C) I often make intuitive or spontaneous decisions.

○ Rarely true=1   ○ Sometimes true=2   ○ Often true=3   ○ Very true=4

D) I freeze up or flip-flop when I try to decide.

○ Rarely true=1   ○ Sometimes true=2   ○ Often true=3   ○ Very true=4

4. Self-Talk

A) I'm often critical or analytical toward myself.

○ Rarely true=1   ○ Sometimes true=2   ○ Often true=3   ○ Very true=4

B) I talk to myself kindly and realistically.

○ Rarely true=1   ○ Sometimes true=2   ○ Often true=3   ○ Very true=4

C) I tend to be idealistic or philosophical in how I reflect.

○ Rarely true=1   ○ Sometimes true=2   ○ Often true=3   ○ Very true=4

D) My inner voice changes a lot—sometimes harsh, sometimes dreamy or absent.

○ Rarely true=1   ○ Sometimes true=2   ○ Often true=3   ○ Very true=4

5. Attention and Focus

A) I focus intensely on one thing but find it hard to shift gears.

○ Rarely true=1   ○ Sometimes true=2   ○ Often true=3   ○ Very true=4

B) I can zoom in or out mentally depending on what's needed.

○ Rarely true=1   ○ Sometimes true=2   ○ Often true=3   ○ Very true=4

C) I think broadly and make creative connections across ideas.

○ Rarely true=1   ○ Sometimes true=2   ○ Often true=3   ○ Very true=4

D) I either hyperfocus and lose track of time or can't focus at all.

○ Rarely true=1   ○ Sometimes true=2   ○ Often true=3   ○ Very true=4

6. Processing Emotions

A) I explain or rationalize emotions rather than feel them.

○ Rarely true=1   ○ Sometimes true=2   ○ Often true=3   ○ Very true=4

B) I let myself feel while also thinking things through.

○ Rarely true=1   ○ Sometimes true=2   ○ Often true=3   ○ Very true=4

C) I often express emotions through art, writing, or metaphor.

○ Rarely true=1   ○ Sometimes true=2   ○ Often true=3   ○ Very true=4

D) I either shut emotions out with logic or get mentally lost in them.

○ Rarely true=1   ○ Sometimes true=2   ○ Often true=3   ○ Very true=4

7. Response to Stress

A) My mind becomes sharp and critical when things go wrong.

○ Rarely true=1   ○ Sometimes true=2   ○ Often true=3   ○ Very true=4

B) I stay mentally clear or pause before reacting.

○ Rarely true=1   ○ Sometimes true=2   ○ Often true=3   ○ Very true=4

C) I tend to "float" or lose track of practical details under pressure.

○ Rarely true=1   ○ Sometimes true=2   ○ Often true=3   ○ Very true=4

D) I bounce between harsh thinking and spacing out.

○ Rarely true=1   ○ Sometimes true=2   ○ Often true=3   ○ Very true=4

8. Memory and Recall

A) I remember facts and sequences clearly but may miss the big picture.

○ Rarely true=1 ○ Sometimes true=2 ○ Often true=3 ○ Very true=4

B) I remember what matters—both details and connections.

○ Rarely true=1 ○ Sometimes true=2 ○ Often true=3 ○ Very true=4

C) I recall impressions or themes more than exact facts.

○ Rarely true=1 ○ Sometimes true=2 ○ Often true=3 ○ Very true=4

D) My memory skips around—I remember odd details and forget key things.

○ Rarely true=1 ○ Sometimes true=2 ○ Often true=3 ○ Very true=4

9. Abstraction vs. Concreteness

A) I prefer clear, real-world examples.

○ Rarely true=1 ○ Sometimes true=2 ○ Often true=3 ○ Very true=4

B) I like both practical examples and big-picture ideas.

○ Rarely true=1 ○ Sometimes true=2 ○ Often true=3 ○ Very true=4

C) I enjoy abstract or theoretical conversations.

○ Rarely true=1 ○ Sometimes true=2 ○ Often true=3 ○ Very true=4

D) I get lost between details and ideas—too vague or too literal.

○ Rarely true=1 ○ Sometimes true=2 ○ Often true=3 ○ Very true=4

10. Thinking Style Under Pressure

A) I narrow things down fast and stick to one clear solution.

○ Rarely true=1 ○ Sometimes true=2 ○ Often true=3 ○ Very true=4

B) I weigh a few solid options before choosing.

○ Rarely true=1 ○ Sometimes true=2 ○ Often true=3 ○ Very true=4

C) I generate lots of ideas and explore different angles.

○ Rarely true=1 ○ Sometimes true=2 ○ Often true=3 ○ Very true=4

D) I either overthink endlessly or jump between too many ideas.

○ Rarely true=1 ○ Sometimes true=2 ○ Often true=3 ○ Very true=4

How to Score Your Head Self Axis Questionnaire

Step 1: Tally Your Scores

Go through your answers and total the points for each letter:

- Each time you rated an A, add the point value you selected (1 = Rarely True, 4 = Very True) to your A total.
- Do the same for B, C, and D responses.
  For example, if you answered Rarely true eight times, that would total 8, Sometimes true eight times would be 16, Often true eight times = 24, Very true eight times = 32.

Best to add this up on a separate piece of paper or in your journal.

Each letter will have a total between 10 (lowest) and 40 (highest).

Your Scores:

　　A = _____　B = _____　C = _____　D = _____

Each letter represents a type of Head Self pattern:

　　A = Analytic-dominant

　　B = Balanced

　　C = Holistic-dominant

　　D = Unstable/Swinging (oscillates between A and C)

Once you're done, proceed to the next section.

Step 2: Interpretation

Find which pattern below matches your scores.

A = 30 or more - Analytic-Dominant Head Self

You tend toward structure, precision, and step-by-step logic. Your strength lies in order and clarity.

What to Support: You may benefit from cultivating flexibility, open-ended thinking, and intuitive trust.

Read: Approaches to Balancing Analytic Mode

B = 30 or more - Balanced Cognitive Style

You fluidly switch between analytic and holistic modes depending on context. This cognitive flexibility is a key resilience trait.

What to Support: Focus on maintaining this integration across different situations.

Read: Approaches for Overall Balance of the Head Self

C = 30 or more - Holistic-Dominant Head Self

You gravitate toward patterns, metaphor, and creativity.

What to Support: You may benefit from developing frameworks and refining details to better ground your ideas and communicate clearly.

Read: Approaches to Balancing Holistic Mode

D = 30 or more - Unstable Cognitive Pattern

You may fluctuate between modes unpredictably—often due to stress, trauma history, or inconsistent learning environments. This pattern may reflect state instability rather than stable preference.

What to Support: Strengthening rhythm and practicing one mode at a time can improve clarity.

Read: Approaches to Balancing Analytic Mode, Approaches to Balancing Holistic Mode

If none of your scores is 30 or more, choose the one that is the highest score. This indicates that you could have a more complex pattern that the interactive form on the website would reveal.

Reflection Prompts (Optional)

› When I'm under pressure, do I tend to narrow my focus—or drift into overwhelm?
› Do I trust my logic more than my intuition—or vice versa?
› What environments help me think clearly? What throws me off?
› Have I ever been criticized for being "too rigid" or "too scattered"?

Balancing the Head Self

The Head Self, which governs both analytical and intuitive thinking, plays a crucial role in how we perceive, process, and respond to the world around us. Achieving balance within the Head Self is essential for clear thinking, effective decision-making, and overall mental well-being.

Below are approaches and therapies that can help bring the Head Self into balance, fostering a harmonious integration between Modes.

Approaches to Balancing Analytic Mode

Creative Practices: Balancing the Head Self isn't just about Analytic Mode thinking—it's also about nurturing creativity and intuition. Creative practices like art, music, writing, or improvisation can activate Holistic Mode thinking, integrating analytical and intuitive processes. These include:

Artistic Expression: Activities like painting or drawing encourage the free flow of creative thought.

Journaling: Writing reflections helps clarify thinking and stimulates creative insights.

Open Monitoring Meditation: Observe thoughts without attachment or judgment, fostering greater flexibility and insight.

Essential Oils

Lavender (Lavandula angustifolia): Gently calms mental overactivity, reduces perfectionism, and helps quiet inner tension. Excellent for easing transitions between task focus and rest

Clary Sage (Salvia sclarea): Encourages emotional clarity and dreamlike insight. Supports letting go of logic and embracing intuitive or symbolic perception.

Ylang-Ylang (Cananga odorata): Softens harsh self-judgment and mental control. Helps reconnect mind and body with feeling states.

Sandalwood (Santalum album): Deepens meditation, slows obsessive thinking, and creates mental spaciousness. Especially good for shifting from linear to holistic mode.

Frankincense (Boswellia carterii): Enhances integration between logical and intuitive centers. Brings a sense of sacred openness and quiet authority.

Acupressure Points

For detailed instructions on technique, timing, and best practices, see the Next Steps *Chapter 23 - Acupressure For Yourself and Others.*

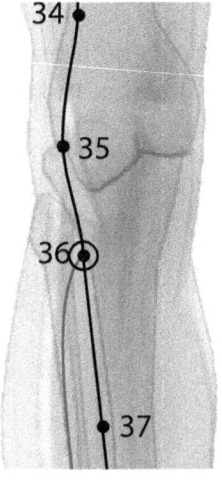

Stomach 36 (Zusanli or Leg Three Miles)

Purpose: Grounds excess energy from the head, supports stamina, and reduces compulsive thinking. Helps balance the upward flow of energy from overthinking by drawing awareness into the body.

Location: Six finger-widths below the kneecap, one finger-width lateral to the shinbone.

How to Use: Press and hold this point for 1-2 minutes on each leg. It provides a sustained increase in energy and can be particularly helpful for physical and mental fatigue.

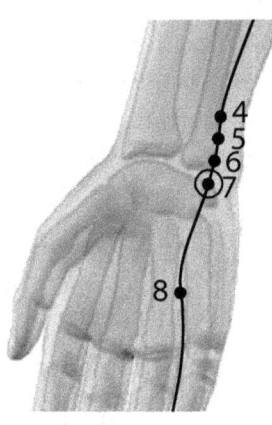

Heart 7 – Spirit Gate (Shenmen)

Opens and protects the "gate" of the Heart—ideal for rebalancing between inward retreat and outward expression.

Location: On the inner wrist crease, to the side of the tendon (flexor carpi ulnaris) toward the middle of the wrist.

Symbolism: Emotional overwhelm
Difficulty expressing or accessing feelings
Calming the Heart and supporting a steady relational presence

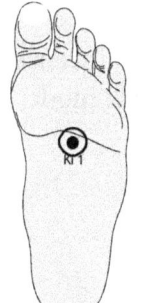

Kidney 1 (Yongquan or Gushing Spring)

Purpose: Ki 1 is the sedation point for the Kidney meridian. It grounds excess energy, drawing it down and helping to calm both the body and mind.

Location: On the sole of the foot, about one-third down from the base of the toes, between the ball of the foot and the center of the heel in the soft area.

How to Use: Apply gentle but firm pressure with your thumb for 1 minute on each foot. This point can be highly effective for calming a racing mind, particularly when paired with Ki 3 for balanced stimulation.

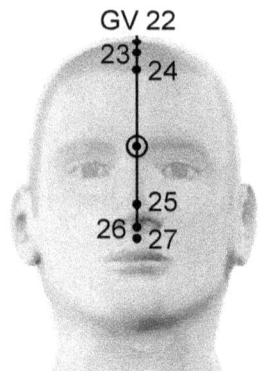

Yintang (Third Eye Point)

Purpose: Helps balance logical and intuitive thinking, easing overactive thoughts and enhancing centered focus.

Location: Midpoint between the eyebrows.

How to Use: Use your fingertip to apply light, steady pressure or small circles for 1–2 minutes.

Vision-Boarding & Symbolic Play

Purpose

This practice is designed to loosen rigid mental patterns by inviting the Holistic Mode—intuition, symbolic thinking, and nonlinear insight—into your awareness. It helps analytic-dominant thinkers visualize goals, feelings, or possibilities in a way that bypasses logic and activates pattern recognition.

What You'll Need

- A large sheet of paper, poster board, or journal spread
- Magazines, images, colored paper, stickers, or digital equivalents
- Scissors, glue, or digital collage app (e.g., Canva, Pinterest, Milanote)
- Optional: music, essential oils (frankincense, clary sage, lavender)

How to Do It

1. Set the Mood

Turn off distractions. Light a candle, apply essential oil (e.g., frankincense or sandalwood), or play gentle music to ease your mind out of task-mode.

2. Breathe and Shift Gears

Take 3–5 deep breaths. Let go of what you "should" be doing or solving.

Say inwardly:

> "I don't need to figure this out. I'm just here to see what wants to emerge."

3. Collect Images Freely

Flip through magazines or image folders and pull anything that speaks to you, even if it doesn't make sense. Don't try to analyze—trust your attraction.

Tip: If your analytic mind kicks in ("What is this for?"), reply: "This isn't for understanding. This is for listening."

4. Create a Spread

Arrange the images on your board. You can group them, place them randomly, or follow shapes/patterns. Add colors, words, or symbols if they arise.

5. Reflect Gently

Once finished, look at the board. Let it "speak" to you before interpreting.

Then, jot down responses to prompts like:

> What themes or patterns do I notice?
>
> What part of me chose these images?
>
> Is this pointing to something I'm ignoring, craving, or becoming?

6. Keep It Visible

Place your board somewhere you'll see it regularly—not as a to-do list, but as a mirror of your deeper self. Update it seasonally if you wish.

When to Use

- After long periods of linear work or decision fatigue
- When you feel disconnected from emotion, intuition, or creative flow
- During major life transitions, or when you're not sure what's next
- When logic fails to solve something that needs symbolic attention

Approaches to Balancing Holistic Mode

Therapies

Neurofeedback: Neurofeedback is a biofeedback technique that trains the brain to regulate its activity, promoting optimal cognitive function. By providing real-time feedback on brainwave activity, neurofeedback helps individuals learn to modulate their cognitive processes, enhancing focus and reducing mental fog. Neurofeedback can be used for:

> **Brainwave Training**: Sessions help train the brain to create more balanced brainwave patterns, improving clarity and focus.
>
> **Self-Regulation**: Neurofeedback enhances the brain's ability to regulate itself, leading to more consistent cognitive balance.

Cognitive Behavioral Therapy (CBT): Cognitive Behavioral Therapy (CBT) is a core approach for balancing the Head Self. CBT focuses on identifying and challenging irrational or biased thought patterns that can lead to negative emotions and behaviors. By reframing these thoughts, CBT helps cultivate a more balanced perspective, improving both analytical and intuitive thinking. Tools include:

> **Thought Records**: Track thoughts, emotions, and behaviors to identify patterns and develop balanced responses.
>
> **Cognitive Restructuring**: Challenge and modify negative or distorted thoughts to support clearer thinking

Focused Attention Meditation

Holistic thinkers often excel at seeing patterns and making intuitive leaps—but may struggle to anchor that insight into concrete action. Focused attention meditation helps train the mind to stabilize on a single object or task, reducing mental drift and increasing follow-through.

How to Practice:

Choose a neutral point of focus, such as your breath, a candle flame, or a word (like "now" or "clarity"). Sit quietly and gently return your attention to that focus whenever your mind wanders. You're not trying to stop thoughts—just to notice when you've left and come back. Start with 5–10 minutes and increase as it feels comfortable.

What it supports:

Builds mental stamina and task completion

Reduces overwhelm from open-ended thinking

Bridges insight with action by strengthening inner structure

Acupressure Points

These points stimulate alertness, integration, and clarity—helping bring structure and verbal orientation into a fluid, pattern-based mindset.

For detailed instructions on technique, timing, and best practices, see the Next Steps *Chapter 23 - Acupressure For Yourself and Others.*

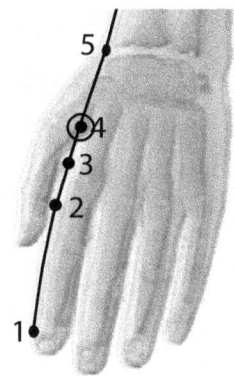

Large Intestine 4 (LI4 – Hegu)

Purpose: Promotes alertness and clears mental fog. Helps transition from diffuse, intuitive awareness into linear thought and verbal processing.

Location: On the back of the hand, in the webbing between the thumb and index finger.

How to Use: Use firm circular pressure with the opposite thumb for 30–60 seconds. Stimulates circulation to the brain and can help break looping or scattered thoughts.

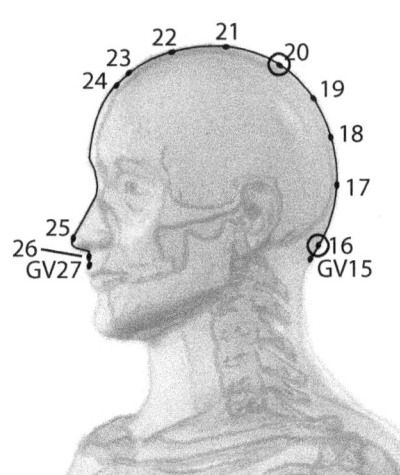

Governing Vessel 20 (GV20 – Baihui - Hundred Meetings)

Purpose: Stimulates mental clarity, focus, and communication between the brain's hemispheres. Supports integration of holistic and analytic processing.

Location: At the crown of the head, on the midline, in line with the tips of the ears.

How to Use: Apply steady pressure with the pads of two fingers or use gentle circular rubbing for 1–2 minutes. Use when you feel mentally scattered or unfocused.

Governing Vessel 16 (GV16 – Fengfu)

Purpose: Enhances cerebral circulation and brings awareness from intuition into structure. Helps link brainstem-level awareness with higher thought.

Location: *(Shown on above chart)* In the hollow just above the spine at the base of the skull, directly on the midline.

How to Use: Press gently upward into the hollow with one or two fingers while breathing slowly for 1 minute. Especially effective when used after GV20.

Essential Oils

Peppermint (Mentha × piperita): Stimulates mental energy, clears brain fog, and increases verbal fluency. Supports transitions from nonlinear thought into structured focus and task completion.

Rosemary (Rosmarinus officinalis): Enhances memory, attention, and cognitive clarity. Helps anchor intuitive insight into linear expression and strengthens analytic sequencing

Memory Training and Logic Puzzles

While Holistic Mode excels at seeing the big picture, it can sometimes bypass the fine details or sequential steps required for implementation. Engaging in memory games, logic puzzles, or verbal-based challenges (like crosswords or language learning apps) helps exercise left-brain circuits and strengthens structure, precision, and sequencing.

Examples to Try:

- Daily crossword puzzles or Sudoku
- Memorizing short passages or poems
- Word games or brain-training apps like Lumosity or Elevate
- Learning simple programming or math problems

What it supports:

    Strengthens verbal fluency and sequential processing

    Trains the mind to track detail without losing sight of context

    Reinforces internal scaffolding for complex ideas

Approaches for Overall Balance of the Head Self

Memory Enhancement Techniques: Memory is a key part of cognitive function, and strengthening memory helps balance the Head Self. Techniques such as mnemonic devices, visualization, and memory exercises can improve retention and recall, supporting both analytical and intuitive processes. Tools include:

> **Mnemonic Devices**: Use acronyms or visualization strategies to help remember information effectively.
>
> **Memory Training**: Exercises designed to strengthen working and long-term memory support overall cognitive health.

Creative Practices: Balancing the Head Self isn't just about Analytic Mode thinking—it's also about nurturing creativity and intuition. Creative practices like art, music, writing, or improvisation can activate Holistic Mode thinking, integrating analytical and intuitive processes. These include:

> **Artistic Expression**: Activities like painting or drawing encourage the free flow of creative thought.
>
> **Journaling**: Writing reflections helps clarify thinking and stimulates creative insights.

Critical Thinking Exercises: Engaging in critical thinking exercises sharpens analytical skills and fosters cognitive balance. These exercises challenge the mind to evaluate information, identify logical fallacies, and think deeply about complex issues, promoting clarity, precision, and insight. This can include:

> **Socratic Questioning**: Ask deep questions to challenge assumptions and explore underlying beliefs.
>
> **Logic Puzzles**: Use puzzles and brainteasers to enhance logical reasoning and problem-solving skills.

Cognitive Flexibility Training: Cognitive flexibility—the ability to adapt thinking in response to new information or changing circumstances—is crucial for a balanced Head Self. Exercises that encourage flexible thinking, such as switching tasks, learning new skills, or approaching problems from different perspectives, can enhance resilience and adaptability. Tools include:

Task Switching Exercises: Practice switching between tasks to improve flexibility.

Learning New Skills: Challenge the brain by learning a new language or musical instrument.

Meditation

Mindfulness meditation enhances cognitive balance by promoting present-moment awareness and reducing mental clutter. This practice allows for clearer observation of thoughts as they arise, preventing over-identification with negative or distracting thoughts. Over time, mindfulness leads to better cognitive flexibility and a balanced integration of analytical and intuitive thought.

Focused Attention Meditation: Concentrate on the breath to calm the mind and sharpen focus. (Better for Holistic Mode Dominant)

Open Monitoring Meditation: Observe thoughts without attachment or judgment, fostering greater flexibility and insight. (Best for Analytic Mode Dominant)

Homeopathic Remedies:

Here's a list of carefully selected homeopathic remedies that support Head Self balance, especially around themes of inward and outward emotional regulation. These remedies can be helpful for emotional sensitivity, relational overwhelm, boundary collapse, and suppressed or frozen feelings—key patterns often seen in Head Self imbalance within the Mind Matrix Model.

A common starting dose is **30c potency, taken 3–4 times per day**. If you notice clear improvement, you may shift to **a single dose of 200c** for deeper, longer-lasting support. For more guidance, see the appendix chapter *Homeopathy: Gentle Remedies for Balance and Health*.

Calcarea Phosphorica: Used for mental fatigue, difficulty concentrating, and feeling overwhelmed.

Lycopodium: Helpful for those struggling with self-confidence and memory.

Gelsemium: Used for performance anxiety and fear of failure, helping enhance cognitive performance under stress.

Essential Oils for the Head Self

Essential oils offer a way to gently shift arousal states through scent. While scientific evidence varies, many people find them soothing or energizing. If you have allergies, respiratory conditions, or other health concerns, approach essential oils with caution and consider consulting an aromatherapy practitioner.

Each of these oils can be used in a diffuser, diluted for topical use (e.g., over the chest or wrists), or simply inhaled from the palms for a quick reset. For more information on using essential oils, see the chapter *Essential Oils—History, Use, and Safety* in the appendix.

Peppermint: Helps improve focus and concentration.

Rosemary: Enhances memory and cognitive performance, ideal for studying or work sessions.

Lavender: Reduces mental stress, allowing for clearer thinking and balance.

Nutritional Support for Cognitive Health

A healthy diet supports cognitive function by providing essential nutrients. Certain foods and supplements can enhance memory, focus, and overall balance.

Omega-3 Fatty Acids: Found in fish and flaxseed, these fats support brain health.

Antioxidants: Foods rich in antioxidants, like berries, protect the brain from oxidative stress.

Choline: Found in eggs and soybeans, essential for brain health and memory.

Acupressure Points for Cognitive Balance

Acupressure can help balance the cognitive mind by enhancing communication between the left and right hemispheres, promoting a harmonious relationship between the Holistic and Analytic Modes, and stimulating cognitive function when needed. Applying gentle pressure to specific points can support mental clarity, focus, and the integration of both logical and intuitive thinking.

For detailed instructions on technique, timing, and best practices, see the Next Steps *Chapter 23 - Acupressure For Yourself and Others.*

For Enhancing Corpus Callosum Function, balancing between the left and right cerebral hemispheres:

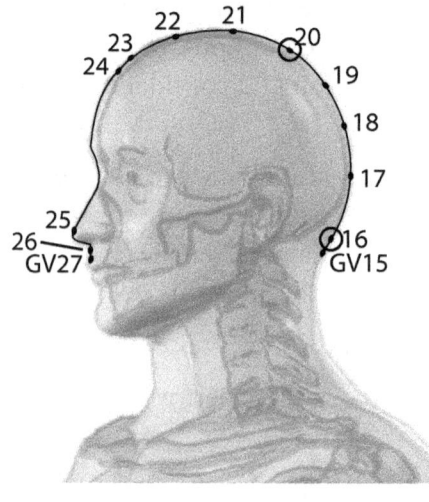

Governing Vessel 20 (GV20 – Baihui, Hundred Meetings)

Purpose: Stimulates mental clarity, focus, and communication between the brain's hemispheres.

Location: At the crown of the head, on the midline, in line with the tips of the ears.

How to Use: Apply steady pressure with the pads of two fingers or use circular rubbing for 1–2 minutes. Supports cognitive integration and whole-brain functioning.

Governing Vessel 16 (GV16 – Fengfu)

Purpose: Enhances cerebral circulation and cross-hemisphere integration.

Location: *(Shown on previous chart)* In the hollow just above the spine at the base of the skull, on the midline.

How to Use: Press gently upward into the hollow for 1 minute while breathing slowly. Especially effective when combined with mindfulness.

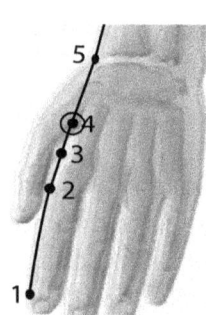

For Balancing the Holistic and Analytic Modes:

Large Intestine 4 (LI4 – Hegu)

Purpose: Supports cognitive flexibility and mental balance across both hemispheres.

Location: In the webbing between the thumb and index finger.

How to Use: Press firmly for 30–60 seconds on each hand. *Avoid during pregnancy.*

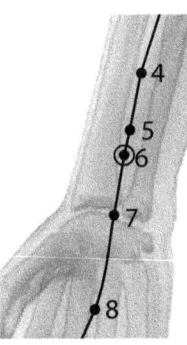

Pericardium 6 (PC6 – Neiguan)

Purpose: Calms the mind, eases anxiety, and supports balanced emotional-cognitive integration.

Location: Three finger-widths above the inner wrist crease, between the two tendons.

How to Use: Press gently and steadily with the opposite thumb for 1–2 minutes. Effective for emotional regulation and mental clarity.

For Increasing Activity of the Analytic Mode (Left Brain):

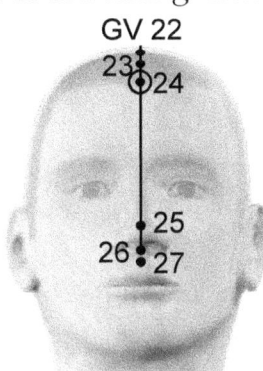

Governing Vessel 24 (GV24 – Shenting)

Purpose: Activates clarity, focus, and detailed thinking.

Location: Just above the midpoint of the forehead, about half an inch into the hairline.

How to Use: Tap or press lightly with a fingertip for 1 minute, ideally while seated upright and focused.

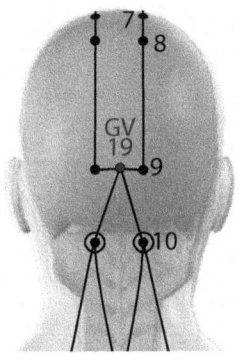

Bladder 10 (BL10 – Tianzhu)

Purpose: Promotes alertness, clarity, and mental strength.

Location: At the base of the skull, two finger-widths out from (lateral to) the spine.

How to Use: Use your thumbs to press upward into both points simultaneously. Useful for centering before mentally demanding tasks.

For Increasing Activity of the Holistic Mode (Right Brain):

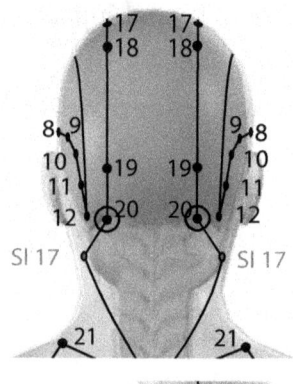

Gallbladder 20 (GB20 – Fengchi)

Purpose: Enhances intuition, creativity, and pattern recognition.

Location: In the hollows on either side of the spine at the base of the skull.

How to Use: Use your thumbs to press upward into the hollows for 1–2 minutes while breathing deeply.

Spleen 6 (SP6 – Sanyinjiao)

Purpose: Fosters emotional balance and holistic insight.

Location: Six finger-widths above the peak of the medial malleolus (inner ankle bone), just behind the shin.

How to Use: Apply steady pressure with your thumb for 1–2 minutes on each leg. *Avoid during pregnancy.*

Using these points can aid in achieving a more balanced and integrated cognitive state, enhancing both mental clarity and flexibility between analytic and holistic approaches. Remember to apply gentle, consistent pressure to each point for 1-2 minutes, while breathing deeply to support relaxation and focus.

Head Self Override Strategies

How to interrupt loops, reset your mental lens, and return to balanced thinking.

When the Head Self is overactivated—whether spiraling into Critic mode or drifting into abstraction—you can't think your way out. These **Override Strategies** are designed to shift your State first, so your mind can follow.

Name the Loop

Say out loud:

> "I'm in a Loop."

This interrupts the trance of overthinking or spiraling and brings the Monarch back online. Even a simple naming brings agency.

Thought Sorting (Externalize It)

Write down the top 3 thoughts on your mind. Label each one:

> *Helpful, Neutral, or Not Mine.*

This helps the Head Self re-engage its filtering function and break out of over-identification.

Cognitive Reset Breath

Inhale for 4 → Hold for 7 → Exhale for 8

This vagal-reset pattern slows the nervous system and helps transition from Critic or Drifter into Synthesizer mode.

Change the Frame (Reframing Prompt)

Ask:

> *Is this absolutely true?*
> *What's another way to see this?*
> *What would I say to someone else who felt this way?*

These questions restore mental flexibility—especially when rigidity has taken over.

Symbol Detox

If you're overwhelmed by meaning or stuck in abstraction (Drifter mode), reduce **symbolic input**: no music, books, or media. Just breath, body, and light movement.

This helps re-anchor the Head Self in direct experience.

Posture Override

Sit or stand upright with your shoulders back and feet grounded.

A collapsed body fuels negative narratives. This simple reset gives the Head Self a new frame to interpret from.

Each of these strategies works **not by fixing the thought**—but by changing the **State** the thought is coming from. The Head Self doesn't need to be silenced. It needs to be rebalanced.

Head Self Fast Reset Meditation

For moments of overthinking, mental overload, or cognitive rigidity.

Length: ~2–3 minutes

Posture: Seated or lying down. Eyes closed or softly focused.

Take a deep breath in…
And a long, slow breath out.

Bring your awareness into your **headspace**—your forehead, eyes, jaw, and scalp.
Notice what you feel there—tension? heaviness? buzz?
Just observe it, without needing to change it.

Let your eyes soften.
Let your jaw unclench.
Let your tongue rest gently in your mouth.

Now, imagine your thoughts as a **sky full of clouds**.
Each thought is a shape—floating.
You don't have to chase them. Just notice them…and let them drift.

With each breath, invite **space** between the clouds.
You're not pushing thoughts away—you're letting them **loosen**.

Feel that space now.
Cool, wide, open.

Breathe in clarity.
Breathe out clutter.

Affirmation:

> *My thoughts are not in charge—I am.*
> *I can loosen the grip of overthinking.*
> *I return to a quiet, open mind.*

Take one more breath and gently return to your day.

Head Self Daily Ritual Meditation

For aligning analytic and intuitive thinking and cultivating clarity.

Length: ~5–8 minutes

Posture: Seated, relaxed. Hands resting on thighs or palms upward.

Close your eyes gently. Bring awareness to your breath.
Let it rise and fall like waves—smooth, even, steady.

Now, picture your mind as a landscape.
It may look like a library…a forest…a quiet ocean.
Whatever comes to you, trust it.

You're going to walk through this mindscape—no rush, just presence.
With each inhale, invite focus and structure.
With each exhale, invite softness and spaciousness.

Inhale – sharpen.
Exhale – soften.

Now place one hand lightly at your forehead.
This is the seat of your Head Self—the keeper of patterns, logic, ideas, and vision.

Ask quietly:

> *"What kind of thinking am I doing today?"*
> *Am I overanalyzing?*
> *Am I disconnected or foggy?*
> *Am I aligned and flowing?*

There's no wrong answer—just awareness.

Now, imagine two streams meeting—one from your left, one from your right.
These are your analytic and intuitive currents.
Watch them merge into a steady river, moving forward together.
Let the breath follow this rhythm:

> Inhale—receive insight.
> Exhale—release rigidity.

Trust the movement. Trust the balance.

Affirmation:

> *I welcome clear, flexible thinking.*
> *My mind is both sharp and spacious.*
> *I trust my capacity to shift and see anew.*

Let your hand fall back to your lap. Take one more breath, feeling both grounded and clear.

When you're ready, gently open your eyes.

Integrating Approaches for Cognitive Balance

Balancing the Head Self often requires a combination of approaches that address the Analytical and Holistic Modes of thinking. By integrating practices that enhance critical thinking, creativity, memory, and cognitive flexibility, you can create a strategy for maintaining clarity and balance.

Whether through mindfulness, neurofeedback, creative practices, or the use of acupressure, homeopathic remedies and essential oils, the key is to find a blend that supports all aspects of cognitive function, leading to a more balanced and effective way of thinking.

Final Thoughts

Your Head Self is a remarkable guide capable of insight, strategy, reflection, and vision. But like any guide, it needs rest, balance, and perspective. When the Analytic Mode dominates, you may lose the thread of meaning or get lost in details and miss the big picture. When the Holistic Mode takes over, you may drift without direction or get lost in a distorted reality.

True cognitive balance comes not from choosing one over the other, but from learning when and how to shift.

This chapter has offered you ways to work with both sides of your Head Self—analytic and holistic, focused and spacious, sharp and soft. As you begin to notice your own mental habits and rhythms, you'll become more skilled at adjusting your cognitive lens—zooming in when precision is needed, and zooming out to see where you are.

Most importantly, you'll begin to see that *thinking is not just a tool, but a landscape.* It is a state of mind that your Monarch can wander around in. One you can move through with greater freedom, curiosity, and care.

The goal isn't perfect clarity, it's flexible clarity. The kind that allows you to return to yourself, again and again, as your mind grows quieter, steadier, and more aligned.

In our next two chapters, we'll take a deeper dive into the State Axis and how to work with both short-term Negative State issues as well as improving your overall State Range.

Chapter Thirteen
The State Axis

"Be still, sad heart! and cease repining;
Behind the clouds is the sun still shining;
Thy fate is the common fate of all,
Into each life some rain must fall,
Some days must be dark and dreary.

~ Excerpt from "The Rainy Day"
by Henry Wadsworth Longfellow

One of the most important aspects of the Mind Matrix is the **State Axis**. We've covered the basics of this and how it interacts with each of the Three Selves, now it's time to get down and dirty with it.

Each of the Selves—**Vital Self, Heart Self** and **Head Self**—has an axis of action that has a wide range of possible states. Each is hugely affected by your overall *mood state* or *state of mind*, the range from "the worst" to "the best." This is the State Axis.

Your nervous system's State exists on a spectrum, ranging from what we call the Positive State (thriving) to the Negative State (survival-focused).

There's also a tipping point between the two—once you cross over into the Negative State, your mind's orientation dramatically shifts, changing how you see yourself, others, and the world around you.

Similarly, when you move back into the Positive State, everything feels more manageable again, and your outlook naturally brightens.

The farther to either Positive or Negative, the stronger the State and its effects but the shift between each is a fundamental shift in perspective.

Your State Range

Positive ▲

State

Negative ▼

The common definition of state, and the one in the Oxford Dictionary of the English Language, is "the particular condition that someone or something is in *at a specific time*." Kind of like the weather on a particular day. But there's really no term in the English language for the range of your overall state of mind *over time*, like an area's *climate* would be to its *weather*.

In the Mind Matrix model, we call that your State Range, or just State with a capital S. Your mood state changes all the time, but there is an overall range of what is normal for you in your day to day life.

Your State Range shapes how you perceive and interact with the world, acting like a filter that colors every thought, emotion, and action. You can think of it as a dimmer switch: when the light is bright, the Positive State, the world feels clear, open, and manageable. When the light dims, the Negative State, everything becomes harder to see, more uncertain, and even threatening.

The Positive State: Thriving

In the Positive State, you feel calm, capable, and connected. Life's challenges may still arise, but you're able to approach them with perspective, resilience, and intentionality. The different aspects of your mind—the Vital Self, Heart Self, and Head Self—work together harmoniously.

When you're in the Positive State:

- You feel safe, both physically and emotionally.
- Your energy is steady, your emotions are balanced, and your thoughts are clear and flexible.
- You have a sense of calm confidence, feeling in control of your actions and open to the world around you.
- Even when things go wrong, you're able to keep perspective, finding solutions or accepting what you can't change without losing your overall sense of contentment.

In this State, the Mind Matrix operates as it was designed to—each Self contributes its strengths, and you thrive as a whole.

The Negative State: Surviving

The Negative State, in contrast, is all about survival. When triggered into the Negative State, your nervous system shifts into reactive mode, often driven by stress, fear, or anxiety. Instead of feeling capable and in control, you may feel overwhelmed and at the mercy of events happening to you.

When you're in the Negative State:

- You see the world through a lens of threat or challenge, making it hard to relax or focus on anything other than survival.
- Your responses tend to be automatic and unconscious, driven by survival mechanisms rather than thoughtful choices.
- You might feel emotionally disconnected, physically tense, or mentally stuck, as if the different parts of your mind are working against each other rather than together.
- This State often results in feelings of being out of control—your thoughts may race, your emotions may overwhelm you, and your body might remain in a high-alert mode long after the perceived threat has passed.

Positive/Balanced State	Negative/Reactive State
Conscious, Centered	Reactive
Egalitarian	Hierarchical
Pleasure Seeking	Distraction/Relief Seeking
Creativity, Engagement	Reactive Actions
Focused on Positives	Focused on Negatives
Spectrum Viewpoint	Binary Viewpoint
Thrive, Flourishing	Survival Orientation
Bountiful	Zero Sum, Never Enough
Awareness/Mindfulness	Vigilance
Discernment	Judgment
Agency, Empowerment	Victimhood
Gratitude	Focused on Lack
Contentment	Discontentment
Love	Fear

How State Affects the Three Selves

Your State—whether the Positive State or the Negative State—directly affects how each of the Three Selves operates.

In the Positive State, the Vital Self is energized and engaged, the Heart Self feels open and connected, and the Head Self is clear and flexible. This alignment allows you to respond to challenges with resilience and creativity.

In the Negative State, the Vital Self might be stuck in overdrive (high alert) or underdrive (fatigue or shutdown), the Heart Self might feel defensive or disconnected, and the Head Self might become rigid, overwhelmed, or unable to process information effectively.

For example, if you're in the Negative State because of an unresolved conflict (Heart Self), you might notice physical tension or a racing heart (Vital Self) and struggle to focus on solutions (Head Self). Similarly, if your Vital Self is depleted due to lack of sleep, it can lead to emotional irritability (Heart Self) and difficulty concentrating (Head Self).

Triggers and Interplay Between the Selves

The switch from the Positive State to the Negative State is often triggered by something in your environment. This could be as obvious as a lion charging toward you, or as subtle as the faint smell of something unconsciously tied to a painful memory—or even your boss's insincere smile.

> *Maria was feeling calm and balanced until a coworker used a dismissive tone similar to her critical parent's voice, instantly triggering feelings of inadequacy and anxiety. By recognizing the trigger, Maria could apply an Override Strategy—brief mindful breathing combined with grounding—to quickly shift herself back toward a Positive State.*

Although these shifts can feel overwhelming, it's important to remind yourself that the Negative State is not permanent. With awareness, persistence, and intentional action you can guide yourself back toward the Positive State, restoring balance and clarity.

Each of the Three Selves can trigger the Negative State:

> The **Vital Self** responds to physical threats, like loud noises or danger, often through fight-or-flight.
>
> The **Heart Self** reacts to emotional pain, such as rejection or loneliness, creating feelings of defensiveness or isolation.
>
> The **Head Self** struggles with mental overwhelm, like unsolvable problems or overwhelm, leading to rigidity or shutdown.

However, the Three Selves don't just trigger the Negative State—they can also work together to restore balance. For example:

- If the **Vital Self** is on high alert, the **Head Self** might step in to assess the situation logically, calming the body through relaxation techniques.
- When the **Heart Self** is triggered by conflict, the **Vital Self** can regulate stress through physical activity like walking or yoga.
- If the **Head Self** feels overwhelmed, the **Heart Self** can provide reassurance through social support, reducing mental strain.

This dynamic interplay between the Selves ensures that even in challenging moments, your mind has the potential to shift back toward the Positive State. Understanding how these triggers and responses interact lays the foundation for exploring a deep understanding of State.

Understanding this dynamic empowers you to notice when one Self is struggling and enlist the others to help restore balance. By recognizing these patterns, you can take actionable steps to guide your Mind Matrix back to the Positive State.

The Fluid Nature of State

State is always fluid—you are never "stuck" in the Positive State or the Negative State permanently. Each moment offers an opportunity to influence your State. By understanding how the Three Selves interact and recognizing the triggers that pull you into the Negative State, you can build the tools to guide yourself back to the Positive State, restoring balance and clarity.

The dynamic nature of the Mind Matrix Model means that the same systems that contribute to imbalance can also bring you back into alignment. Whether it's calming your Vital Self, addressing emotional pain in your Heart Self, or clearing mental clutter in your Head Self, each part of the Mind Matrix Model has the power to help you restore balance and thrive.

> *Buddhist Psychology and the Nature of State*
>
> *In Buddhist psychology, the concepts of dukkha and sukha offer profound insight into what we call State in the Mind Matrix Model.*
>
> ***Dukkha***, *often mistranslated simply as "suffering," more accurately refers to a pervasive sense of dissatisfaction or dis-ease. It includes obvious suffering, but also the subtler sense that something is missing or off. It closely mirrors what we describe as the Negative State—a state of disconnection, fear, or internal conflict.*
>
> ***Sukha***, *in contrast, means ease, well-being, or the felt sense of harmony. It reflects the Positive State—where the three selves are integrated, your nervous system is regulated, and your experience feels open, coherent, and empowered.*
>
> *For more information on how the Mind Matrix Model aligns with Buddhist Psychology, see the chapter in the Next Steps section of the website, Buddhism and the Mind Matrix Model—*
> *mmm.tips/next*
> *You'll need to sign up for access.*

Emotions in Relation to the Three Selves and States

Emotions are the bridge between the internal and external worlds, dynamically engaging the Vital Self, Heart Self, and Head Self. Each Self plays a distinct role in generating, contextualizing, and processing emotions, creating a layered and interconnected experience.

Understanding how emotions arise and function within the Three Selves, as well as how they shift between the Positive and Negative States, provides a framework for emotional awareness and integration.

We covered the Self-State interaction in each Self chapter, but they are included here as well, along with their diagrams.

The Vital Self: Instinctive Survive- and Thrive-Based Emotions

The Vital Self governs the body's core survival mechanisms and produces emotions that are *immediate, reactive, and physiologically driven.* These emotions are tied to primal instincts and ensure physical safety and balance.

Core Emotions:

Fear: Triggers fight, flight, or freeze in response to danger.

Anger: Mobilizes energy to confront obstacles or threats.

Disgust: Protects the body by avoiding harmful substances or situations.

Satisfaction/Satiety: Signals that basic needs (e.g., hunger, thirst, rest) have been met, fostering a sense of calm and restoration.

Relaxation: Indicates safety, allowing the body to recover and conserve energy.

Thriving: Reflects Vitality, energy, and readiness to engage with opportunities and challenges.

Characteristics:

Fast, reflexive, and deeply tied to physical sensations.

Often binary (e.g., safe/unsafe) and focused on immediate needs.

Vital Self and State:

Positive State: Positive emotions like satisfaction, relaxation, and thriving emerge when the body's needs are met and the parasympathetic system is activated.

Negative State: Negative emotions like fear or anger dominate when the body perceives a threat, amplifying arousal and reactivity.

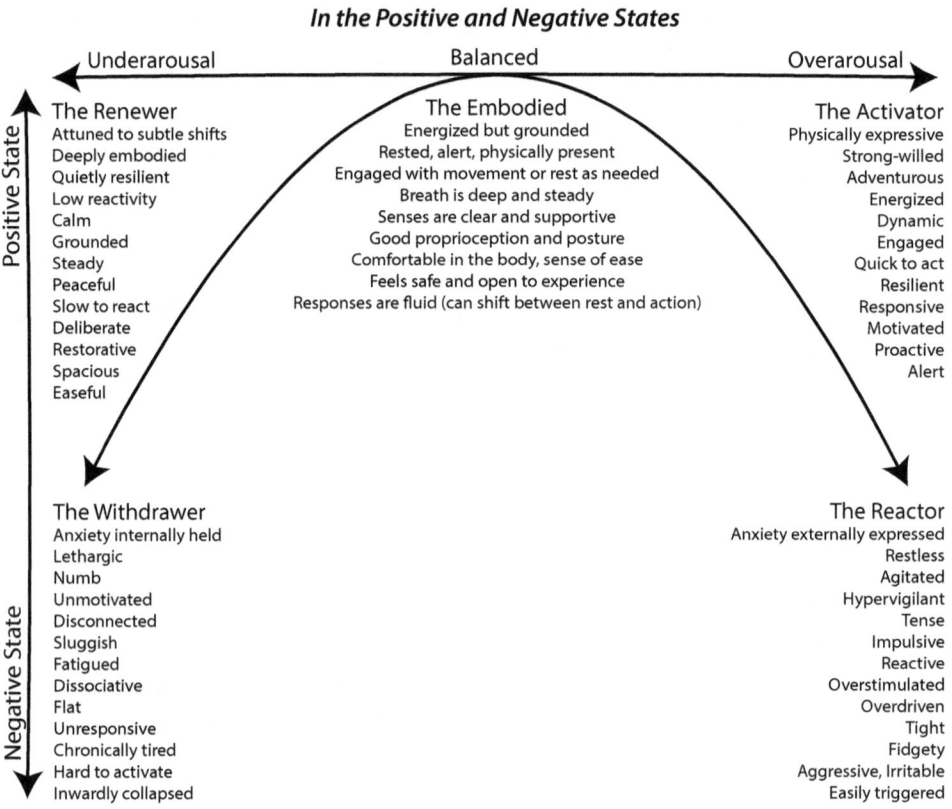

Vital Self
In the Positive and Negative States

The Heart Self: Relational and Contextual Emotions

The Heart Self manages emotions related to relationships, social interactions, and attachments. These emotions are more nuanced and contextual, shaping how we connect with others and navigate the social world.

Core Emotions:

Love/Attachment: Fosters connection and intimacy.

Empathy/Compassion: Allows resonance with others' emotions and experiences.

Shame: Signals a breach in social or relational expectations, encouraging repair.

Guilt: Motivates accountability and ethical behavior in relationships.

Joy: Strengthens social bonds and celebrates shared experiences.

Characteristics:

Context-dependent, involving social norms, cultural values, and relational dynamics.

Often intertwined with the Heart Self scripts we follow in our relationships.

Heart Self and State:

Positive State: Positive emotions like love and joy arise from secure attachments and mutual connection, broadening relational engagement.

Negative State: Negative emotions like shame and guilt can dominate, narrowing relational focus and triggering protective behaviors like withdrawal or appeasement/fawning.

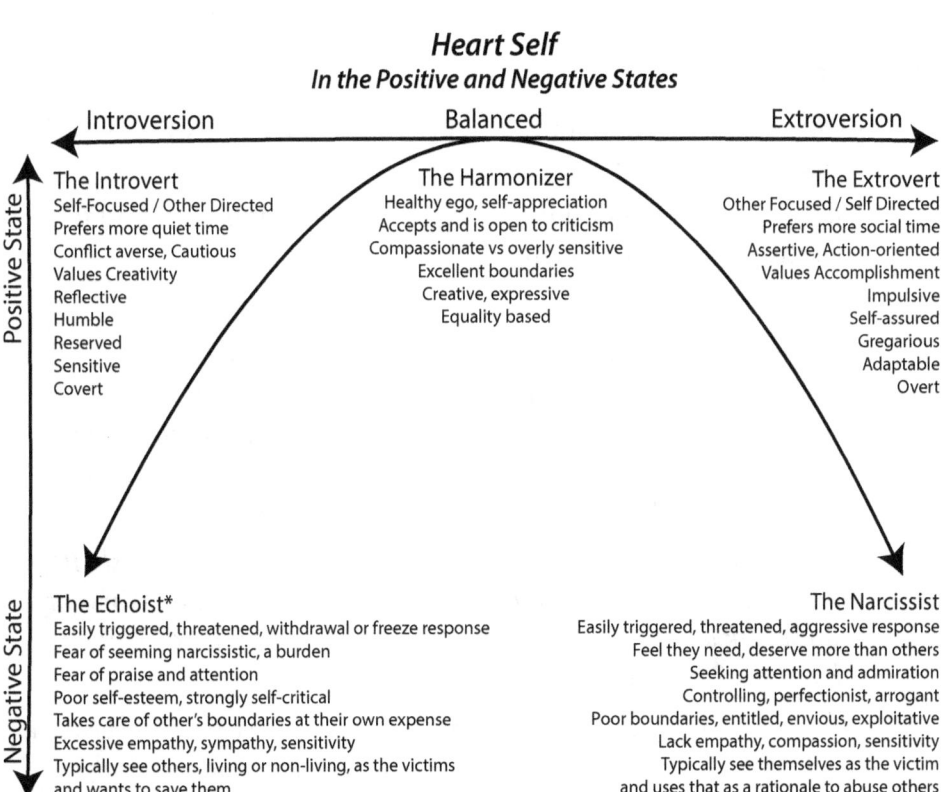

Heart Self
In the Positive and Negative States

Introversion — Balanced — Extroversion

The Introvert
Self-Focused / Other Directed
Prefers more quiet time
Conflict averse, Cautious
Values Creativity
Reflective
Humble
Reserved
Sensitive
Covert

The Harmonizer
Healthy ego, self-appreciation
Accepts and is open to criticism
Compassionate vs overly sensitive
Excellent boundaries
Creative, expressive
Equality based

The Extrovert
Other Focused / Self Directed
Prefers more social time
Assertive, Action-oriented
Values Accomplishment
Impulsive
Self-assured
Gregarious
Adaptable
Overt

The Echoist*
Easily triggered, threatened, withdrawal or freeze response
Fear of seeming narcissistic, a burden
Fear of praise and attention
Poor self-esteem, strongly self-critical
Takes care of other's boundaries at their own expense
Excessive empathy, sympathy, sensitivity
Typically see others, living or non-living, as the victims and wants to save them

The Narcissist
Easily triggered, threatened, aggressive response
Feel they need, deserve more than others
Seeking attention and admiration
Controlling, perfectionist, arrogant
Poor boundaries, entitled, envious, exploitative
Lack empathy, compassion, sensitivity
Typically see themselves as the victim and uses that as a rationale to abuse others

* Term coined by Dr. Craig Malkin

The Head Self: Evaluative and Reflective Emotions

The Head Self processes emotions that arise from meaning-making, reflection, and evaluation. These emotions often involve abstract thinking and long-term perspectives.

Core Emotions:

- **Pride**: Positive State pride reflects on achievements and reinforces self-worth. Negative State pride is used as a defense.
- **Regret**: Arises from analyzing past actions and their consequences.
- **Hope**: Centers on imagining positive future outcomes.
- **Awe**: Combines reflection with a sense of wonder about something greater.
- **Frustration**: Signals a cognitive block or unmet expectation.

Characteristics:

- Deliberative, slower to emerge, and tied to thoughts and beliefs.
- Involves evaluating actions, outcomes, and possibilities.

Head Self and State:

Positive State: Emotions like hope and awe inspire creativity and broaden perspective.

Negative State: Emotions like regret and frustration can lead to cognitive rigidity, narrowing thought patterns.

> **Unsustainable Highs: When Motivation Backfires**
> *Modern culture often confuses activation with motivation. Motivational speakers push people into high-arousal Positive States. While this can feel inspiring in the moment, it often creates an artificially elevated State that the system cannot maintain.*
>
> *Motivational hype mimics a kind of nervous system sugar rush. It feels good, but it doesn't build long-term State Regulation. Worse, it can shrink a person's State Range by creating internal expectations that they should always feel "fired up" to succeed.*
>
> *In contrast, true regulation means learning to move flexibly between high and low arousal, inward and outward focus, and the analytic and holistic modes of the mind.*

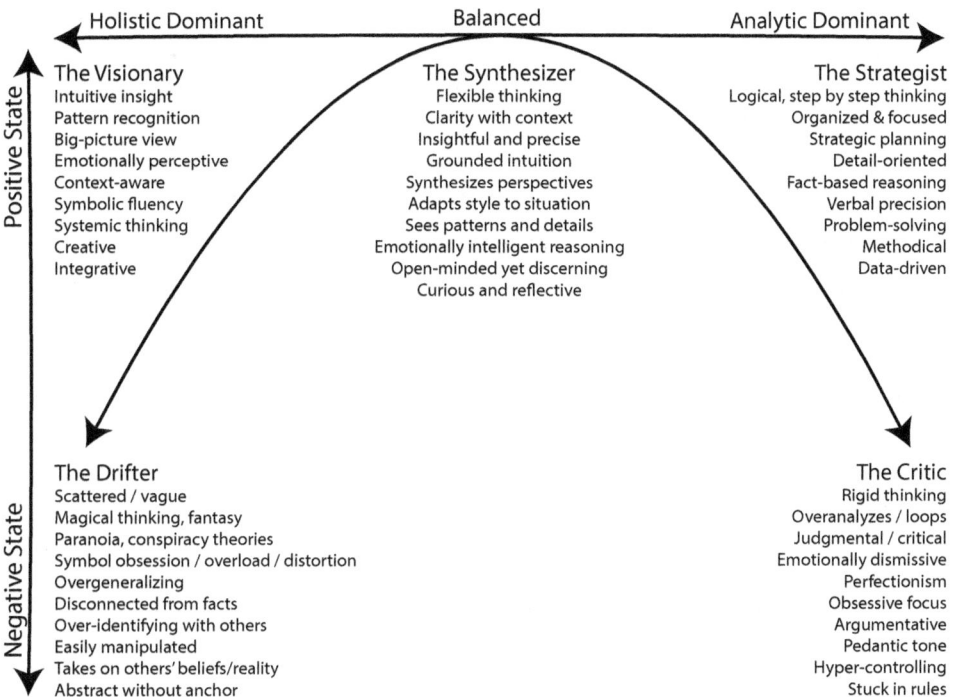

Interplay of the Selves in Emotional Experience

Emotions rarely exist in isolation within a single Self. Instead, they arise from the dynamic interplay between the Vital, Heart, and Head Selves. For example:

Fear (Vital Self) → Anxiety (Head Self): Fear triggers a Vital response, but the Head Self's reflection on potential threats can prolong it as anxiety.

Love (Heart Self) → Satisfaction (Vital Self): Relational love can evoke physical relaxation and satiety, reinforcing the connection.

Awe (Cognitive Self) → Goosebumps (Vital Self): A reflective realization can trigger a physical sensation, deepening the impact.

Physical Sensations and Their Role in Emotion

Physical sensations are inseparable from emotions, providing a *somatic foundation* that enhances, contextualizes, and often triggers emotional experiences. These sensations are mediated by the Vital Self but inform the Heart and Head Selves.

How Physical Sensations Enhance Emotions:

Amplification of Emotional Intensity:
- A pounding heart makes fear feel more urgent.
- Goosebumps heighten the sense of awe or inspiration.

Reinforcement of Emotional Meaning:
- A warm sensation in the chest enhances feelings of love or empathy.
- A physical "wash" of relaxation reinforces relief or satisfaction.

How Physical Sensations Contextualize Emotions:

Connecting the Body to the Experience:
Sensory feedback (e.g., tightness in the stomach) helps ground emotions in the body, making them tangible and harder to ignore.

Providing Relational Cues:
Subtle sensations like leaning toward someone or averting gaze guide relational dynamics and emotional expression.

How Physical Sensations Trigger Emotions:

Bottom-Up Processing:
A sudden physical stimulus (e.g., a cold breeze or loud sound) can trigger an emotional response like alertness, fear, or excitement.

Somatic Memory:
Physical sensations tied to past experiences (e.g., the warmth of sunlight recalling a happy memory) can evoke strong emotions in the present.

Emotions and the State Axis

The Positive and Negative States profoundly influence how emotions are processed and experienced across the Selves:

Positive State:

- Emotions are balanced, integrated, and adaptive.
- Positive emotions like love, hope, and awe dominate, broadening awareness and fostering connection.
- Sensory responses (e.g., goosebumps, relaxation) enhance emotional depth and meaning.

Negative State:

- Emotions are fragmented, rigid, and reactive.
- Negative emotions like fear, shame, or frustration dominate, narrowing focus and triggering protective responses.
- Physical sensations may feel overwhelming or disconnected, amplifying distress.

Cutting Out the Middleman

When we're in pain—physical, emotional, or mental—our instinct is often to look outside ourselves for relief. We think, "If only I had more money, a better relationship, a new job, or a different body, then I'd feel better." This is the Middleman illusion: the belief that external changes are the true cause of happiness or peace.

But this way of thinking keeps us trapped in a cycle of waiting to truly live a fulfilling life for the possibility of a better future. We wait for circumstances to change, for others to behave differently, for life to align just right before we let ourselves feel content or free. The Mind Matrix Model offers another path: cutting out the middleman.

Instead of chasing external solutions, we go straight to the source—State.

Your State determines how you experience everything. A Positive State doesn't mean your life is perfect. It means you have the inner clarity, regulation, and emotional capacity to meet challenges with creativity, resilience, and meaning. A Negative State, by contrast, filters everything through a lens of fear, scarcity, and pain, even if nothing is objectively wrong.

When you learn to regulate your State, you gain direct access to what you were hoping those outer changes would give you: calm, joy, connection, clarity, empowerment, and peace.

In this sense, State becomes the gateway to real, lasting transformation.

In the Mind Matrix Model, this is a core principle: you don't have to wait for your life to change to feel better, you can begin by changing your internal conditions first.

State Magnets

Sit up and focus now, I'm going to give you a powerful tool to manage your State. And understand how we get trapped in the Negative State. I would say this one section is worth the price of admission.

> *When my mother was teaching me to drive, she said something that truly caught my attention. "Don't look at the side of the road in order to keep from driving too far on the side, focus on where you want to go.* ***Where you look is where you drive.****"*

The same principle applies to life. **Wherever you place your focus—emotionally, mentally, energetically—that's where your system steers.** This isn't just true of actions, but of thoughts, feelings, and State.

In the Mind Matrix Model, we call these State Magnets. Your focus acts like a magnetic pull on your system, drawing your thoughts, emotions, and body responses toward whatever you're locked onto. When you're anxious and hyper-focused on what might go wrong, you're magnetizing yourself into a more intense Negative State. When you're dwelling on past mistakes, you're reinforcing feelings of shame or regret and deepening your Heart Self's dysregulation. Even subtle habitual focuses, like scanning for threats or constantly rehashing a grievance, can become powerful Negative State Magnets.

Here's the paradox: we often focus most on the things we want to get away from. But this keeps them at the center of our awareness, like staring at the ditch while trying not to crash into it. The body tenses, the mind narrows, and the State destabilizes. Without realizing it, we're driving straight toward what we fear or dread.

The solution isn't denial or toxic positivity. It's choosing your magnet wisely. This is the power of the Reflective Catalyst, the conscious part of you that can ask, "Where do I actually want to steer?"

Let's review the different attributes of the Positive and Negative States:

Positive/Balanced State	Negative/Reactive State
Conscious, Centered	Reactive
Egalitarian	Hierarchical
Pleasure Seeking	Distraction/Relief Seeking
Creativity, Engagement	Reactive Actions
Focused on Positives	Focused on Negatives
Spectrum Viewpoint	Binary Viewpoint
Thrive, Flourishing	Survival Orientation
Bountiful	Zero Sum, Never Enough
Awareness/Mindfulness	Vigilance
Discernment	Judgment
Agency, Empowerment	Victimhood
Equanimity, Gratitude	Focused on Lack
Contentment	Discontentment
Love	Fear

Each of these terms can act as a State Magnet, drawing you into either the Positive or Negative State.

For example, *gratitude*. Most people think of gratitude as a result of circumstances—a kindness offered, a lucky break, the appreciation for someone or something in your life. But evoking a feeling of gratitude moves you toward the Positive State. It's actually a way of caring for yourself. The deeper and more powerful the gratitude, the stronger the magnetic pull toward positivity.

Try it now. Close your eyes and think of something or someone you are deeply grateful for. Imagine that you are breathing that deep feeling of gratitude in and out through your heart. I'll wait here until you're done.

Welcome back! If you were able to truly focus on gratitude, you will have felt your State shift. This is true of all of the Positive State attributes. You can change your State by focusing on pleasure, creativity, bountifulness, awareness, discernment vs. judgment, empowerment, contentment and love.

And, unfortunately, the opposite is also true.

One Insult, a Thousand Echoes

There's an old story from the Buddhist tradition:

A man is walking through a village when a stranger insults him—harsh words, an unfair judgment. The moment passes, and the stranger is gone.

But the man cannot let it go.

He replays the insult in his mind all day. He lies awake that night, hearing it again. He imagines what he should have said. He feels shame, anger, confusion. Days pass, then weeks. He tells others about the insult, trying to get validation or clarity. Still, it churns.

Eventually, a wise friend says to him:

"The stranger insulted you once. But you have insulted yourself a thousand times."

Focusing on the negative attributes of State evokes the Negative State. For this poor fellow, focusing on anger, hurt and shame immersed him in the Negative State. Each mental replay isn't neutral—it reinforces the Head-Heart Loop, dragging his system deeper into the Negative State.

Perhaps this is familiar to you, times when you've been unable to let go of some perceived insult or actual harm received at the hands of a person lost in the Negative State.

Once you're in the Negative State, the world shifts. You see only the negatives. Looking back at your past, you see the painful periods and the disappointments. Thinking about the future, you picture only frustration, sadness, hopelessness. Which just further feeds the Negative State. Your State becomes self-generating. When you are in the Negative State, all you see are reasons to be in the Negative State. When in the Positive State, you see all the reasons to be present, positive and even grateful.

The Positive and Negative States are right next to each other, like two sides of a coin. What flips it is not your situation, but your focus, moving you toward one or the other.

> ### The Samurai and the Monk
>
> This story is from the Zen Buddhist tradition.
>
> *A fearsome samurai once came to a humble monastery and demanded to be taught the difference between heaven and hell.*
>
> *The old monk looked at him calmly and said,*
>
> *"Why should I teach you? You're dirty. You smell. Your sword is rusty and your mind dull. You're a disgrace to the warrior class."*
>
> *The samurai turned red with rage. Trembling, he drew his sword and raised it above the monk's head.*
>
> *The monk looked up at him and said softly,*
>
> *"That is hell."*
>
> *The samurai froze.*
>
> *In a single moment, he understood: his fury, his ego, his loss of control—that was hell. He dropped his sword, fell to his knees, and bowed low in gratitude, tears in his eyes for this gentle monk willing to risk his life to impart such a lesson.*
>
> *The monk then smiled wide, saying,*
>
> *"And that is heaven."*

Practices that promote a Positive State often seem simple, but they're profound in their effects:

- **Gratitude:** Focusing on what you are grateful for shifts perception toward abundance and presence.
- **Creativity:** Engaging in the process of creation brings engagement, flow, and self-expression.
- **Mindfulness:** Staying present in the current moment interrupts reactive loops and anchors you in awareness.
- **Equanimity:** Being content with your life, even during challenging times, supports emotional steadiness and perspective.
- **Love**—toward self, others, and life itself—rebuilds trust in connection.

Reflections Through the Mind Matrix

This is a story of State, and the power of the Monarch to awaken within a moment of activation.

The samurai's Vital Self was flooded with adrenaline: fight-or-flight, eyes narrowed, sword raised. His Heart Self was engulfed in shame and insult, fueling rage in the Vital Self. His Head Self was hijacked by a binary Script: dominate or be dishonored.

In a single line, the monk mirrors it all back with clarity. And in that flash of recognition—not suppression, but awareness—the samurai shifts from reactive to reflective.

That's the moment the Monarch awakens. That's what a State Shift feels like: the difference between hell and heaven, in a single breath.

Now, where would you rather spend your life?

Because you do have a choice. But only when you're in the Positive State. Otherwise the choice is made for you by your old patterns.

Discerning Positive and Negative Orientation

One stumbling block you'll need to watch out for:

A negative orientation often masquerades as a positive one. On the surface, it may look like a goal, a desire, or a hope, but underneath, it may be rooted in aversion, fear, or escape. For example:

> *"I wish I were rich!"*

At first glance, this sounds like a forward-moving intention. But in most cases, it's actually a reaction, a desire to escape financial stress and avoid discomfort, or feel worthy in a culture that links money with identity.

The question to ask is, am I focusing on moving toward something I want, or trying to escape from something I don't want?

If you use affirmations, this distinction is essential. An affirmation that's rooted in a negative won't take you where you truly want to go.

Signs of Negative Orientation in Disguise

You can often detect a negative orientation by noticing:

- The underlying emotion: Is it fueled by anxiety, envy, shame, or desperation?

- The imagery: Is it a fantasy of being "finally safe" or "finally admired," rather than a grounded vision of purpose?
- The narrative tone: Is there a sense of "then I'll be okay" implying that you aren't okay now?

In the Mind Matrix Model, this kind of thinking often reflects:

A Head Self stuck in future fantasy or fear-based planning

A Heart Self seeking approval or belonging through external symbols

A Vital Self trying to discharge stress through imagined relief

Transforming Orientation: From Escape to Intention

Instead of trying to escape discomfort, you can shift the same desire into a Positive Orientation by naming what it truly seeks.

Negative Orientation:

"I wish I were rich so I could stop worrying." (Head Loop + Vital stress + Heart shame)

Positive Orientation:

"I want to move toward bountifulness so I can create a life rooted in open-hearted generosity and calm." (A Monarch intention guided by clarity and care.)

It's the same outer goal, but the internal posture is entirely different. One is rooted in reaction, the other in reflection.

Quick Test: Is This Desire Positive or Negative?

Ask yourself:

Is this moving toward meaning, or away from discomfort?

What feeling do I imagine this goal will "fix"?

Which of my Three Selves is most activated in this desire—and what does it actually need?

When the Monarch pauses to ask these questions, it can turn reactive loops into reflective choices and help the entire system orient toward true alignment, not just momentary relief.

Final Thoughts

Emotions connect the Vital, Heart, and Head Selves like threads in a living tapestry. They help us make sense of our experiences, not just through thoughts, but through the felt language of the body and heart.

The physical sensations of the Vital Self often provide the groundwork for how emotions arise. A racing pulse, a tight chest, a sudden heaviness—these are early signals that ripple upward through the Heart and Head Selves. The Heart Self adds meaning. The Head Self interprets, assigning understanding.

But all of these layers are filtered through one crucial lens: your State.

We are constantly being triggered into the Negative State by outdated Sentries—patterns that were once helpful, even essential, but are no longer serving us.

When you're in a Positive State, emotions feel easier to understand, express, and regulate. When you're in a Negative State, they can feel overwhelming, distorted, or stuck. That's why State Shift is such a powerful tool. Because when your State changes, your entire emotional experience can shift with it.

Through the power of the Monarch's Reflective Catalyst, once you bring an unconscious Sentry into conscious awareness, you can begin to change it. And each Sentry transformed is a shift toward the Positive State.

By learning how to recognize when you're triggered and intentionally shifting your State, returning to awareness, you gain access to more resilience, clarity, and compassion across all Three Selves.

In the next chapter, we'll explore exactly how to do that, starting with fast, in-the-moment strategies to help you reset, and moving into deeper practices that gradually shift your State Range toward the Positive over time.

Chapter Fourteen
Working with State

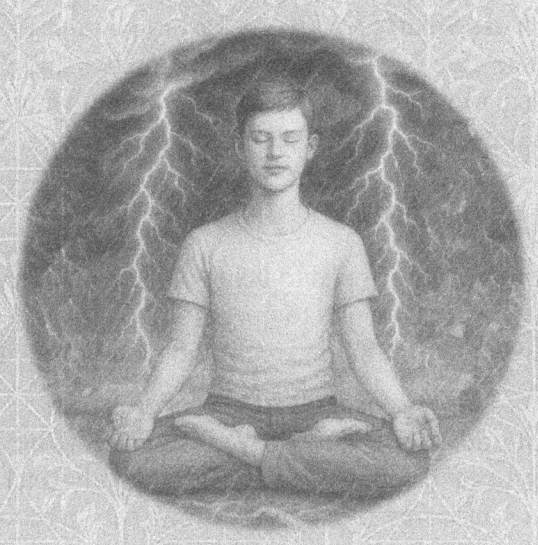

"Hope" is the thing with feathers -
That perches in the soul -
And sings the tune without the words -
And never stops - at all -

And sweetest - in the Gale - is heard -
And sore must be the storm -
That could abash the little Bird
That kept so many warm -

I've heard it in the chillest land -
And on the strangest Sea -
Yet - never - in Extremity,
It asked a crumb - of me.

~ "Hope" is the thing with feathers
  by Emily Dickinson

This chapter provides tools to shift your State, either rapidly in acute moments of dysregulation (Fast Override Strategies) or through ongoing practices that gradually improve your overall resilience and stability (Deep Override Strategies).

> **Fast Override Strategies** are quick interventions you can use immediately during moments of distress or dysregulation, such as breathing exercises, sensory grounding, or acupressure.

> **Deep Override Strategies** involve sustained practices—like meditation, regular exercise, nutritional adjustments, and somatic therapies—that expand your State Range, strengthen your nervous system, and help maintain long-term balance.

State Axis Questionnaire

Below is a questionnaire designed to help you determine your typical State patterns—whether you tend to operate in a Balanced (Positive) or Reactive (Negative) State, and how easily you shift between them.

You can also access a downloadable PDF version of the form as well as an interactive version by visiting the Mind Matrix Model website. You'll need to register if you haven't yet. You can sign up for free access by scanning the QR code or visiting this short link:

https://mmm.tips/state

The interactive form can be used to chart your progress over time, and includes many combination patterns that reveal more complex dynamics.

Instructions

For each question, choose the option (Rarely true, Sometimes true, Often true, Very true) that best describes your typical experience—not what you wish were true. Don't overthink it. Go with your first honest reaction.

Use a journal, notes app, or form field to track your responses.

If you are keeping a journal, this is a good time to write your responses down there so you can check up on how you're doing later. Otherwise just grab a piece of paper or a screen device to track your answers.

> **Note:** *This is not a medical test, but a self-reflection tool designed to help you explore approaches for improving your quality of life.*

1. When something stressful or disappointing happens:

A) I immediately go into worst-case thinking or emotional shutdown.
○ Rarely true=1   ○ Sometimes true=2   ○ Often true=3   ○ Very true=4

B) I stay grounded and respond with perspective.
○ Rarely true=1   ○ Sometimes true=2   ○ Often true=3   ○ Very true=4

C) I get thrown off at first, but I usually come back to myself pretty quickly.
○ Rarely true=1   ○ Sometimes true=2   ○ Often true=3   ○ Very true=4

D) I never know how I'll react—sometimes I collapse, other times I overreact.
○ Rarely true=1   ○ Sometimes true=2   ○ Often true=3   ○ Very true=4

2. When I'm under pressure:

A) I get overwhelmed, anxious, or numb.
○ Rarely true   ○ Sometimes true   ○ Often true   ○ Very true

B) I can handle stress without losing access to calm or clarity.
○ Rarely true   ○ Sometimes true   ○ Often true   ○ Very true

C) I get tense but can usually recover with a break or support.
○ Rarely true   ○ Sometimes true   ○ Often true   ○ Very true

D) I often feel like I'm holding it together until something small pushes me over.
○ Rarely true=1   ○ Sometimes true=2   ○ Often true=3   ○ Very true=4

3. When something unexpected disrupts my plans or rhythm:

A) I feel disoriented, frustrated, or thrown off for a long time.
○ Rarely true=1   ○ Sometimes true=2   ○ Often true=3   ○ Very true=4

B) I adjust pretty easily and move forward.
○ Rarely true=1   ○ Sometimes true=2   ○ Often true=3   ○ Very true=4

C) I might get flustered at first but usually adapt without much trouble.
○ Rarely true=1   ○ Sometimes true=2   ○ Often true=3   ○ Very true=4

D) I feel like my system can't find its footing again after I'm thrown off.
○ Rarely true=1   ○ Sometimes true=2   ○ Often true=3   ○ Very true=4

4. When I feel emotionally activated (angry, anxious, ashamed, etc.):

A) I lose perspective and it's hard to think clearly.
○ Rarely true=1   ○ Sometimes true=2   ○ Often true=3   ○ Very true=4

B) I can stay present with the emotion without getting lost in it.
○ Rarely true=1   ○ Sometimes true=2   ○ Often true=3   ○ Very true=4

C) I feel it strongly, but I can self-regulate fairly quickly.
○ Rarely true=1   ○ Sometimes true=2   ○ Often true=3   ○ Very true=4

D) I either get flooded or totally numb—there's not much in between.
○ Rarely true=1   ○ Sometimes true=2   ○ Often true=3   ○ Very true=4

5. When I reflect on how I've handled challenges this year:

A) I've often reacted in ways I regret or didn't feel in control of.
○ Rarely true=1   ○ Sometimes true=2   ○ Often true=3   ○ Very true=4

B) I've been able to stay relatively steady, even when things were hard.
○ Rarely true=1   ○ Sometimes true=2   ○ Often true=3   ○ Very true=4

C) I've had ups and downs, but I always found my way back.
○ Rarely true=1   ○ Sometimes true=2   ○ Often true=3   ○ Very true=4

D) I've felt unsteady or stuck in cycles I couldn't quite shift.
○ Rarely true=1   ○ Sometimes true=2   ○ Often true=3   ○ Very true=4

6. When I'm having a peaceful or joyful moment:

A) I often feel like something bad is about to happen.
○ Rarely true=1   ○ Sometimes true=2   ○ Often true=3   ○ Very true=4

B) I can let myself enjoy it and trust the experience.
○ Rarely true=1   ○ Sometimes true=2   ○ Often true=3   ○ Very true=4

C) I enjoy it but sometimes feel a little wary of it fading.
○ Rarely true=1   ○ Sometimes true=2   ○ Often true=3   ○ Very true=4

D) I don't really experience that kind of peace or joy very often.
○ Rarely true=1   ○ Sometimes true=2   ○ Often true=3   ○ Very true=4

7. When I feel overwhelmed or uncomfortable:

A) I distract myself with work, screens, or staying busy to avoid it.
○ Rarely true=1   ○ Sometimes true=2   ○ Often true=3   ○ Very true=4

B) I pause, feel what's happening, and respond intentionally.
○ Rarely true=1   ○ Sometimes true=2   ○ Often true=3   ○ Very true=4

C) I use things like walking, talking, or music to help shift.
○ Rarely true=1   ○ Sometimes true=2   ○ Often true=3   ○ Very true=4

D) I either ignore it completely or get lost in it without meaning to.
○ Rarely true=1   ○ Sometimes true=2   ○ Often true=3   ○ Very true=4

8. When strong emotions come up:

A) I shut them down or override them so I can keep going.
○ Rarely true=1   ○ Sometimes true=2   ○ Often true=3   ○ Very true=4

B) I allow the emotion to move through without taking over.
○ Rarely true=1   ○ Sometimes true=2   ○ Often true=3   ○ Very true=4

C) I feel it fully and then shift using grounding or breath.
○ Rarely true=1   ○ Sometimes true=2   ○ Often true=3   ○ Very true=4

D) I go between avoiding the feeling and getting overwhelmed by it.
○ Rarely true=1   ○ Sometimes true=2   ○ Often true=3   ○ Very true=4

9. When I get dysregulated/knocked off balance:

A) I stay stuck for hours or days before I can reset.
○ Rarely true=1   ○ Sometimes true=2   ○ Often true=3   ○ Very true=4

B) I notice it and can usually shift myself back fairly quickly.
○ Rarely true=1   ○ Sometimes true=2   ○ Often true=3   ○ Very true=4

C) I need time and tools, but I come back to baseline.
○ Rarely true=1   ○ Sometimes true=2   ○ Often true=3   ○ Very true=4

D) I either suppress it or spiral in it—it takes a lot of effort to return.
○ Rarely true=1   ○ Sometimes true=2   ○ Often true=3   ○ Very true=4

10. Overall, my internal climate (mood, energy, sense of safety):

A) Often feels heavy, tense, or disconnected, even on neutral days.
○ Rarely true=1   ○ Sometimes true=2   ○ Often true=3   ○ Very true=4

B) Feels steady, open, and responsive most of the time.
○ Rarely true=1   ○ Sometimes true=2   ○ Often true=3   ○ Very true=4

C) Fluctuates depending on stress, but I usually recover.
○ Rarely true=1   ○ Sometimes true=2   ○ Often true=3   ○ Very true=4

D) Feels fragile or easily disturbed—like I'm always managing something under the surface.
○ Rarely true=1   ○ Sometimes true=2   ○ Often true=3   ○ Very true=4

How to Score Your State Axis Questionnaire

Step 1: Tally Your Scores

- Go through your answers and total the points for each letter:

    Each time you rated an A, add the point value you selected (1 = Rarely True, 4 = Very True) to your A total.

- Do the same for B, C, and D responses.
    For example, if you answered Rarely true eight times, that would total 8, Sometimes true eight times would be 16, Often true eight times = 24, Very true eight times = 32.

Best to add this up on a separate piece of paper or in your journal.

Each letter will have a total between 10 (lowest) and 40 (highest).

Your Scores:

    A =   B =   C =   D =

Each letter represents a type of State pattern:

    A = Negative State dominant

    B = Positive State dominant

    C = Adaptive / temporary dysregulation

    D = State instability / fragility

Once you're done, proceed to the next section.

Step 2: Interpretation - Single Pattern

Find which pattern below matches your scores.

High A - Negative State Dominant / Collapse or Reactivity

This pattern is if your results include A 30 or above and B, C and D 20 or below.

You may be living in a chronic Negative State—where stress, shutdown, or overreaction are frequent defaults. You might feel foggy, tense, depleted, or stuck in worst-case thinking. This is often a sign that your system isn't getting the recovery time it needs, or that trauma has shaped your baseline State.

What to support: Daily override strategies (breath, grounding, regulation), safe physical practices, and building a slow return to trust in rest, joy, and perspective.

High B - Resilient State Range / Positive State Dominant

Read this if your results are B=30 or above and A, C and D=20 or below.

You live mostly in a grounded, flexible State. You're able to feel stress or emotion without being consumed by it, and return to center without force. Your Monarch likely stays online even when challenged.

What to support: Keep rhythms steady, continue emotional check-ins, and use your State stability to help regulate other Selves when needed.

Read: Ch. 5: Stress, Anxiety & Depression; Ch. 6: Working with Stress, Anxiety and Depression

High C - Adaptive but Stress-Sensitive State

Read this if your results are C=30 or above and A, B and D=20 or below.

You respond to stress with a degree of reactivity, but you have tools and awareness that help you recover. You may spend more time in the transitional zone between Positive and Negative State.

What to support: Strengthen pre-regulation habits (e.g., transitions, rest before burnout), and refine your ability to recognize early dysregulation signs. You're close to resilience—but may need to slow down more than you think.

Read: Ch. 5: Stress, Anxiety & Depression; Ch. 6: Working with Stress, Anxiety and Depression

High D - State Fragility / Instability

Read this if your results are D 30 or above and A, B and C 20 or below.

Your State may be easily tipped by internal or external triggers, and your system may not recover consistently. This suggests a narrow or reactive State Range, often formed by developmental trauma, chronic stress, or unrepaired shock. You might swing between shutdown and overload, or feel like your internal climate is hard to trust.

What to support: Rhythm, containment, relational repair, and practices that restore baseline safety over time (like orienting, bilateral movement, somatic co-regulation). This is not a failure—just a sign your nervous system needs more protection and pacing.

Read: Ch. 5: Stress, Anxiety & Depression; Ch. 6: Working with Stress, Anxiety and Depression

If none of your scores is 30 or more, choose the one that is the highest score. This indicates that you could have a more complex pattern that the interactive form on the website would reveal.

Optional Reflective Prompts

Use these to explore your results:

- What does it feel like in my body when I shift into the Negative State?
- What helps me come back?
- Which State pattern shows up most under relational stress? (Heart Self) Under physical exhaustion? (Vital Self) When obsessed or overwhelmed? (Head Self)
- What's one cue I could start noticing that says, "My State is shifting"?

Next Steps Based on Your Score

- **Inward-Focused:** Explore tools in **Inward-Focused State Pattern** on page 248, like grounding, heart-opening herbs, and expressive therapies.
- **Outward-Focused:** Go to the section **Outward-Focused State Pattern** on page 255. It includes supports such as boundary-toning remedies, reflective journaling, and grounding herbs or oils.

> **Balanced:** Jump to **Balanced Orientation** on page 261, with gentle adaptogens, secure attachment practices, and restorative rituals.

While it's not inherently unbalanced to lean more inward or outward, extreme tendencies in either direction or too much instability and bouncing between states can create challenges. In certain situations, having the flexibility to shift between inward and outward focus can be beneficial.

Additionally, as we'll explore in the state chapter, the farther out you are on this axis, the more vulnerable you may be to the Negative State and instability.

Understanding your position within the Heart Self can offer valuable insights into your social behaviors, emotional regulation, and interpersonal relationships, supporting your work toward a balanced state.

> *Note: While these questionnaires are a helpful tool for self-assessment, it's important to recognize that we may not always be the best judges of our own tendencies. Our perceptions can be influenced by biases or blind spots.*
>
> *To gain a more accurate understanding, it can be very helpful to have someone who knows you well—like a partner, close friend, family member, or colleague—answer the questions about you. Their perspective can provide additional insights and help paint a clearer picture of your social and emotional patterns.*

Shifting Your State

Your State, or more specifically your State Range, is the range that is normal to you—the overall climate your system is operating in between Oh yes! and Ouch!

Sometimes what you need is fast relief: a breath, a scent, a touchpoint that brings you back to the present. You may also decide you need a deeper rebalancing: changing your rhythms, feeding your system differently, or working with long-term patterns that shape how you respond to life. This chapter gives you both—short-term interventions and long-term strategies—to help you regulate your State and expand your State Range over time. Whether your system is frozen, agitated, scattered, or overwhelmed, the tools here are designed to help you shift your State.

Understanding State Loops

State Loops or just Loops, are recurring patterns that lock your system into a limited range of reactivity. Each Self has its own Loop, and these often reinforce one another.

We're going to spend an entire chapter going over Loops and how to get out of them using Overrides, but here we're going to lay out the groundwork of how these work and how to use some basic overrides to get out of a Loop.

> - **Vital Loop:** The body gets stuck in patterns of hyperarousal (fight/flight) or hypoarousal (freeze/shutdown), or bouncing between the two. This Loop often resists cognitive input and requires somatic (meaning body sensation level) intervention.
> - **Heart Loop:** Emotional overwhelm or withdrawal becomes repetitive. Feelings of shame, abandonment, or relational fear can dominate and spiral into social disconnection or dependency.
> - **Head Loop:** Overthinking, rigidity, rumination, or dissociation. Often reinforced by trying to "figure things out" while in a dysregulated (also known by its technical name, *discombobulated*) state.
> - **Cascading Loops:** One Self's dysregulation pulls others in. Example: an anxious body (Vital) triggers fear of abandonment (Heart), which then fuels catastrophic thinking (Head).

Breaking a Loop usually can be done by shifting the most activated Self first, or engaging the least activated Self to create leverage.

Working with Inward, Outward, and Balanced State Orientations

Your orientation—whether more inward, outward, or balanced—shapes how you regulate your State and how you respond to both stress and support. This isn't about personality type—it's about where your attention naturally goes under pressure and what strategies resonate most when you're trying to restore balance.

Inward-Focused State Pattern

When you're inward-focused, you tend to internalize experiences. You may pull away from external input to protect your system, but can get stuck in loops of overprocessing, emotional suppression, or physical shutdown. You may also feel overwhelmed by external demands and prefer internal safety or solitude, even when dysregulated.

When you're inward-focused, your system tends to pull inward under stress—into silence, collapse, mental loops, or freeze. Override strategies for this pattern should gently stimulate and support safe expression.

What to watch for:

› Collapsing inward during stress (freeze, fatigue, dissociation)

› Emotional processing without expression (overthinking, shame spirals)

› Difficulty reaching out or asking for help

Fast Overrides for Inward-Focused States

Energizing Breathwork

Stimulating breath (e.g., "breath of joy" or deep belly inhales with quick exhales) helps interrupt dissociation or internal collapse.

Sighing Out Breath + Stretch: Inhale deeply while raising arms overhead; exhale with a strong audible sigh while folding forward or shaking hands. Repeat 3x.

Voice Activation

Humming or softly vocalizing tones (e.g., "mmm," "om") helps stimulate the vagus nerve and move energy outward.

Try reading something aloud—preferably a poem, prayer, or affirmation that feels warm or grounding.

Object Focus Externalization

Hold and describe an object out loud: texture, color, memory. This helps externalize inner attention.

Bonus: Use a small object (stone, leaf, tool) and speak a wish, frustration, or truth into it—then place it somewhere visible.

Temperature Shift + Movement

> Splash cold water on your face or arms and immediately follow with brisk, rhythmic movement (e.g., shaking, marching in place, wrist rolls).
>
> Stimulates circulation and prevents energy from becoming stuck.

Connection Pings

> Send a short message to a safe person. Even a simple "thinking of you" or "can I share something?" reorients outward and invites co-regulation.

Deep Overrides for Inward-Focused Patterns

Movement-Based Expression

> Qigong or gentle yoga that includes reaching outward, twisting, and breath-coordinated movement.
>
> Aim for 10–20 minutes daily to reawaken body engagement and expressive potential.

Creative Externalization

> **Daily expressive journaling:** ("Here's what I'm feeling. Here's what I wish I could say.").
>
> **Visual arts:** paint, collage, or color—not to be good, but to externalize what's stuck.

Morning Activation Ritual

> Light candle, open window, and speak a one-word intention aloud. Then move for 2 minutes (even walking in place or shaking).
>
> This builds a habit of showing up visibly, even in small ways.

Co-Regulated Contact

> Plan brief, safe social contact before it's urgent—short calls, silent co-working, or voice note exchanges.
>
> Helps shift the loop from isolation into presence, without requiring full vulnerability.

Therapeutic Approaches

Somatic Experiencing (SE): Helps restore physical presence and boundary awareness through gentle tracking of body sensations and incomplete defensive responses.

Expressive Arts Therapy: Encourages emotional and relational self-expression through image, sound, and movement—especially helpful when verbalization feels difficult.

Internal Family Systems (IFS): Helps map and engage with internal voices, especially frozen or exiled parts that tend to dominate when inward-focused.

Group Therapy (with safety): Offers a structured relational field to explore safe externalization of internal states.

Diet and Nutritional Support

Warming, grounding foods: Soups, stews, root vegetables, cooked greens with ghee or olive oil.

Regular meals: Eat every 3–5 hours to prevent blood sugar dips that worsen fatigue or fog.

Spices: Use cinnamon, ginger, turmeric, or garlic to gently activate digestive and circulatory systems.

Morning protein: Stabilizes energy and anchors the Vital Self.

Nutritional Supplements

Vitamin B-complex (methylated): Supports energy metabolism and nervous system function, especially for fatigue + low drive.

Iron or ferritin check: Especially for menstruating individuals or those with anemia, as iron deficiency can mimic collapse, fatigue and cognitive fog.
Best form of iron is ferrous bisglycinate (also known as iron bisglycinate chelate)), which is well-absorbed and gentle on the stomach. For optimal uptake, take it with vitamin C.
Avoid ferrous fumarate and iron oxide—while they may raise blood iron levels, they are poorly utilized by the body and more likely to cause constipation or GI discomfort.

CoQ10 or NAD+: Support mitochondrial energy in cases of deep fatigue or burnout.

Adaptogens: Rhodiola or Asian ginseng (in small doses) can provide activating support if constitutional heat is low. Avoid if you have high anxiety.

Magnesium glycinate or threonate: Calms the nervous system without sedation; excellent for sleep and high reactivity. Magnesium threonate crosses into the brain easily, so it's better for neurological issues or sleep problems.

Herbs

Tulsi (Holy Basil): Gently uplifting and balancing; increases emotional clarity and supports energetic movement.

Eleuthero (Siberian ginseng): Activates core energy without pushing the system into overdrive.

Rose (petal or tincture): Opens the Heart, encourages receptivity, and gently softens suppression.

Milky oat seed: Restores depleted nerves after prolonged inward contraction.

Homeopathy

Pulsatilla: For gentle, inward types who become emotionally withdrawn, weepy, or fearful of rejection.

Silicea: For highly sensitive individuals who tend to hide or collapse inward under social or emotional stress.

Baryta Carbonica: For deep insecurity and social inhibition—particularly when there's fear of being seen.

Ignatia: For unresolved grief, emotional suppression, or feeling "stuck" internally.

Essential Oils

Sweet Orange: Gently energizing and uplifting; supports mood and confidence without overstimulation.

Ginger: Warming and vitalizing; useful when energy is low or somatic numbness is present.

Cinnamon: Gently stimulates the system and supports blood flow and focus.

Rose Otto: Softens emotional rigidity and helps bridge inwardness with relational receptivity.

Use oils in a diffuser or diluted on pulse points. Morning diffusion of sweet orange + ginger is ideal for lifting fog or inertia.

Acupressure Points

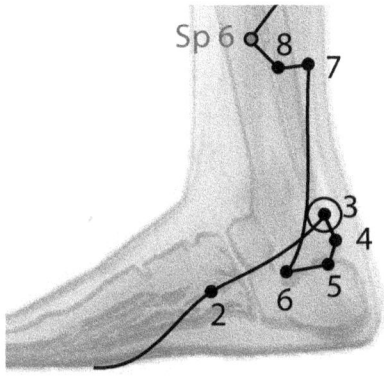

Kidney 3 (Taixi or Great Stream)

Purpose: Ki 3 strengthens the foundational energy of the body, supporting physical recovery, vitality, and emotional resilience. It is ideal for inward states of depletion, fatigue, and collapse.

Location: Inside of the ankle in the depression between the medial malleolus (inner ankle bone) and Achilles tendon.

How to Use: Apply steady pressure with your thumb for 1–2 minutes on each ankle. Breathe slowly as you press. Especially helpful in the morning or when energy is low.

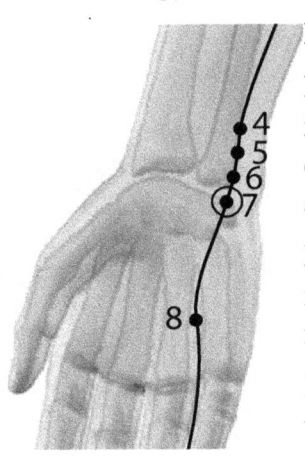

Heart 7 (Shenmen or Spirit Gate)

Purpose: Ht 7 calms the mind, soothes irritability, and reduces emotional agitation, especially during periods of high arousal or emotional suppression.

Location: On the inner wrist crease, at the radial (thumb) side of the tendon of the pinky finger.

How to Use: Apply gentle pressure with your thumb or fingertip, holding for 1–2 minutes on each wrist. This point helps ease mental tension and supports emotional stability and expression.

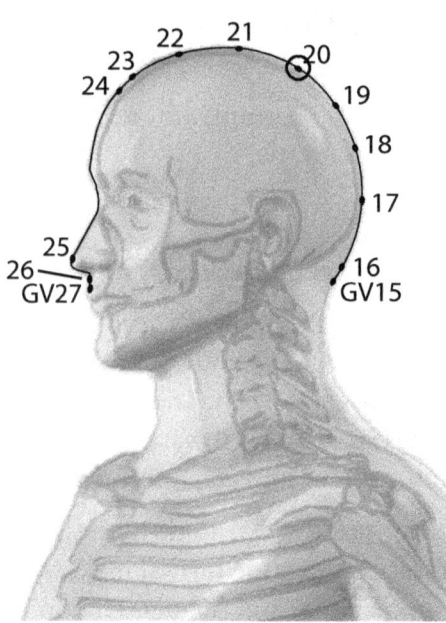

Governing Vessel 20 (Baihui or Hundred Meetings)

Purpose: GV 20 lifts energy upward when the system feels collapsed or foggy. It supports mental clarity, alertness, and reconnects the Vital and Head Selves.

Location: At the crown of the head, on the midline, approximately at the midpoint between the tips of the ears.

How to Use: Lightly tap or massage in a circular motion for 30–60 seconds. Especially useful when feeling heavy, low, or checked out.

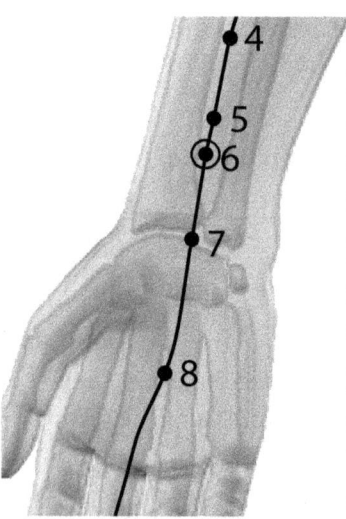

Pericardium 6 (Neiguan or Inner Gate)

Purpose: Calms anxiety, supports emotional circulation, and helps ease the grip of inward emotional entanglement. Excellent for bridging internal tension with external presence.

Location: Four finger-widths above the inner wrist crease, between the two tendons on the underside of the forearm.

How to Use: Massage gently with your finger or thumb in small circles for 1–2 minutes. Use during journaling, processing emotions, or before connecting socially.

Guided Meditation: "Breath as Bridge" (5–6 min)

This meditation helps gently re-engage the outer world through sensation and breath.

Begin in a seated or supported posture.

Close your eyes or soften your gaze.

Feel the ground beneath you. Let it hold you.

Inhale slowly…imagine breath rising like warm light through your chest.

Exhale gently…as if sighing into the world.

As you breathe, say inwardly:

"With each breath, I return to presence."

Bring awareness to the sounds around you. Noticing without flinching.

Bring awareness to your skin, your breath, your body in space.

Say inwardly:

"It's safe to be here. I am in the world."

End by opening your eyes and anchoring in your surroundings for 30 seconds.

Outward-Focused State Pattern

When you're outward-focused, your energy flows toward people, tasks, and external feedback. This can bring momentum and responsiveness—but under stress, it may lead to overstimulation, overcommitment, or avoidance of inner signals. You may seek distraction instead of introspection and swing into anxiety or burnout.

When you're outward-focused, your system scans the environment for input, stimulation, or reassurance. Under stress, this can become overextension, anxiety, or disconnection from inner cues. Override strategies for this pattern should focus on containment, boundary-building, and internal attunement.

What to watch for:

› Restlessness, overworking, or compulsive helping

› Avoiding quiet, alone time, or internal discomfort

› Emotional dysregulation from excessive social input

Fast Overrides for Outward-Focused States

Box Breathing + Hand on Heart

Inhale 4, hold 4, exhale 4, hold 4.
Do this with a hand over your chest or sternum. Feel containment.
Imagine the breath is smoothing the edges of your awareness inward.

Boundary Reset Touch

Sit with your back to a wall. Cross your arms or place one hand on opposite shoulders or thighs.
Repeat: "I'm here. This is my space."

Window-Gaze Pause

Look at something far away (out a window, down a hallway) for 30 seconds while breathing slowly. It signals your system that you are safe and don't need to track everything.

Drop the Anchor

Stand or sit. Inhale and press your feet into the floor. Exhale and imagine sending your awareness down through your body.
Use the cue: "Down, not out."

Stillness in Motion

Instead of pacing or spiraling outward, pick one intentional motion—like stirring tea, brushing hair, or organizing one drawer—and do it slowly. Containment in motion.

Deep Overrides for Outward-Focused Patterns

Reflective Rituals

Use a small journal structure daily: "What did I feel today?" / "What did I avoid?" / "What do I need?"
Build capacity for internal space by making it predictable and safe.

Digital Boundaries

Designate 1–2 hours daily as a no-screen zone. Use that time for rest, reading, or sensory grounding.

Containment Practices

Weighted blankets or compression wraps during downtime.
Structured reflection before bed: "What's mine? What can I release?"

Nature Anchoring

Visit the same place in nature once a week. Pay attention to how it changes. Let that mirror your own shifts—slower, cyclical, less reactive.

Outward-Focused State Pattern: Modalities and Approaches

When your system leans outward, it may orient to others, tasks, or stimulation for safety. Under stress, this can lead to overextension, reactivity, anxiety, or emotional dispersal. The goal is not to shut down your relational energy, but to strengthen your capacity for internal grounding, containment, and clear emotional boundaries.

Therapeutic Approaches

Polyvagal-Informed Therapy: Helps increase vagal tone and support co-regulation while reducing chronic sympathetic activation (fight/flight).

Dialectical Behavior Therapy (DBT): Strengthens emotional regulation and teaches boundary-setting without emotional suppression.

Mindfulness-Based Cognitive Therapy (MBCT): Combines cognitive tools with awareness practices to interrupt over-engagement and looping thoughts.

Narrative Therapy: Helps externalizers reorganize meaning and reduce emotional reactivity without losing relational flow.

Diet and Nutritional Support

Stabilizing, slow foods: Complex carbs (quinoa, root vegetables), warm grains, protein-rich snacks.

Reduce stimulants: Cut back on caffeine, sugar, and spicy or overly salty foods if you're feeling emotionally volatile.

Hydration focus: Especially for outward types who "forget" to nourish internally—room temperature or warm water preferred.

Regulation tip: Try herbal teas (tulsi, lemon balm, or reishi) in the afternoon or after social contact to slow momentum.

Eat sitting down: Don't multitask. Use meals as built-in slowing rituals.

Key Nutritional Supplements

Magnesium glycinate or threonate: Calms the nervous system without sedation; excellent for sleep and high reactivity. Magnesium threonate crosses into the brain easily, so it's better for neurological issues or sleep problems.

L-Theanine: Reduces sympathetic arousal while supporting mental focus; ideal during workdays or travel.

GABA precursors: For individuals prone to anxiety, over-talking, or racing thoughts. Precursors include Taurine, L-Theanine (also found in green tea).

Glycine: Works synergistically with GABA to calm the nervous system and improve sleep quality, especially in those who feel too "wired" to rest.

Omega-3 fatty acids (EPA dominant): Support mood regulation and decrease systemic inflammation linked to reactivity.

Vitamin B-complex: Especially important if you're burning energy fast without recharging adequately.

Herbs

Passionflower: Soothes mental and emotional overactivity, especially in extroverts with looping thoughts.

Skullcap (Scutellaria lateriflora): Grounds excess nervous energy without dulling awareness.

Reishi mushroom: Nourishes the Heart and slows the pace of reactivity, especially in socially sensitive individuals.

Holy Basil (Tulsi): Supports mood regulation and helps rebuild a healthy rhythm between giving and restoring.

Homeopathy

Phosphorus: For socially vibrant, empathic people who burn out easily or become overly open and porous.

Lachesis: For expressive types who suppress emotion until it bursts; helps regulate intensity and fear of emotional confinement.

Nux Vomica: For overachievers prone to anger, frustration, or collapse when pushed too far. Helpful for irritability masked by productivity.

Sulphur: For highly verbal, mentally overstimulated individuals who become scattered, exhausted, and irritable.

Gelsemium: For anticipatory tension and social performance anxiety.

Essential Oils

Vetiver: Deeply grounding, ideal for soothing overstimulation and helping the system return to inner awareness.

Sandalwood: Softens mental and emotional overactivity while promoting clear focus.

Patchouli: Reconnects attention to the body and encourages presence.

Myrrh: Brings energy downward and stabilizes emotional excess.

Frankincense: Enhances breath awareness and spaciousness in high-output minds.

Use these oils in evening baths, pre-sleep rituals, or diffused during solo time. Vetiver and sandalwood are especially helpful in quiet transitions (e.g., turning off devices).

Acupressure Points

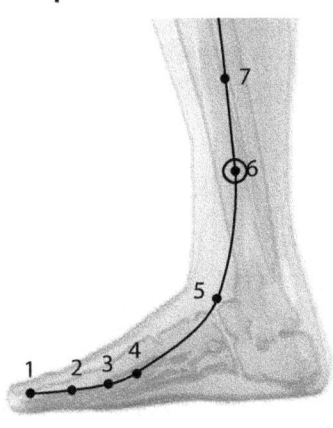

Spleen 6 (Sanyinjiao or Three Yin Intersection)

Purpose: Anchors the nervous system, reduces emotional reactivity, and harmonizes the Vital and Heart Selves. Especially helpful for tension that shows up as worry, over-efforting, or people-pleasing.

Location: On the inside of the lower leg, about four finger-widths above the inner ankle bone, just behind the shinbone.

How to Use: Apply firm, slow pressure for 30-45 seconds. Breathe deeply and allow tension to melt downward.

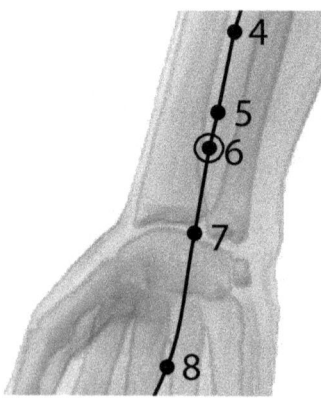

Pericardium 6 (Neiguan or Inner Gate)

Purpose: Supports emotional containment, helps reduce anxiety and emotional flooding from relational triggers.

Location: Four finger-widths above the inner wrist crease, between the tendons.

How to Use: Massage with slow, circular pressure. Use before challenging conversations or to calm post-social fatigue.

Kidney 1 (Yongquan or Gushing Spring)

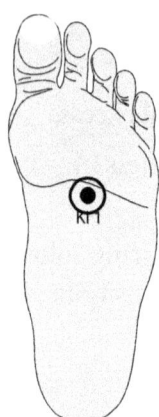

Purpose: Draws energy down from the head, calms agitation, and reconnects the body's lower energy centers—excellent for grounding extroverted overactivation.

Location: On the sole of the foot, one-third down from the base of the toes, between the ball of the foot and the center of the arch.

How to Use: Apply firm pressure with the thumb for 30–60 seconds, or rub in small circles. Use after long periods of social or mental stimulation.

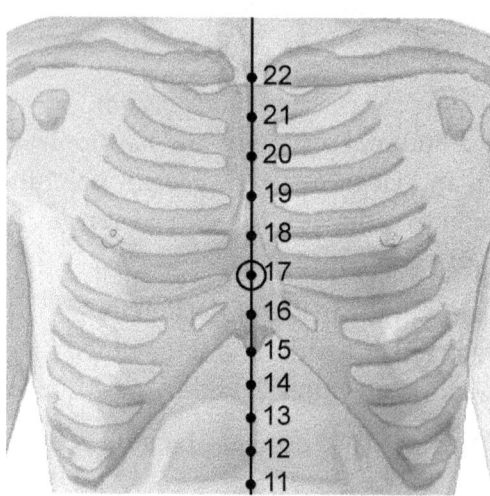

Conception Vessel 17 (Shanzhong or Chest Center)

Purpose: Opens the chest, calms emotional urgency, and restores balance to outwardly activated Heart energy.

Location: At the center of the sternum, midway between the nipples.

How to Use: Place the palm over the point and take 3–5 deep breaths. This works well as a settling practice after speaking or social over-engagement.

Guided Meditation: "Return to Center" (7 min)

This practice helps outward-focused individuals slow down and re-anchor attention inward.

Sit or lie down with eyes closed. Place your hands over your heart or belly.

Feel the contact. Feel your breath move beneath your hands.

Inhale for 4…exhale for 6.

As you breathe, say inwardly:

> *"My center is here."*

Let your awareness slowly gather from outside—social roles, digital noise, things undone.

Call it back.

> *"Return."*

Visualize your breath like soft light, gathering threads of attention and weaving them gently inward.

Let the outer world recede just for now. Let yourself belong to yourself again.

Close with three grounding breaths. When ready, open your eyes and pause before re-engaging.

Balanced Orientation

If you scored evenly across State responses or tend to fluctuate fluidly, you likely have a balanced orientation—able to go inward or outward as needed. But even balanced types have blind spots. Your task is often about maintaining rhythm, not over-extending into either extreme.

Balanced individuals can access both inward and outward strategies—but risk losing center when pulled too far in either direction. Overrides here should focus on maintenance, micro-adjustments, and subtle regulation rhythms.

What to watch for:
- Subtle tipping into over-adapting (pleasing, over-attuning)
- Losing personal rituals or boundaries under external pressure
- Overestimating your regulation capacity and skipping recovery

Fast Overrides for Balanced Orientation

3-Breath Integration

Breath 1: Feel your feet (Vital Self)

Breath 2: Feel your heart/chest (Heart Self)

Breath 3: Observe your thoughts (Head Self)

Let the Monarch step in and name what's most active.

Shoulder Reset + Still Point

Roll shoulders forward and back 3x.

Then place one hand on your sternum and pause. Breathe. Listen inwardly: "Am I too far out or too far in?"

Self-Check Affirmation

Say out loud: *"What do I need?"* then listen for the first sensation—not answer—your body gives. Use it as your compass.

Switch Anchor

If you're over-activated, place hands on thighs and exhale.

If you're shut down, rub your hands together or lightly tap your chest until energy returns.

Environment Tune-Up

Shift lighting, sound, or scent. Small sensory edits can reorient your State quickly.

Deep Overrides for Balanced Patterns

1. Rhythmic Rituals

Maintain daily check-in routines: morning intention, midday breath or walk, evening reflection.

Don't wait for disruption—regulate in advance.

2. Adaptogenic Support

Use herbs like eleuthero, rhodiola, or holy basil to support flexibility across fluctuating demands.

These herbs support balance without sedation or stimulation.

3. Mixed-Mode Practices

Alternate expressive (talking, journaling) with integrative (breath, meditation) modalities.

Try a weekly combo like yoga + journaling + mindful cooking.

4. Seasonal Adjustments

Track what throws you off: weather, daylight shifts, sleep changes. Create seasonal toolkits (e.g., light therapy in winter, hydration in summer) to protect your baseline.

5. Symbolic Anchors

Use a meaningful object or image that represents center and coherence. Keep it visible. Touch or look at it daily.

Balanced Orientation State Pattern: Modalities and Approaches

If you have a balanced State orientation, you likely shift with some ease between inward and outward focus. But balance doesn't mean immunity—over time, external demands, accumulated micro-stressors, or subtle dysregulation can wear away your resilience. You may find yourself pulled into over-adaptation, subtle self-abandonment, or quiet depletion. The goal is maintenance, micro-correction, and rhythm, not perfection.

Therapeutic Approaches

Mindfulness-Based Cognitive Therapy (MBCT): Strengthens the reflective capacity of the Head Self while maintaining awareness of emotional and somatic cues.

Craniosacral Therapy: Gently supports subtle shifts and clears held tension in high-functioning systems with quiet dysregulation.

Hakomi Therapy: Integrates mindfulness with somatic awareness and memory processing; ideal for clients who appear well-regulated but struggle with depth shifts.

Relational Therapy: For those who struggle to assert needs while appearing adaptable; this approach supports clarity and congruence in boundary repair.

Diet and Nutritional Support

Cycle-based nourishment: Align meals with your daily rhythm—lighter meals when energy is high, denser meals when slowing down.

Mood-supportive foods: Include omega-3s, leafy greens, and foods rich in tryptophan and magnesium (e.g., seeds, bananas, legumes).

Anti-inflammatory baseline: Limit refined oils and excessive dairy or gluten if they subtly affect your energy or mood.

Stabilizing hydration: Warm teas or mineral broths in the evening can soothe the system without sedation.

See the Next Steps Chapter 22 - Dietary Guide for more information.

Key Nutritional Supplements

Magnesium glycinate or threonate: Gentle support for sleep, tension, or emotional drift. Magnesium threonate crosses into the brain easily, so it's better for neurological issues or sleep problems.

B-complex with methylated B12 and folate: Maintains stable mood and energy across daily State transitions.

Adaptogenic blends: Support subtle flexibility and prevent low-grade burnout—ashwagandha + rhodiola is a good balance blend.

L-Tyrosine (when depleted): Supports dopamine pathways if motivation or cognitive stamina begin to decline.

See the Next Steps chapter, Nutritional Supplements Guide, for more info.

Herbs

Holy Basil (Tulsi): Restorative and emotionally balancing—good for maintaining middle ground and navigating mild overwhelm.

Lemon Balm: Calms emotional noise without sedating; supports reflective processing.

Rhodiola: Increases adaptability and mental clarity under mild strain.

Milky Oat Seed: Nourishes resilience and rebuilds nervous system tone during cumulative stress.

Homeopathy

Calcarea carbonica: For those who carry hidden inner tension under calm exteriors—useful when groundedness gives way to stuckness or overwhelm.

Natrum Muriaticum: Supports emotional openness and fluidity when emotional self-protection hardens.

Phosphorus: Helps maintain openness and empathic flow when sensitivity starts tipping into depletion.

Ignatia: Use when balanced individuals hit a sharp emotional rupture and can't fully "get over it."

Sulphur: For mental overactivity that begins to pull attention away from embodiment.

Essential Oils

Frankincense: Supports deep breathing and quiet integration; balances all three Selves and promotes inner reflection.

Clary Sage: Helps regulate emotional fluctuations, especially when pulled between focus modes.

Lavender: Stabilizes nervous system without dulling clarity—ideal for end-of-day wind-down.

Cedarwood: Strengthens boundaries and helps restore energy without overly sedating.

Use oils in daily transitions—waking, working, decompressing, and sleep. Rotate weekly to avoid habituation.

Acupressure Points

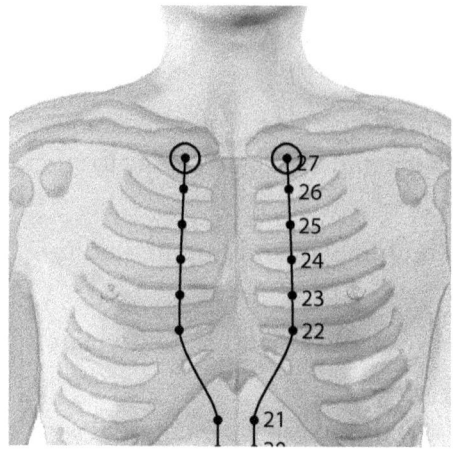

Kidney 27 (Shufu or Shu Mansion)

Purpose: Opens chest, regulates breathing, and helps reset rhythm between inward and outward shifts. Especially useful when emotional energy feels subtly stuck or unexpressed.

Location: Just below the clavicle on either side of the sternum, near the shoulder joints.

How to Use: Massage gently in a circular motion for 30–60 seconds while breathing into the chest.

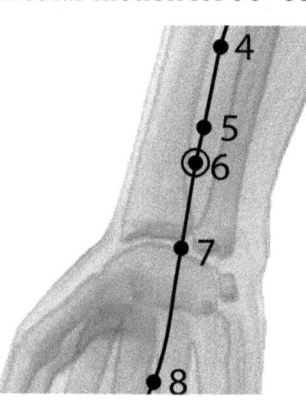

Pericardium 6 (Neiguan or Inner Gate)

Purpose: Balances emotional circulation and nervous system tone—especially helpful for people who tend to stay "in the middle" until they suddenly drop.

Location: Four finger-widths above the inner wrist crease, between the tendons.

How to Use: Hold gently for 1–2 minutes or rub in small circles.

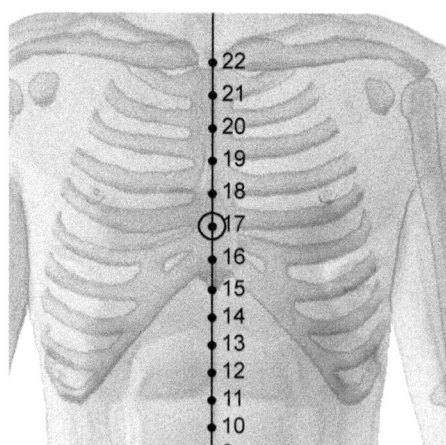

Conception Vessel 17 (Shanzhong or Chest Center)

Purpose: Opens emotional flow and helps reconnect you to intention, especially when you've gone too long without centering.

Location: At the center of the sternum, four finger-widths from the bottom of the sternum.

How to Use: Press gently while breathing slowly into your chest. Use with affirmations or during guided intention-setting.

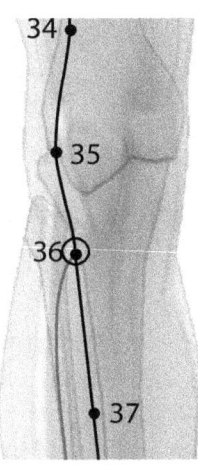

Stomach 36 (Zusanli or Leg Three Miles)

Purpose: Restores vitality and mental clarity; balances energy and supports mood when mildly depleted or subtly dysregulated.

Location: Four finger-widths down from the bottom of the kneecap, one finger-width lateral to the shinbone.

How to Use: Press deeply and firmly for 30 seconds to 1 minute. Excellent morning point or midday reset.

Guided Meditation: "Rhythm Within" (6–7 min)

This meditation strengthens awareness of your internal rhythm so you can return to center before imbalance accumulates.

Sit comfortably. Place one hand on your belly, the other on your chest.

Close your eyes and breathe slowly. Inhale 4…exhale 6.

Feel your breath as a wave. Let it rise and fall.

Now ask: "What part of me is leading right now?" Vital…Heart…Head?

Don't fix it—just notice.

Inhale:

"I'm listening."

Exhale:

"I'm returning."

Imagine a slow pulse beating at your core—not rushed, not still.

Let it guide you to your natural pace.

Stay here, breathing with your rhythm, for a few more moments.

When ready, open your eyes and ask:

"What would nourish my rhythm today?"

Integrating Your Orientation with Your State Pattern

These orientations aren't static—they shift based on context and level of dysregulation. In the Positive State, your natural orientation becomes a gift. In the Negative State, it can become a trap. For example:

- An inward-focused person in the Positive State becomes reflective, intuitive, and centered. In the Negative State, they may collapse inward and isolate.
- An outward-focused person in the Positive State is engaged, vibrant, and attuned. In the Negative State, they may become frantic, reactive, or scattered.
- A balanced person in the Positive State can fluidly respond to any moment. In the Negative State, they may feel pulled in too many directions and lose coherence.

The goal isn't to become one type or another—but to build awareness and flexibility across all three.

Final Thoughts: You Can Shape Your State

State is not fixed. It is fluid, dynamic, and responsive to what you do, how you relate, and what you believe is possible. The idea that "this is just how I am" is often a product of repeated dysregulation, not a truth about you.

You don't need to control every thought or perfectly balance your system to heal. You only need enough awareness to notice when you're shifting off-center, and enough self-compassion to try something different.

Override Strategies aren't shortcuts or bypasses—they're invitations. Each breath, each grounding point, each reflective practice is a door that leads you back to yourself. Sometimes the door is small. Sometimes it's hard to find. But it's always there.

The more familiar you become with your personal State Range, the more you'll recognize the early signs of contraction—and the more options you'll have to return to coherence. Over time, these micro-adjustments accumulate into lasting change. This is how State becomes not just a reaction, but a terrain you learn to inhabit wisely.

You don't have to feel good to begin.

You just have to begin.

Chapter Fifteen

Balance Between the Selves

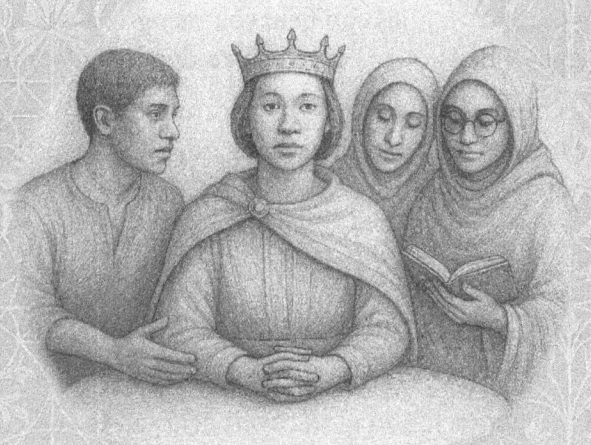

*Your inner world
   is not a thing,
   but a becoming*

*Not a fixed picture,
   but a dance
   by the many kinds of you—*

*Those that you know,
Those you know well,
and those you do not, yet*

~ The Self
   by Sam McClellan

Integration vs. Domination

In the Mind Matrix Model, balance between the Vital Self (safety), Heart Self (comfort), and Head Self (integrity) is essential for a stable, adaptable mind.

However, there are times when one or two Selves dominate the third, either reinforcing each other in the Positive State (based on values and strengths) or in the Negative State (driven by fear, avoidance, or aggression).

Understanding these dynamics can help you recognize when your system is in balance versus when you're being overridden by one or more Selves.

As the conscious mind, the Monarch's role is to serve as a wise council leader attuning to each Self, and preventing any single one from overriding the others out of fear or urgency.

When the Selves Work in Balance

In a healthy state, the Three Selves operate in dynamic equilibrium, adjusting to circumstances without completely overriding one another.

> **Vital Self** provides a foundation of physical safety and energetic regulation.
>
> **Heart Self** ensures connection, empathy, and emotional balance.
>
> **Head Self** guides integrity, logic, and thoughtful decision-making.

Example: You're asked to take on a major project at work. Your Vital Self assesses whether you have the energy, your Heart Self considers the relational dynamics of saying yes or no, and your Head Self determines if it aligns with your long-term goals.

If all three Selves are in balance, you can make a grounded decision.

The Positive State Qualities of the Three Selves

When balanced, each Self contributes to a thriving, healthy mindset:

> **Vital Self → Safety & Resilience**: A sense of groundedness, energy regulation, and physical security.
>
> **Heart Self → Comfort & Connection**: The ability to form healthy relationships, experience joy, and navigate emotions effectively.

Head Self → Integrity & Clarity: The capacity for rational thinking, ethical decision-making, and maintaining perspective.

In the Positive State, the Three Selves support each other, creating a flexible and responsive approach to life.

The Negative State Qualities of the Three Selves

When in the Negative State, each Self manifests a primary form of imbalance:

Vital Self → Fear: Fight-flight-freeze responses, hypervigilance, survival-driven reactions.

Heart Self → Shame: Rejection sensitivity, social withdrawal, people-pleasing, self-worth issues.

Head Self → Rigidity/Distortion: Overanalyzing, obsessive thoughts, paranoia, catastrophizing, black-and-white thinking.

Why Rigidity or Distortion?

The Head Self determines our view of reality, based on the internal model of reality we are running. In the Positive State, the Head Self offers clarity, perspective, and integrative thinking. It flexibly moves between detailed analysis and broad insight. But in the Negative State, it can become imbalanced in one of two directions—either overly analytic or overly holistic—losing the ability to adapt, reflect, or access truth clearly.

Analytic Mode Imbalance (Overthinking, Rigid Logic, Control)

This mode narrows awareness, focusing excessively on structure, logic, and dissection. It can lead to:

Overanalyzing: Obsessing over details, second-guessing every decision, and getting stuck in loops of "figuring it out."

"If I can just understand every angle, I'll finally feel safe."

Rationalization: Using logic defensively to justify actions or beliefs that don't align with deeper values.

"I know it's not ideal, but here's why it makes sense..."

Black-and-White Thinking: Reducing reality into extremes—right or wrong, good or bad—without room for nuance.

"Either I succeed or I'm a failure."

Catastrophizing: Projecting the worst-case scenario based on logical projection, often fueled by internal fear.

> "This one mistake means everything will fall apart."

Paranoia and Hypervigilance: Constructing complex interpretations where threat or betrayal is imagined in innocent cues.

> "They haven't replied—something must be wrong."

Holistic Mode Imbalance (Diffuse, Overly Symbolic, Unbounded)

This mode sees patterns and possibilities, but without grounding, it can slip into confusion or magical thinking:

Magical Thinking: Believing that thoughts, symbols, or synchronicities are inherently predictive or causal.

> "I thought about her this morning, and she texted, so I must be psychic."

Over-Association: Drawing overly broad or emotionally charged connections between unrelated things.

> "This always happens when I wear this color. It must be bad luck."

Spiritual Bypass: Using abstract or spiritual concepts to avoid grounded emotional work or conflict.

> "It's all just energy, so I don't need to feel my anger."

Loss of Boundaries Between Ideas: Everything blends into everything else—difficulty organizing thoughts, prioritizing, or communicating clearly.

> "I just have this big feeling and can't explain it—but everything feels connected and overwhelming."

Idealization: Seeing people, situations, or ideologies in an overly romanticized light, ignoring flaws or risks.

> "They're perfect! They just get me, even though we barely know each other."

Restoring Balance in the Head Self

When the Head Self is balanced, it uses both Analytic Mode and Holistic Mode as tools, each supporting the other. A flexible Head Self can both structure ideas clearly and see patterns and meaning, grounding imagination with reason and softening rigid logic with insight.

When Two Selves Override the Third

Imbalances happen when two Selves reinforce each other while suppressing the third. This can occur in both the Positive State (driven by values and strengths) or the Negative State (driven by fear and survival instincts).

Vital + Heart Overriding Head (Integrity)

Positive State Pattern: Grounded Empathy

You prioritize connection and physical well-being over rigid rule-following.

> *Example: You might take a spontaneous vacation despite work obligations, valuing relaxation and connection.*

Negative State Pattern: Fearful Avoidance

You suppress your voice to avoid conflict, even when integrity matters.

Fear (Vital Self) + Fear of rejection (Heart Self) = Avoiding confrontation even when integrity (Head Self) says to speak up.

> *Example: Staying silent about an ethical concern at work due to fear of job loss and social rejection.*

Head + Heart Overriding Vital (Safety)

Positive State Pattern: Purposeful Sacrifice

You push past physical discomfort to serve a higher cause—prioritizing ideals and social responsibility over personal comfort.

> *Example: Activists, teachers, or leaders often push through exhaustion to serve a greater cause.*

Negative State Pattern: Rational Override

You ignore your body's signals to meet perceived obligations or social pressure—rigid logic (Head Self) + Social pressure (Heart Self) = Ignoring physical limits.

> *Example: Pushing yourself to complete work despite exhaustion because you feel responsible and don't want to let others down.*

Head + Vital Overriding Heart (Comfort)

Positive State Pattern: Strategic Focus

You emphasize discipline and objectivity, setting aside emotional distractions—prioritizing discipline and rationality over emotional indulgence.

> *Example: A scientist or strategist might focus solely on objective reality, dismissing emotional distractions.*

Negative State Pattern: Detached Survival

You cut off from emotional needs or relationships to focus on efficiency or control—survival instincts (Vital Self) + Rational detachment (Head Self) = Neglecting emotional needs or relational dynamics.

> *Example: A person making a financial decision that prioritizes efficiency and survival, even if it damages their relationships.*

> ## Catching the Override in Real Time
>
> Sometimes the override happens before you realize it. Here are quick "tells" and in-the-moment questions to help bring awareness back to center:
>
> **You feel physically exhausted but still say yes** → Ask: *"What does my Vital Self need right now?"*
>
> **You're about to apologize—again—but feel resentful inside** → Ask: *"Is my Heart Self overriding my integrity?"*
>
> **You've been working for hours and suddenly feel shaky or numb** → Ask: *"Has my Head Self forgotten my body?"*
>
> **You're going silent instead of raising a concern** → Ask: *"What would each Self say if it had a voice here?"*
>
> Let the Monarch pause and call a council. Even a few seconds of curiosity can shift your course.

Restoring Balance Between the Selves

Recognizing when two Selves are dominating can help restore balance:

Vital Self Needs Support? Check in with your body. Are you ignoring rest, nutrition, or basic needs?

Heart Self Needs Support? Acknowledge emotions and relational needs. Are you withdrawing, suppressing, or over-accommodating others?

Head Self Needs Support? Engage critical thinking and reflection. Are you making impulsive choices based on fear or emotional discomfort?

The key to balance is *integration*—allowing all three Selves to inform decisions without any single one taking over. By regularly checking in with all three, you ensure that your boundaries, decisions, and emotional health remain in harmony.

As the conscious mind, you the Monarch play a key role in this balance. *You must learn to act not as a judge, but as a skilled facilitator—listening to the needs of each Self without letting any single one dominate out of urgency or fear.* By returning to this reflective center, you can avoid being pulled off course by reactive dynamics and instead allow all three Selves to participate meaningfully in your decision-making.

For addressing specific Self, state, or anxiety issues, consult the appropriate chapter for deeper exploration and practical techniques.

Modalities for Rebalancing the Selves

Different healing modalities are more effective depending on which Self is most imbalanced. Here's a quick reference guide:

Self Most Affected	Best-Suited Modalities	Focus
Vital Self	Somatic therapies, breathwork, acupuncture, massage, TRE (Tension/Trauma Release Exercises), movement practices (yoga, qigong, tai chi)	Restore energy balance, process trauma held in the body

Self Most Affected	Best-Suited Modalities	Focus
Heart Self	Emotion-focused therapy, Internal Family Systems (IFS), expressive arts therapy, safe group work, attachment repair, EMDR (for relational trauma)	Rebuild trust, co-regulation, emotional expression, boundaries
Head Self	Cognitive-behavioral therapy (CBT), narrative therapy, mindfulness-based cognitive therapy, psychoeducation, inquiry work (e.g., The Work by Byron Katie)	Shift rigid thought patterns, integrate multiple perspectives, restore cognitive flexibility

Many approaches address more than one Self. The key is to notice where the imbalance lives and choose methods that speak to that layer of the Self.

Guided Meditation: The Council Within

This meditation helps you reconnect to all three Selves and invite them into inner harmony.

Begin by finding a comfortable position, sitting or lying down. Let your breath arrive slowly, without trying to change it. Just observe.

Bring your awareness to your body — your muscles, your posture, the weight of gravity. This is the home of your Vital Self.

Ask gently: *"What do you need right now to feel safe?"*

Listen. It may speak through sensations — tightness, calm, a desire to stretch or rest.

Now shift your attention to your heart center — the chest, the throat, the subtle emotions underneath your day. This is your Heart Self.

Ask: *"What are you feeling right now? What do you need to feel loved, connected, or understood?"*

Simply witness what arises, without judgment.

Finally, bring your focus to your mind — your thoughts, your inner commentary, your imagination. This is the Head Self.

Ask: *"What thoughts are looping or loud?"*

Then ask: *"What truth is trying to emerge beneath them?"*

Now picture all three Selves — Vital, Heart, and Head — coming together in a circle, like trusted advisors around a table. You are the Monarch, the reflective center.

Imagine them sharing gently. Each speaks in turn. Each is heard. No one is silenced or overpowered.

Let the council rest in quiet presence. Let your breath anchor you as their wisdom integrates.

When you're ready, thank each Self. Gently open your eyes, and bring that sense of balance with you.

Affirmation:

I honor each part of me—body, heart, and mind—and lead with compassion, clarity, and balance.

Selves Balance Homework: Know Your Cues

"Before you can shift your state, you have to recognize where you are."

Each of your three Selves has different signals when it's in the Positive State (balanced) or Negative State (dysregulated). Learning to recognize these early cues gives you the power to respond rather than react.

Use this worksheet to track what each Self looks and feels like for you in both states.

Vital Self – Body & Energy

Your Vital Self speaks through sensation and physical behavior. This table helps you recognize how your body communicates when you're thriving versus when you're in survival mode. Tuning into these cues is often the first step in restoring balance.

State	Body Sensations	Energy Levels	Physical Behaviors
Positive State (thriving, balanced)	e.g., relaxed jaw, deep breaths	e.g., steady, calm, energized	e.g., fluid movement, restful sleep
Negative State (tense, survival mode)	e.g., clenched stomach, shallow breath	e.g., wired or exhausted	e.g., restlessness, collapse, poor sleep

Heart Self – Emotion & Connection

The Heart Self reveals itself through emotional tone, relationships, and internal dialogue. This table outlines what connection and disconnection look like in your system, helping you identify when you're emotionally open—or when you're reacting from hurt.

State	Emotional Tone	Relational Cues	Self-Talk
Positive State (open, connected)	e.g., gratitude, warmth	e.g., enjoying company, feeling seen	e.g., "I'm enough," "I can handle this"
Negative State (hurt, reactive)	e.g., shame, resentment	e.g., avoiding people, over-apologizing	e.g., "They don't care," "I messed up again"

Head Self – Thought & Perception

The Head Self reflects how you think, focus, and make meaning. This table shows the difference between flexible clarity and distorted loops, making it easier to catch when your thoughts are helping—or hijacking—your sense of perspective.

State	Thought Patterns	Focus Style	Internal Narratives
Positive State (clear, balanced)	e.g., flexible, creative	e.g., steady, big-picture	e.g., "Let's try this," "There's more than one way"
Negative State (rigid, distorted)	e.g., looping, worst-case	e.g., scattered or hyperfocused	e.g., "Nothing will work," "It's all on me"

Integration Prompts

Once you've identified how each Self shows up in both Positive and Negative States, it's time to bring that awareness into real life. These prompts help you reflect on your patterns, catch early cues before they escalate, and notice which override dynamics tend to run the show. Use them as a weekly check-in—or anytime you feel out of sync.

Which Self do you notice most easily? _____

Which cues do you tend to miss until it's too late?

_____

What's one early cue you'll watch for this week in each Self?

Vital: _____

Heart: _____

Head: _____

Which of the override combinations (Vital + Heart, Head + Heart, Head + Vital) feels most familiar to you? How has it shown up in your life recently? Put a check by the one, or if more than one, number them by importance from least to most.

Vital + Heart: _____

Head + Heart: _____

Head + Vital: _____

Matching Cues to Override Strategies

"Once you recognize a cue, the next step is knowing what to do with it."

Now that you've identified what Positive State and Negative State look like in your Vital, Heart, and Head Selves, use this worksheet to match those states with override strategies that help you shift.

Choose one or two override tools for each Self. These can be physical, emotional, cognitive, or relational — the goal is to restore balance in the Self that's struggling.

Vital Self Override Plan

Your body is usually the first to signal that you're slipping into a Negative State—but it's often the easiest to ignore. This section helps you spot physical cues early and choose a simple override strategy to shift your energy or calm your system. These don't need to be dramatic—sometimes a few deep sighs or a walk outside can change everything.

Cue You Noticed	Negative State Reaction	Override Strategy
e.g., jaw tension, shallow breath	*e.g. feeling wired but tired*	*e.g. 3 deep sighs + brisk walk outside*

Other Override Options:
- Shaking out limbs
- Acupressure: Ki1, Sp6
- Warm bath or cold rinse
- Grounding in nature
- Yoga, tai chi, qigong, or slow stretching
- Breath: 4–7–8 or box breathing

Heart Self Override Plan

When the Heart Self tips into shame, fear, or disconnection, it can feel overwhelming—or like you're disappearing. This table helps you name emotional cues and relational reactions, then match them with tools that bring comfort, connection, and presence back online.

Cue You Noticed	Negative State Reaction	Override Strategy
e.g., wanting to hide or over-apologize	*e.g., Shame spiral or social shutdown*	*e.g., Call a safe person + 5-min heart meditation*

Other Override Options:

- Eye contact with a trusted person
- Soothing voice self-talk ("I see you, I've got you")
- Journaling or writing a letter to your younger self
- Physical affection (hug, hand on heart)
- Singing or toning with emotional release
- Co-regulation: sitting quietly near someone calm

Head Self Override Plan

The Head Self can spiral quickly—whether into loops, catastrophizing, or complete shutdown. This section helps you track the early signs and apply gentle cognitive or creative resets. Sometimes, interrupting a loop is as simple as doodling, reframing, or naming what's true.

Cue You Noticed	Negative State Reaction	Override Strategy
e.g., thought loops or catastrophizing	*e.g., "Nothing will work" spiral*	*e.g., 5-minute focus shift + doodling patterns*

Other Override Options:

- 5-sentence reality check ("What are 5 facts I know?")
- Mind map a challenge with colors or shapes
- Reframe: "What would I say to a friend?"
- Movement + music to disrupt rigid focus
- Read or listen to something beautiful or inspiring
- Tapping or bilateral stimulation (e.g., EMDR, butterfly hug)

> The **Butterfly Hug** *is a simple self-soothing technique often used in trauma therapy (like EMDR) to promote emotional regulation and a sense of safety.*
> *How to do it:*
> *Cross your arms over your chest so that each hand rests on the opposite upper arm or shoulder—like forming butterfly wings.*
> *Gently tap one side, then the other, in a slow, alternating rhythm (left–right–left–right).*
> *Breathe slowly as you do this, allowing your nervous system to settle. It's commonly used to help people ground themselves during emotional distress or to integrate positive experiences.*

Integration Journal Prompt

After experimenting with different override strategies, it helps to reflect on what actually worked—and why. Use this prompt to track your wins, notice patterns, and fine-tune your responses over time. The more you understand what shifts you, the easier it becomes to choose it again.

Which override strategy helped most this week — and why do you think it worked?

Final Thoughts: The Art of Inner Alignment

Each of your Three Selves—Vital, Heart, and Head—has its own rhythm, its own wisdom, and its own impulse to protect you. Sometimes that protection looks like collapse; sometimes it looks like overdrive. The Vital Self might freeze—or it might charge forward in a panic. The Heart Self might retreat into shame—or overextend itself in pursuit of connection. The Head Self might go silent and foggy—or spin up into overanalysis and control.

This is the dance of imbalance—not one of failure, but of adaptation. These Selves step up when they believe they must take the wheel, often because the others have gone offline or the system has entered the Negative State.

But healing is not about suppressing these impulses—it's about listening to them, honoring them, and helping them work *together*.

Integration happens when:

    The Vital Self knows when to rest *and* when to rise.

    The Heart Self knows how to feel deeply *and* how to express clearly.

    The Head Self knows when to analyze *and* when to let go.

Balance isn't about keeping everything equal. It's about *relational intelligence* within yourself—understanding when one Self needs to lead and when it needs to yield. It's about helping the overprotective Head Self loosen its grip, supporting the flooded Heart Self with containment, and calming the overactive Vital Self without silencing its instincts.

When these Selves stop competing and start collaborating, you begin to operate from a deeper kind of wisdom—the kind that adapts, rather than reacts. This is the role of the Monarch: not to control with force, but to guide with clarity and trust.

You are not meant to live in one mode. You are meant to move between them with grace.

And every time you recognize a loop, use an Override, or simply pause and re-center—you're practicing that grace.

Balance isn't a static destination. It's a living, responsive practice. And the more you walk this path, the more your system learns to walk with you.

Chapter Sixteen
Loops and Overrides

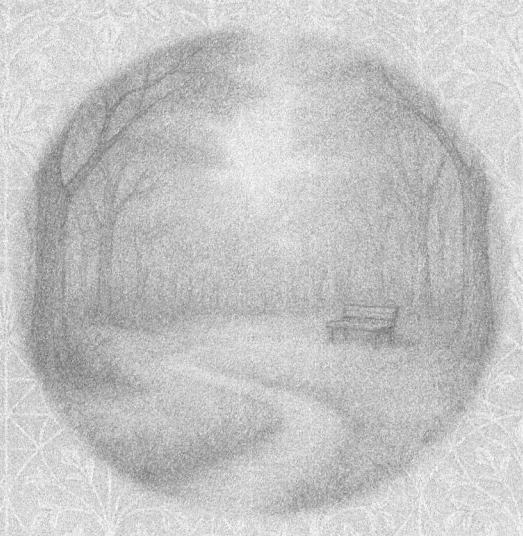

*Be patient toward all that is unresolved in your heart
and try to love the questions themselves,
as if they were locked rooms or books written
in a foreign language.*

*Do not seek the answers now.
They cannot be given to you
because you would not yet be able to live them.*

*The task is to live everything.
Live the questions now.
Perhaps, gradually, without even noticing,
you will live your way into the answer.*

~ Rainer Maria Rilke
  from Letters to a Young Poet, Letter Four

Introduction: The Power of Loops and Overrides

A Loop is a self-perpetuating pattern of thought, emotion, or behavior that reinforces itself, often making it feel inescapable. Some Loops are short-term and habit-based, while others are trauma-driven, deeply wired into the nervous system. Loops can feel like fate—repeating cycles that define who you are or how life works. But in truth, they're just patterns. And patterns can be changed.

Overrides are interruptions to Loops, helping to break automatic patterns and shift states. While mild Loops can often be overridden quickly, trauma-based Loops require deeper interventions, as they originate from survival-based responses. Once you identify the Loop, you can begin to match it with the right kind of override: breathing, movement, a boundary, a reframing.

Over time, this practice of interrupting and rerouting Loops builds something powerful: State flexibility. Instead of being dragged from one reaction to the next, you begin to choose. You recover faster. You gain perspective. And eventually, you rewrite the pattern altogether.

This chapter explores different types of Loops, how trauma influences them, and offers tools for effective overrides for the Self most affected.

Differentiating General Loops from Trauma-Based Loops

Not all Loops are trauma-based. Some are habitual and reinforced by culture, while others are nervous system imprints from past experiences.

General Loops (Conditioned, Non-Trauma-Based)

Culturally Reinforced Loops:

> Productivity addiction → Overworking → Burnout → Repeat
>
> Social media dopamine cycles → Craving → Checking → Brief relief → More craving

Cognitive Habit Loops:

> Procrastination → Avoidance → Increased stress → More procrastination
>
> Overthinking → Mental exhaustion → Difficulty deciding → More overthinking

Overrides for General Loops:
Behavioral disruption
Changing routines to break automatic responses

Behavioral disruption targets the Loop at the level of habit and external triggers. It's about interrupting patterns before they can run their course.

Examples:

- Turning off notifications for social media to stop doom-scrolling or comparison Loops.
- Taking a different route home to avoid environmental cues linked to stress responses.
- Switching your morning sequence—shower before breakfast instead of after—to create novelty and shake loose rigid momentum.
- Moving your workspace to a new location when stuck in a productivity or procrastination Loop.
- Setting a "pattern breaker" alarm mid-day to check in: "Am I Looping right now?"

Cognitive Reframing

Challenging distorted beliefs that reinforce the Loop.

Cognitive reframing helps the Head Self pause and reassess what story is being told—and whether it's still true or helpful. You may find at first that a part of you rebels at the "lie" of reframing something in a positive way (pushback), but that will pass if you persist.

Examples:

- Instead of "I always mess things up," try: "That didn't go how I wanted, but I'm learning and adjusting."
- Using the phrase "I'm having the thought that…" to create distance from a Looping narrative.
- Replacing "This always happens" with: "What are three times this *didn't* happen?"
- Asking yourself: "What would I say to a friend with this thought?"
- Practicing spectrum thinking: "Where am I on a scale of 1–10 right now, and what would a 5 look like?"

Somatic Reset

Moving the body to create a new physiological state.

When a Loop is reinforced by your internal state—tense, collapsed, frozen—changing that state physically helps the whole system shift.

Examples:

- Shaking out your limbs or bouncing on your heels to release built-up adrenaline.
- Doing 3 rounds of 4–7–8 breathing (in for count of 4, hold for 7, out for 8) to activate the parasympathetic nervous system.
- Going for a 10-minute walk, especially in nature, to shift both body and perception.
- Holding a cold object (ice cube, metal spoon) to ground out of dissociation or rumination.
- Lying on your back with legs up a wall to reset the nervous system if overwhelmed or drained.
- Doing 1–2 minutes of yoga, tai chi, gentle Qigong, or stretching to integrate body, breath, and awareness.

Trauma-Based Loops (Autonomic Nervous System Imprints)

Vital Self Loops (Survival-Based Patterns):

Overarousal Loops: Hypervigilance → Anxiety → Startle response → More hypervigilance

Shutdown Loops: Numbing → Avoidance → Isolation → More numbing

Heart Self Loops (Shame & Attachment-Based Patterns):

Shame Loops: Self-criticism → Withdrawal → Social isolation → Reinforced shame

Fawn Response Loops: Over-apologizing → Over-accommodating → Feeling drained → More fawning

Head Self Loops (Rigid Thought Patterns):

Obsessive Loops (Analytic Mind): Overanalyzing → Decision paralysis → Fear of mistakes → More overanalyzing

Conspiratorial Loops (Holistic Mind): Seeing hidden patterns → Paranoia → Disbelief in all information → Reinforced distrust

Overrides for Trauma-Based Loops:

For Vital Self hyperarousal: Vagus nerve activation, grounding techniques, acupressure.

> **Description:** When the Vital Self is locked in anxiety or fight-or-flight, the body stays on high alert. This Loop may include racing thoughts, muscle tension, irritability, or panic.
>
> **Support Strategies:** Activate the vagus nerve through breathwork (e.g., 4-7-8 or humming), engage in grounding techniques like cold water on the hands or 5-4-3-2-1 sensory tracking (see the sidebar on the next page), or use acupressure (See Points for Calming High Anxiety/Arousal on page 133).

For Vital Self body-level depression or shutdown: Slow, gentle movement, breathwork, nature to increase engagement.

> **Description:** This freeze response results in collapse, dissociation, or numbness. You may feel disconnected, foggy, or unable to initiate action.
>
> **Support Strategies:** Use slow, gentle movement (e.g., rocking, swaying), breath practices including deep breaths which, while difficult at first, antidote the freeze response, or nature-based re-engagement (sunlight, walking barefoot) to bring Vital energy back online.

For Heart Self shame-based Loops: Self-compassion, co-regulation, journaling.

> **Description:** These Loops are driven by feelings of unworthiness, internalized rejection, or harsh self-judgment. Often rooted in early relational trauma, they erode the Heart Self.
>
> **Support Strategies:** Practice self-compassion techniques (e.g., hand on heart with soothing phrases), co-regulation (e.g., spending time with someone with whom you are emotionally attuned), or expressive journaling to externalize the shame story and rewrite it with empathy.

For Heart Self fawn response Loops: Boundary-setting practice, assertiveness training, body awareness.

> **Description**: This Heart Self response to perceived threat involves chronic people-pleasing, over-accommodation, or loss of personal boundaries to avoid conflict or disapproval. Rather than fighting, fleeing, or freezing, the Heart Self tries to maintain connection by minimizing its own needs. It is often a survival adaptation to early relational danger.
>
> **Support Strategies**: Use boundary-setting scripts and assertiveness exercises to rebuild autonomy. Practice saying "no" in low-stakes settings and track bodily sensations of guilt or anxiety that arise. See *Chapter 19 - Setting Healthy Boundaries* for more.

For Head Self obsessive Loops (Analytic mode dominant): Cognitive defusion, structured flexibility exercises.

> **Description**: The mind becomes stuck in repetitive thinking—often trying to find certainty, solve unresolvable problems, or control perceived threats. The Head Self is overactivated, often to avoid emotion or uncertainty.
>
> **Support Strategies**: Use **cognitive defusion** techniques where you step back from your thoughts by labeling them (e.g., "I'm having the thought that..."), scheduled "worry time" (a limited 15 minute period each day to focus on your worries), or structured flexibility practices like choosing random variations in routine to disrupt rigidity.

For Head Self conspiratorial Loops (Holistic mode dominant): Reality-testing, widening perspectives.

> **Description**: These Loops form around mistrust, suspicion, or a perceived need to uncover hidden truths. Often rooted in betrayal trauma or prolonged dysregulation, they can involve patterns of black-and-white thinking, projection, or narrative control especially when the Head and Heart Selves are in protective overdrive.
>
> **Support Strategies**: Use **reality-testing exercises** (e.g., "What are five alternative explanations?"), and practice **widening perspective** by exposing yourself to multiple viewpoints, grounding in present-moment context, and inviting input from trusted, regulated voices. Restoring nuance and flexibility helps soften the rigidity and fear driving the Loop.

5-4-3-2-1 Sensory Tracking

This is a great Fast Override that is included in this section, but is really a helpful grounding tool for all Selves and State.

This classic grounding technique helps you exit a Loop by anchoring your awareness in the present moment through your five senses.

How to Do It:

Slow down. Take a deep breath. Then name aloud or silently:

5 things you can see
(Look around. Notice color, shape, movement, contrast.)

4 things you can touch
(Feel your clothing, the chair beneath you, your breath in your hands.)

3 things you can hear
(Internal or external—your breath, ambient sounds, background noise.)

2 things you can smell
(If nothing stands out, notice the absence—or inhale something nearby.)

1 thing you can taste
(A sip of tea, the aftertaste in your mouth, or just awareness of your tongue.)

Why It Works:

Each Self gets something it needs:

*The **Vital Self** grounds in body-based, physical input.*

*The **Heart Self** softens through gentle redirection and safety signals.*

*The **Head Self** is invited out of abstraction into concrete experience.*

Use it when you feel unmoored, overwhelmed, or trapped in a repeating thought-emotion Loop. It's simple, portable, and powerful.

***Tip:** If you can't access all five senses, just do what you can. The goal is presence, not perfection.*

How Each Self Experiences Loops and Overrides

Vital Self Loops & Overrides

When the Vital Self is stuck in a Loop, it often plays out as physical or energetic dysregulation. These Loops are rooted in the body's instinctive survival responses—fight, flight, freeze—and tend to bypass conscious thought altogether. They may show up as tension, hypervigilance, restlessness, numbness, or collapse. Because these Loops live in the body, somatic overrides are essential.

Fight/Flight Loops

Pattern: Hyperawareness → Startle response → Overreactions → More hyperawareness

These Loops emerge when the nervous system is stuck in high gear. You may feel jumpy, irritable, unable to settle, or like you're always on edge. Even small stimuli (a noise, a facial expression, a change in tone) can set off a cascade of physiological and emotional reactivity.

Override Strategies:

- **Grounding exercises** – Feel your feet on the floor, press your palms together, or hold a weighted object. These send safety signals to the body.
- **Breathwork** – Use calming breath patterns such as 4–7–8 or long exhales (e.g., inhale for 4, exhale for 6–8) to signal a downshift in arousal.
- **Bilateral stimulation** – Cross-crawl tapping, EMDR butterfly hug, or rhythmic walking help reset the nervous system and reorient you in the present moment.

Freeze Loops

Pattern: Dissociation → Avoidance → Emotional numbness → More dissociation

Freeze Loops occur when the body responds to overwhelm or helplessness by shutting down. You may feel disconnected from your body, exhausted, spacey, or unable to take action—even though you want to. The Loop deepens as inaction leads to more shame, inertia, or collapse.

Override Strategies:

- **Sensory activation** – Use temperature (cold water, scented oils), textured objects, or stimulating music to gently wake the system.
- **Movement** – Start with small, rhythmic actions like swaying, stretching, or rocking to begin thawing the freeze. Avoid intense exercise initially—it can feel too jarring.
- **Vagus nerve stimulation** – Try humming, chanting, gargling, or long vocal exhalations to engage the parasympathetic system from the bottom up and encourage safe re-engagement.

Heart Self Loops & Overrides

When the Heart Self becomes dysregulated, Loops often revolve around relational insecurity—especially shame, people-pleasing, or emotional withdrawal. These Loops tend to reinforce negative beliefs about worth, connection, and belonging. Since the Heart Self operates relationally, many of the most effective overrides involve compassion, boundaries, and co-regulation.

Shame-Based Loops

Pattern: Feeling unworthy → Withdrawing → Confirming negative beliefs → More withdrawal

This Loop begins when a moment of perceived rejection, failure, or disconnection activates internalized shame. You might start pulling back from others, telling yourself you're too much—or not enough. That withdrawal deepens the story that you don't belong, making it harder to reach out or show up authentically.

Override Strategies:

- **Self-compassion practices** – Try placing a hand over your heart and saying: "This is hard, but I am still worthy." Use phrases that soften your inner tone.
- **Reframing core beliefs** – Gently question the narrative: "Is it true that I'm unlovable…or am I in a shame Loop?"
- **Co-regulation** – Seek out safe, affirming connection (a text, eye contact, being near someone calm) to help reset the Heart Axis from outside in.

Fawn Response Loops

Pattern: People-pleasing → Resentment → Exhaustion → More people-pleasing

This Loop arises when the Heart Self bypasses its own needs to maintain perceived safety or approval. You say yes to avoid conflict or rejection, but then feel depleted or unacknowledged. Instead of addressing the imbalance, the pattern reinforces itself—more pleasing, less presence.

Override Strategies:

- **Small boundary-setting practices** – Start with "micro-no's," like "I'll need to think about that" or "Not today." Practice with people you feel safest with.
- **Track resentment** – Use it as a signal: "Where did I abandon myself here?"
- **Daily check-ins** – Ask, "What do I need emotionally today that I might be bypassing?"

Head Self Loops & Overrides

Head Self Loops arise when cognition becomes rigid, distorted, or hyperactive. These Loops can emerge from either mode of thinking—analytic or holistic—and often involve the Head Self trying to impose control on discomfort or ambiguity. Over time, they disconnect you from clarity, presence, and perspective.

Obsessive Loops (Analytic Mind)

Pattern: Fixation on details → Fear of imperfection → Paralysis → More fixation

This Loop often shows up as perfectionism, overanalysis, or the inability to "let it go." It may feel like you're just being thorough—but really, the Head Self is trying to manage fear through excessive control. The more you focus, the more overwhelmed you become.

Override Strategies:

- **Cognitive flexibility training** – Try choosing between two "good enough" options without optimizing. Or practice letting someone else make the decision.
- **Thought labeling** – Say, "I'm noticing a perfection Loop" to break identification.

- **Creative interruption** – Doodle, collage, or do a 5-minute "messy draft" to disrupt precision pressure.

Conspiratorial Loops (Holistic Mind)

Pattern: Hyperconnection of patterns → Distrust of sources → More isolation → Reinforced paranoia

This Loop stems from overextended holistic thinking—linking symbols, meanings, and events in ways that feel intuitive but increasingly distorted. It often emerges when emotional vulnerability (especially betrayal) hasn't been metabolized. Trust is replaced with vigilance, and nuance collapses into certainty.

Override Strategies:

- **Critical thinking exercises** – Ask: "What evidence would disprove this belief?" or "What's another possible explanation?"
- **Perspective widening** – Intentionally expose yourself to differing, non-threatening viewpoints (e.g., memoirs, documentaries, dialogue).
- **Restore safety first** – When mistrust is active, cognitive interventions work better after some grounding or Heart Self regulation.

Recognizing Your Loop & Choosing an Override

Step 1: Identify Your Dominant Loop

- Are your Loops physiological (body-based)? → Vital Self override needed.
- Are your Loops emotional and relational? → Heart Self override needed.
- Are your Loops cognitive and belief-driven? → Head Self override needed.

Step 2: Select the Right Override

Fast Overrides: Good for mild Loops (e.g., cold exposure, deep breathing, bilateral tapping).

Deep Overrides: Needed for trauma-based Loops (e.g., DBR, EMDR, memory reconsolidation, somatic therapy).

Strengthening the Override System for Long-Term Change

How to Make Overrides More Effective Over Time

- **Consistency is key:** Small, repeated overrides train the nervous system to shift states more easily.
- **Override stacking:** Combining techniques enhances effectiveness (e.g., movement + breathwork + cognitive reframing).
- **Self-awareness practice:** Tracking triggers and state shifts builds better override intuition.

Reflection Question:

Which Loop do you notice most in your life? What is one override technique you can try today?

Final Thoughts: Breaking Free from Automatic Patterns

As stated above, Loops can feel like fate—repeating cycles that define who you are or how life works. But in truth, they're just patterns. And patterns can be changed.

Breaking free doesn't require perfect awareness or instant transformation. It begins with noticing: *Am I in a Loop? Which Self is Looping? What's the thought, feeling, story or sensation that keeps pulling me back?*

Once you identify the Loop, you can begin to match it with the right kind of override: a breath, a movement, a boundary, a reframe.

Over time, this practice of interrupting and rerouting Loops builds something powerful: State flexibility. Instead of being dragged from one reaction to the next, you begin to choose. You recover faster. You gain perspective. And eventually, you rewrite the pattern altogether.

This chapter has offered tools to understand and override Loops at the level of the Vital, Heart, and Head Selves. But Loops don't just live in sensation, emotion, or thought—they're also shaped by symbols. The metaphors we carry. The meanings we assign. The mental maps we live inside.

In the next chapter—***Symbols as the Architects of Perception***—we'll explore how symbols silently shape your reality, how distorted or inherited symbols reinforce negative Loops, and how conscious symbolic work can become a profound tool for transformation and healing.

Chapter Seventeen

Symbols as the Architects of Perception

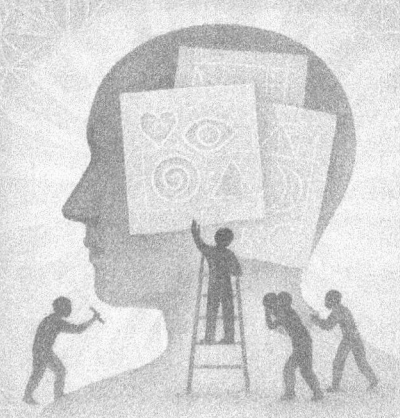

*To see a World in a Grain of Sand
And a Heaven in a Wild Flower,
Hold Infinity in the palm of your hand
And Eternity in an hour.*
~ Excerpt from Auguries of Innocence
 by William Blake

Introduction: The Power of Symbols

Symbols shape our perception, influencing how you experience the world on conscious and unconscious levels. Whether a national flag, a personal memento, or an archetypal image from mythology, symbols act as shortcuts for meaning, triggering emotional, cognitive, and physiological responses.

While symbols exist externally, their true power comes from the meaning we attach to them, and this attachment is shaped by our personal experiences, cultural conditioning, and unconscious associations.

This chapter explores how symbols influence each Self, how trauma can cause symbols to trigger automatic Negative State shifts, and how conscious engagement with symbols can shape perception and State regulation, greatly improving your lived experience.

How Symbols Influence Each Self

Vital Self: Physical & Instinctual Reactions to Symbols

The Vital Self interprets symbols on a deeply physiological level, often bypassing conscious awareness. Symbols associated with safety or threat can trigger immediate bodily responses through the fight, flight, or freeze mechanisms.

Here are some examples:

- **Safety:** The warmth of sunlight on skin or the scent of baking bread may create an instant sense of well-being, signaling the body that all is well.
- **Threat:** A flashing emergency light, the sound of yelling, or even the sterile white of a hospital hallway may cause the Vital Self to contract or brace—sometimes before you even know why.
- **Grounding:** The weight of a familiar blanket or the repetitive sound of ocean waves can signal "safe to rest," gently activating the rest promoting parasympathetic nervous system.
- **Activation:** A ringing bell before a performance or the sound of a whistle before a race can mobilize energy, activating a readiness state on the Vital Axis.

Heart Self: Symbols as Emotional & Experiential Anchors

The Heart Self assigns meaning to symbols through personal experiences, social bonds, and emotional associations. These symbols often become anchors for connection, memory, or belonging. They can carry both comforting and painful emotional weight, and may differ drastically from person to person based on relationship history.

- **Relational Symbols:** A worn-out sweater from a lost loved one, a wedding ring, or a child's drawing taped to the fridge can each become a portal to connection and emotion.
- **Experiential Symbols:** A surfer's board isn't just a tool, it's an emotional extension of their identity and freedom. A musician might hold the same connection to a particular guitar.
- **Cultural Symbols:** A flag in a window may trigger a sense of safety and belonging for some, while evoking discomfort or fear for others based on their social context.
- **Triggers:** The sight of a Thanksgiving dinner table may invoke a feeling of warmth and safety, but for someone estranged from their family it may evoke sadness or shame, rather than warmth.

Head Self: Symbolic Processing in the Analytic & Holistic Minds

The Head Self processes symbols through meaning-making, but how it does so depends on whether the Analytic Mode or Holistic Mode is dominant.

Analytic Mode:

- Breaks down symbols into categories or historical context.
- Uses symbols to explain, reference, or label rather than evoke.
- Often filters out emotional or unconscious resonance.

    Example: A historian studying a coat of arms might focus on its heraldic structure and time period rather than its meaning to the person who wore it.

    Example: A scientist may view the ouroboros (a snake eating its own tail) as an outdated alchemical symbol, missing its metaphorical depth.

Holistic Mode:
- Perceives symbols intuitively, as metaphors or archetypes.
- Sees relationships between symbols across domains—dreams, art, personal mythologies.
- Pulls symbolic meaning from sensation, emotion, and pattern more than fact.

  Example: The image of a spiral may evoke a sense of growth, recursion, or spiritual evolution without needing to define it.

  Example: A dream of a key might be understood not just as access, but as inner readiness for transformation—something "unlocking" within.

Symbols, Trauma, and State Shifts

Symbols can become trauma triggers when they are associated with negative past experiences. A traumatic event imprints meaning onto a symbol, turning it into an automatic State activator.

> **Example:** A person who experienced rejection as a child may react strongly to symbols of exclusion (e.g., a closed door, an ignored text message), instantly shifting into Negative State shame or withdrawal.

Media, propaganda, and cultural conditioning can use symbols to reinforce fear-based States.

> **Example:**
> News outlets, political campaigns, or even advertising can repeatedly associate specific colors, music, or imagery with fear, danger, or threat. A flashing red alert banner with dramatic music on a news channel can become a conditioned symbol of crisis, even when the content is mundane. Over time, exposure to this kind of symbolic pairing can trigger a subtle but chronic Negative State, keeping the nervous system in low-level vigilance, anxiety, or division.

Personal symbolic associations can unknowingly keep someone in chronic emotional loops.

> **Example:** A person struggling with self-worth may unconsciously surround themselves with symbols of failure (unfinished projects, reminders of past mistakes), reinforcing the Negative State.

Media Saturation & Symbolic Overload

The unconscious—especially the Vital and Heart Ministers—often can't tell the difference between real and symbolic threats. When we're constantly exposed to fear, anger, and emotionally charged images in the news, on social media, or on entertainment media our nervous system stays on high alert.

Even if the Head Self understands it's "just a show" or a dramatic headline, the Vital Self may still react as if it's a real threat. The Heart Self can also respond emotionally—feeling fear, sadness, or anger—even when we know, logically, that what we're seeing isn't happening to us directly.

Over the past seventy years, our experience of the world has changed. First came radio, then television, then cable TV, and now the internet. These changes didn't just bring more information, they changed the way we take in the world. Today, we're surrounded by symbols, sounds, and images designed to grab our attention and keep us watching.

I like to describe this as a shift from "the world at large" being based on our own first-hand experience to a version of reality that's shown to us, *mostly through screens*. In contrast, our actual lived environment has become what I call "the world at small," playing a smaller and smaller role in shaping what we perceive as real.

Our focus—and with it, our sense of environment and reality—has shifted from the local world around us to an artificial reality shaped by media. And that reality is designed primarily around the needs of large corporations that need to engage us, and keep us engaged, in order to make money.

The Advent of Agony Advertising

As television took hold in the mid-20th century, advertising quickly evolved from simple product announcements to highly emotional, psychologically driven messaging. Advertisers realized they weren't just selling goods—they were selling identities, solutions, and feelings. This gave rise to what in the advertising business is called **agony advertising**: a strategy where the viewer's discomfort is deliberately triggered—through fear, shame, or insecurity—and the product is then offered as the cure.

It was no longer just "here's what this product does," but "here's what's wrong with you or your life without it."

This model works by creating a quick, sharp Negative State trigger activating the Vital Self's sense of threat, or the Heart Self's fear of rejection or failure. The Head Self, now unsettled, looks for resolution, and the commercial provides it. *You're too old, too heavy, too tired, too poor, too out of step, not good enough in some way, and this skin cream, cool car, or laundry soap will fix it.* Even happiness was reframed as something needing external purchase.

Over time, commercials began using emotionally charged music, symbolic imagery, and fast-paced edits to bypass rational thought and speak directly to unconscious vulnerabilities. The goal wasn't to inform, it was to create a moment of discomfort just long enough to tell you that buying would make you feel better.

News As Manipulation

News has increasingly utilized the same tools as advertising in order to capture and keep our attention.

Before the late 1960s, news was seen as a public service. The "Big Three" TV networks—ABC, CBS, and NBC—aired short news programs with minimal advertising. The goal was to inform, not entertain.

That changed in 1968 with the launch of 60 Minutes, a weekly news magazine show that mixed storytelling with journalism. It was a hit. Soon other networks followed, and news began to turn into entertainment that made money.

Then came cable television. More channels meant more competition. In 1980, CNN introduced 24-hour news. But with nonstop coverage came a new problem: if viewers got bored, they could just change the channel. To prevent that, networks started making stories feel more urgent using dramatic music and visuals, fast-paced reporting, and emotional commentary. This approach was called sticky programming because it made viewers want to keep watching.

But from a nervous system perspective, it wasn't just overstimulating, it was addictive. The constant novelty, urgency, and emotional charge hijacked our attention systems and trained our minds to seek more of the same, even when it left us anxious or drained.

The internet made competition even more intense. In 1992, there were only around 50 websites; by the year 2000, there were over 17 million.

More and more, people were turning to the web instead of television. Social media followed, giving everyone a voice—but also overwhelming us with opinions, images, and emotional content. Suddenly, anyone could act like a news source, and the competition for attention exploded.

To stand out in the noise, many media outlets shifted toward opinion-based news. Fox News led this trend in the late 1990s, and by 2002, it had passed CNN in ratings. This new style of news focused less on facts and more on emotion, identity, and outrage. *It didn't just report what happened, it told you how to feel about it.* This model kept viewers glued to the screen, but it came at a cost: it increased division, reactivity, and symbolic overload.

The result is our current society, where more and more we are turning against our fellow citizens and voting for the people who most trigger us.

The High-Stimulation Trap: How Media Rewires Our Attention and State

Most modern media is designed to be activating. Fast cuts, flashing graphics, dramatic sound cues, and emotionally charged content don't just keep us engaged, they keep us activated and triggered.

From a nervous system standpoint, this means we're spending more time in a state of subtle (or not-so-subtle) fight-or-flight activation. Over time, this constant stimulation changes how our brain functions. It shortens attention spans, weakens our ability to stay with slower or subtler experiences, and leaves us more easily distracted and restless.

Neurologically, for many of us it raises the Vital Self's baseline arousal level, which makes us more prone to anxiety, emotional reactivity, and difficulty regulating our State.

We start to crave the very kind of stimulation that's dysregulating us—more drama, more violence, more action—without realizing what we've lost in the process.

As discussed in Chapter 6, *Stress, Anxiety, and Depression*, chronic stress often leads to anxiety. And the higher the anxiety level, the more uncomfortable it becomes to slow down and release that stress. Instead, we turn to coping strategies—most often distraction or suppression. Media in its current form offers both.

The Nervous System and Symbolic Overload

Dysregulating, overly dramatic media doesn't just share ideas, it uses symbols to trigger emotional reactions. It repeats powerful images, phrases, and voices that feel important, even if the actual meaning is unclear. These symbols can overwhelm the nervous system.

- The Vital Self responds to loud voices, fast cuts, and dramatic visuals as if they are urgent or involve real danger, activating the body's fight-or-flight response.
- The Heart Self reacts to the emotional tone of the story, getting caught up in feelings of fear, anger, grief, or belonging.
- The Head Self, overwhelmed by the flood of information and its effect on the Vital and Heart Selves, may shut down, go rigid, or fall into black-and-white thinking.

Over time, this constant flood of emotional content reshapes how we relate to the world. A hat, a flag, or a news headline may no longer feel like a symbol of an idea. They feel like a signal of who is safe and who is not, who is "us" and who is "them."

This is symbolic overload. It's not just too much information, it's too many emotional triggers happening too fast, bypassing our ability to reflect or respond calmly. Our systems become trained to react rather than reflect. ***The result is more fear and hate, more division, and more disconnection from ourselves and from each other.***

We are living in what is arguably the safest time in human history, and people feel more mortal fear than ever. It's not right.

The Media Diet

As I said, our perception of the world around us has gone from being entirely based on what we perceive in our local world, to being mostly an artificial reality based on the larger world portrayed in our screens.

Along with that, the Selves—primarily the Vital Self—are constantly tracking the perceived level of threat.

If your overall experience of the world is that it's filled with danger and threats, your nervous system will orient more toward danger. It will become much more vulnerable to the Negative State even if most of that information and experience is coming through a screen.

When Symbols Rewrite Culture – The Fiji Television Study

In the late 1990s, a striking real-world experiment unfolded on the island of Viti Levu, Fiji, offering one of the most vivid demonstrations of how symbols introduced through media can rapidly reshape cultural norms and personal health.

The Study:

Led by medical anthropologist Dr. Anne Becker, researchers examined what happened when television was introduced to Fijian society for the first time in 1995. Traditionally, Fijian culture had celebrated fuller body types and emphasized communal eating and strong social bonds. Eating disorders were virtually unknown.

By 1998, just three years later, everything had changed.

15% of girls reported inducing vomiting to lose weight.

74% said they felt "too fat."

83% said television had influenced how they saw their bodies.

"Beverly Hills 90210" and other Western shows had become powerful symbolic role models, associating thinness with status, beauty, and success.

Why It Matters in the Mind Matrix:

The Heart Self—especially in adolescence—is shaped by emotional meaning and relational modeling. When a symbol (like the body type of a TV character) becomes linked to acceptance, status, or belonging, it bypasses logic and begins to shape identity. The Head Self may rationalize this shift: "If I looked like that, I'd be more respected."

Meanwhile, the Vital Self may begin responding with physiological stress, food restriction, or even shutdown in response to internalized threat.

This study is now a landmark example of how symbolic imagery—especially when emotionally charged—can override cultural values and rapidly reshape individual behavior and group norms. It reminds us that symbols don't just reflect our world; they can rewire it.

I call the input of information from screens your **media diet,** *and just like the food you eat, what you ingest through your screen deeply affects you.*

If you eat highly processed foods with lots of sugar, salt, and spices, everything healthy starts tasting bland and boring. Similarly, if you are constantly feeding your mind overstimulating media content, you desensitize your internal system to subtlety, making calm, presence, and genuine connection feel dull or unsatisfying. Just like your taste buds, your mind can lose its ability to appreciate the richness of simple, nourishing experiences.

But you can change that. Shift your media diet toward calmer, more human stories and issues. Start focusing more on the world at small—the people and the places around you—and less on screens. And you can enrich your environment with symbols that evoke a Positive State.

Reducing Symbolic Overload

In a world saturated with media, reducing symbolic overload isn't just about turning off the news. It's about consciously shaping the symbolic environment your nervous system is exposed to every day.

Our minds are constantly interpreting symbols, whether we're aware of it or not. And those symbols—whether a siren, a news show, a comment thread, or a social media ad—affect the Vital, Heart, and Head Selves in powerful ways.

We often forget that we can choose the symbolic landscape we live in. Reducing symbolic overload isn't just about blocking negative input, it's about intentionally using symbols to regulate your State, support your Selves, and shift perception toward grounded presence and resilience.

To reduce symbolic overload, we can take three complementary steps:

Limit Exposure to Negative Symbolic Inputs

This means being intentional about what you allow into your mind, especially through screens. Every headline, photo, facial expression, and color palette carries symbolic meaning. Some symbols are neutral or uplifting, but many modern media sources rely on threat-based, fear-inducing, or identity-challenging symbols that trigger dysregulation.

Examples:

- Doom-scrolling before bed exposes your Vital Self to a flood of micro-threats: disasters, violence, social collapse. Even if you're not consciously distressed, your body registers it.
- Watching emotionally charged political commentary activates the Heart Self's sense of tribalism or shame, while putting the Head Self into defensive or rigid thinking loops.
- Social media comparison cycles, especially images of curated success, wealth, or perfection can activate scripts of inadequacy or failure, even if they're only glanced at for seconds.
- Endlessly watching television shows and movies play out scenarios that are designed to distract us from our feelings and trigger our negative emotions—anger, fear, shame, betrayal, etc.

Make your phone or tablet a safe place

- Remove or hide triggering apps from your home screen.
- Unfollow accounts that provoke fear, anger, or shame without resolution.
- Replace late-night screen time with something grounding or physical, like stretching or listening to calming music.
- Use filters, ad blockers, or browser extensions that help reduce sensationalist headlines or autoplay videos.

Curate Your Environment with Supportive Symbols

The key to reducing symbolic overload isn't just to eliminate symbols, but to repattern the symbolic field you live in. Your nervous system is constantly asking, "What does this mean?" If the answer—over and over—is "danger," "not enough," or "you don't belong," then dysregulation becomes the baseline.

But if your surroundings begin to say, "you are safe," "you matter," and "there is beauty," the Selves respond. The Vital Self settles, the Heart Self softens, and the Head Self regains clarity.

Once you remove or reduce draining inputs, work to fill your environment with symbols of safety, balance, and meaning, the kinds of cues your nervous system needs to stay in a Positive State.

This doesn't mean ignoring problems or "positive thinking." It means feeding your system with symbols that reflect what you're building toward, not just what you're afraid of.

Examples:

- **Art and imagery:** Hang visuals that evoke calm, beauty, strength, or awe. This could be a painting that reminds you of stillness, a photo of a loved one, or a landscape that makes you sigh when you look at it.
- **Natural objects:** Stones, shells, leaves, water bowls, candles—simple objects that carry sensory grounding and symbolic resonance with life, cycles, and stillness.
- **Sound environments:** Replace background TV or social noise with nature sounds, instrumental music, or calming spoken word. The symbolic meaning of sound—such as birdsong or gentle drumming—can shape the Heart Self's emotional climate.
- **Personal tokens:** A gift from a mentor, a childhood keepsake, a handwritten note from someone who loves you, all serve as emotional anchors that remind you of belonging and wholeness.
- **Ritual objects:** A journal placed near your bed, a mug used for tea and reflection, or a small altar space with meaningful items all serve as regular symbolic invitations to return to balance.

Use Ritual & Symbolic Action to Reinforce State Shifts

Symbols come alive when they are connected to rituals—small, intentional actions repeated often that carry meaning and generate a Positive State. Rituals reinforce neural pathways and reshape how we associate objects, actions, and spaces.

Ritual doesn't have to be spiritual or dramatic. It can be as simple as how you start your day or how you slow down at night.

Examples:

- A morning journaling practice that turns a blank page from a symbol of overwhelm into one of clarity and opportunity.
- Lighting a candle or changing your clothes at the end of the workday as a way of marking a State Shift telling your body it's safe to downshift.

- Placing your hand on your chest during stress as a symbolic act of self-soothing and presence.
- Reading a passage or poem from a favorite book out loud.
- Taking a walk on a familiar path in nature.
- Drinking a cup of tea while sitting in a favorite spot, maybe listening to soothing music or reading something meaningful.

These actions teach your nervous system: this symbol now means safety, clarity, connection.

Reflection: Mapping Your Symbolic Field

Your symbolic environment is talking to you all the time. The question is, what is it saying?

Take a moment to look around your space with fresh eyes. Not just what's there, but what it represents to your unconscious:

- Do your walls and shelves reflect beauty, strength, peace or pressure, clutter, and chaos?
- Are your screens filled with reminders of connection and creativity or anxiety, competition, and comparison?
- Which objects feel like "you" and which feel like leftovers from someone else's version of your life?

Reflection Exercise:
> *Look around your space. What symbols dominate your environment? Do they bring peace and connection, or do they reinforce stress and negativity?*
> *What is one symbolic shift you can make today?*

Final Thoughts: Symbols as Keys to Consciousness

Symbols are more than decoration. They are the deep architecture of perception—the inner maps we follow without realizing we've memorized them. When those maps are distorted by trauma, culture, or inherited beliefs, they become triggers that shape our lives in ways that seem inevitable. But when symbols are brought into awareness, they become tools of transformation.

> *So many changes are possible when we stop seeing ourselves as helpless victims of our past and our present situations, and begin seeing the many ways we unconsciously hold ourselves back.*
>
> *When you learn to observe normally unconscious triggers consciously, that makes it possible to use the Monarch's power of the Reflective Catalyst to reshape them—to override old Scripts, soften limiting beliefs, and access deeper sources of wisdom.*

You've now explored how the Mind Matrix Model works with symbols not just to interpret meaning, but to shift experience. You've seen how distorted symbols can reinforce loops, how archetypal images can awaken dormant parts of the Self, and how consciously reframing the meaning of your symbols for each of the Three Selves can change your sense of what's possible.

You now know that you can invest your home and your work environments with positive symbols as a way to regulate and balance yourself and counterbalance the effects of media, making it easier to be content and mindful.

In the next chapter—**Self and Other**—we'll turn our attention to how the Self begins to form through relationship. Just as symbols shape perception, early interactions shape identity. You'll explore the foundations of **Self-Other Differentiation**, and how our first experiences of connection and separation write the emotional blueprints we carry into every part of life.

Chapter Eighteen
Self and Other

I celebrate myself, and sing myself,
And what I assume you shall assume,
For every atom belonging to me as good belongs to you.
I loafe and invite my soul,
I lean and loafe at my ease observing a spear of summer grass…
…(I am large, I contain multitudes.)
I concentrate toward them that are nigh, I wait on the door-slab.
Who has done his day's work? who will soonest be through with his supper?
Who wishes to walk with me?

~ Excerpt from Song of Myself
  by Walt Whitman

Differentiation Across the Three Selves

We often hear the term "self-improvement" for working on ourselves. But in the Mind Matrix Model, there's a deeper question: what is the Self we're trying to improve? And perhaps, how do we negotiate around where we end and someone else begins?

This chapter introduces a key concept that underlies the entire Mind Matrix Model: *Self-Other Differentiation*. It's the developmental process of learning to be a "me" in a world of "other," and it plays out differently across each of the Three Selves—Vital, Heart, and Head. When it goes well, it builds resilience, clarity, and connection. When it's disrupted, we struggle to stay balanced, especially in relationships or under stress.

Let's look at how this process unfolds.

Self-Other Development: A Spiral Through the Selves

The process of self-development in childhood unfolds in three distinct but overlapping stages, each aligned with one of the Three Selves. In each phase, there is an initial period of connection or merging that creates a sense of safety, followed by increasing levels of separation, exploration, and independence.

Rather than a straight line, this process moves in a spiral pattern. Within the larger developmental arc of each Self, there are smaller spirals related to stages of separation and reconnection in the development of Self-Other Differentiation. These spirals within the overall spiral pattern help build the child's confidence and resilience.

Early on, however, the return to connection can feel intense or even frantic, especially if the separation was challenging or unexpected.

SPIRAL OF SELF-OTHER DEVELOPMENT

CONNECTION / SEPARATION

Head
(~2–12+ years)
Cognitive and ideological boundaries

Heart
(~9 months–3 years
Emotional and relational boundaries

Vital
(~1–12 months)
Safety and physical boundaries

In these moments, what the child needs most is reconnection, reassurance, and a sense that they're still safe. Through this process of practicing separation and reconnection over time, the child learns to trust that they are safe and cared for.

> ### Separation-Individuation in Developmental Psychology
> *In Margaret Mahler's theory of child development, the Mind Matrix Model process of Self-Other Differentiation is called Separation-Individuation Theory where, over time, the child gradually develops object constancy, or a stable internal sense of the caregiver's presence, and a growing confidence in their own selfhood.*
> *The smaller spirals in the diagram on the left are divided into connection and separation. In Separation-Individuation Theory they are described as practicing (separation and exploration) and rapprochement (return and reconnection).*

Vital Stage (1–12 months)

This stage is about safety and physical differentiation.

- Infants begin to separate from the caregiver's body through mobility, sleep-wake rhythms, and response to signals they generate such as hunger or discomfort.
- A healthy Vital Self begins with the experience: "I am in a body, and I am safe in this world."

Heart Stage (9 months–3 years)

Emotional and relational patterns emerge: joy, shame, longing, defiance.

- Children experiment with closeness and separation ("No!"), forming the basis for emotional boundaries.
- Success here allows for: "I have feelings and needs, and they can be met without losing love."

Head Stage (2–12+ years)

Children begin to form internal stories, moral frameworks, and abstract categories.

- Differentiation now includes mental independence: "I can think differently than you and still belong."
- Healthy development here supports curiosity, flexibility, and tolerance of difference.

Adolescent Self-Development: The Second Spiral

Of course, development doesn't end in early childhood. In fact, preteens and teenagers go through a second spiral of development where the relatively concrete childhood model formed in early life is broken down and replaced with a more abstract adult model. Just like baby teeth fall out to make room for permanent ones, early patterns of self and other give way to more complex, mature ones.

This phase can be intense, dramatic, and unpredictable—but also necessary. While Self-Other Differentiation continues, this stage is primarily about self-identity, along with growing autonomy and awareness:

Vital Self - Tweens to Early Teens (Approx. 8–14 years):
Physical transformation begins with the onset of puberty. The body changes rapidly—often awkwardly—and hormonal surges can dysregulate the system. Adolescents must learn to inhabit a new physical form and manage fluctuations in energy, appetite, and sleep.

This is the foundation for adult embodiment. Not just surviving in a changing body, but learning to live inside it with growing presence and awareness.

Heart Self - Early to Mid Teens (Approx. 12–18 years):
Social connection becomes paramount. Friendships, crushes, peer approval, and rejection all take on new emotional weight. Teens develop powerful relational yearnings and fears, and often swing between emotional openness and self-protective withdrawal.

This is where relational scripts from childhood are tested and either rewritten or reinforced. Teens begin experimenting with closeness, boundaries, identity, and emotional repair.

Head Self - Late Teens - Early Adulthood (Approx. 15–28 years):
Abstract thinking blossoms. Teenagers and young adults begin to recognize systems, hypocrisy, and ideological contradictions, and often develop a passionate (and sometimes rigid) sense of what's right or just. This stage isn't just "teen rebellion," it's the natural unfolding of cognitive individuation.

Young people test limits, question inherited beliefs, and try on worldviews as they construct their own internal frameworks. The prefrontal cortex—the part of the brain responsible for judgment, planning, and long-term decision-making—has finished most of its structural development in the mid to late 20's, however many people don't experience full integration of these capacities until the early 30's.

If this second spiral is well supported—with appropriate but not burdensome boundaries, space for mistakes and messiness, and room for honest conversation—the adolescent can emerge with a strong sense of their own identity and the physical, emotional, and cognitive tools of an adult self, grounded in a stable foundation for future growth.

If, on the other hand, the stressors they face are excessive or developmentally inappropriate, they may struggle to shift from a childhood model of the world to a more mature, flexible adult one. Cognitive psychology has found that people in a Negative State cannot update their internal model of reality. As a result, they may retain a rigid or immature worldview, only partially supplemented by learned social norms or abstract reasoning. In short, others may experience them as immature or lacking the depth of understanding expected of adults.

Not every adolescent receives the support they need during this crucial period. But even if this spiral wasn't fully completed, it can be revisited later through insight, care, and intentional healing. While the process may be more complex in adulthood, growth is still possible for developing a more resilient and integrated self.

These two developmental stages are followed by three others—midlife, senior and elderly, each of which is less dramatic than the first two but still follow the same progression of Vital–Heart–Head Self progression.

Developmental Axes Across the Three Selves

Each Self expresses development through its own axis of functioning. Here's how they work:

Vital Self Axis:

> **Internal Focus**: Aware of bodily needs, inner rhythms, and proprioception.
>
> **External Focus**: Attuned to sensory input, environmental threats, or social energy.
>
> **Balance**: Able to shift between inner awareness and environmental responsiveness.

Heart Self Axis:

> **Introversive**: Inwardly reflective, emotionally sensitive, attuned to others' needs.

Extroversive: Expressive, assertive, and energized by relational engagement.

Balance: Comfortable with solitude and connection; attuned but not over-attuned.

Head Self Axis:

Holistic Mode: Pattern-based, big-picture, intuitive.

Analytic Mode: Detail-oriented, logical, linear.

Balance: Can shift between modes depending on the task or context.

When Development is Interrupted

If development is interrupted at any stage, identity and differentiation can become unstable or rigid. These disruptions can show up as either an internal pattern (collapse, fusion, over-merging) or an external pattern (defensiveness, over-separation, domination).

Vital Self Disruption

Collapse / Fusion (Underarousal Mode)

The person struggles to feel clearly where their body ends and the world begins. They may have a vague or shifting sense of physical boundaries, difficulty detecting internal cues (such as hunger, fatigue, or pain), or become emotionally passive or frozen under stress.

This can also manifest as physical awkwardness or accident-proneness, especially when the body is not fully mapped in awareness.

These patterns often develop in early environments where bodily safety or attunement was inconsistent, intrusive, or absent.

Examples:

A child who grew up in a chaotic or neglectful home might learn to dissociate from their body as a survival strategy. As an adult, they may struggle with chronic fatigue, poor proprioception(awkwardness), or a tendency to "check out" during conflict.

This person might not notice they're in physical discomfort until it becomes overwhelming—skipping meals, ignoring pain, or staying in overstimulating environments too long.

Hypervigilance / Over-Separation (Overarousal Mode)

Here, the Vital Self is always on guard. The person is highly sensitive to sounds, smells, or movement, and tends to perceive others' presence as intrusive or overwhelming. Their posture may be tense, breath shallow, and movement rigid.

This is often rooted in early environments that felt unsafe or unpredictable, or where the child had to act aggressively to get their needs met.

Examples:

A teen who grew up with a volatile caregiver might tense up every time someone enters a room, even if they know logically there's no threat.

Someone with sensory defensiveness may find certain noises or touch so overwhelming that they avoid social settings altogether, retreating to hyper-controlled environments.

Heart Self Disruption

Over-Merging / Entanglement (Echoist Mode):

The emotional boundaries for this person are too thin. They can tend to absorb others' moods, feel responsible for everyone's feelings, and find it nearly impossible to say no. Their identity can blur in relationships, and they may confuse closeness with self-erasure.

This often develops in childhood environments where the child's sense of safety depended on managing the emotional states of others—whether through emotional enmeshment, parental instability, punitive control, or the child's reality being overridden or denied. To stay safe, they learned to monitor, adapt to, or disappear beneath others' needs and narratives.

Examples:

A friend becomes anxious and suddenly you're anxious too without knowing why. You start trying to fix their problem before they even ask.

You feel intense guilt for declining a favor, even if you're exhausted or overcommitted.

Over-Separation / Defensive Control (Narcissist Mode):

Here, the person maintains emotional distance and control as a defense against vulnerability. They may dismiss or devalue emotional connection, present a polished or superior persona, or engage relationally only on their own terms.

Beneath the surface, this pattern often reflects early emotional betrayal, engulfment, or invalidation—experiences where the child's emotional truth was unsafe, ignored, or punished. To protect themselves, they learned to prioritize self-image, minimize relational dependence, and avoid being emotionally known.

At its core, this form of over-separation is not about confidence—it's about protection from emotional injury that once felt unbearable.

Examples:

A partner expresses an emotional need, and you respond by changing the subject, offering critique, or positioning yourself as the more reasonable or self-sufficient one.

You prefer relationships where you're admired or depended on, or where you are the leader, but feel uncomfortable when others try to get close to your inner emotional world.

Head Self Disruption

Over-Identification / Lack of Boundaries (Holistic Mode):

The Head Self becomes overly porous, especially in social or ideological settings. The person takes on the beliefs, opinions, or logic of others without inner filtering, leading to anxiety, confusion, or loss of personal perspective.

This often develops in environments where disagreement was unsafe, where someone else strongly enforced their own reality view, or where approval was tied to conformity.

Examples:

In group discussions, you quickly adopt the group's opinion, then feel unsettled or unclear afterward, wondering if it's really what you think.

You often leave conversations with stronger personalities and feel mentally foggy or like you've lost your footing.

Rigidity / Mental Isolation (Analytic Mode):

The thinking mind becomes a fortress. The person relies on rigid logic, black-and-white reasoning, or intellectual control to avoid emotional discomfort or complexity. They may dismiss other viewpoints, micromanage outcomes, or get stuck in obsessive loops.

This can emerge from environments where thinking was a primary form of safety, or where nuance was not modeled or tolerated.

Examples:

You compulsively research every possible option before making a decision, then second-guess it anyway.

When someone challenges your beliefs, you instinctively push back or withdraw, rather than exploring the discomfort or ambiguity together.

How the Vital Self Sets the Baseline Orientation

While Self-Other Orientation shows up differently in each of the Three Selves, the direction of the system as a whole is usually deeply influenced by the earliest stage of development: the Vital Self. This early wiring—formed through nervous system patterns, physical safety, and primal connection—sets a foundational tone for how the entire personality leans.

In infancy, before language or emotional memory, the brainstem and sensory body are already learning: *Do I need to act out to get my needs met? Do I feel safe when I'm quiet? Does the world come to me, or do I need to go to it?*

These patterns form what we might call a default orientation toward self or other, inward or outward, that will color how later Selves emerge even if their experiences are quite different.

Because of this, it's relatively common to see patterns where all three Selves align with the initial Vital Self orientation, whether an internal, external, or balanced tilt.

Common Self-Other Patterns

Finding Self-Other balance doesn't mean standing exactly in the middle all the time. It's about understanding your natural tendencies, noticing when they serve you—and when they don't—and learning how to flex.

Here are a few patterns you might recognize:

The Self-Leaner

> You're more internally driven, and have trouble with energy and momentum - Vital Self underarousal mode.

- You are sensitive and value space and solitude - Heart Self introversive mode.
- You enjoy creativity and beauty, and can get lost in a project - Head Self holistic mode.

Try this:

Balance immersion with anchoring. Try setting small physical rituals like stretching before and after creative work, or checking in with your body every hour.

Create space to share your ideas with someone who will listen without needing you to linearize or explain them fully, just to stay connected as you go deep.

The Other-Leaner

- You're highly responsive to the external world and often operate in a state of high energy, staying focused on tasks, performance, or constant activity - Vital Self overarousal mode.
- You're quick to act, lead, or offer solutions but may overlook your own inner signals in the process - Heart Self extroversive mode.
- You feel most steady when things are moving, structured, or under control, but struggle to slow down, soften, or let yourself be fully seen - Head Self analytic mode.

Try this:

Practice pausing before you respond, especially in conversations or when tension rises. Instead of solving or structuring the moment, ask: What am I feeling underneath this impulse to manage or fix?

Create space for stillness—short breaks, quiet walks, or breath-based practices—and watch how your internal voice begins to emerge.

The Flipper (Oscillating)

- You swing between high and low energy, from drive and activity to fatigue or shutdown – Vital Self imbalance.
- You alternate between feeling completely self-reliant and urgently needing connection or reassurance – Heart Self oscillation.
- Your thinking flips between rigid, overfocused problem-solving and scattered, symbolic or emotional interpretations, making it hard to settle into one clear perspective – Head Self mode switching.

Try this:

Start tracking when and how you flip. Just a sentence or two each day: What set it off? What helped you come back? Notice if certain people or situations consistently pull you toward one pole.

Use rhythm—meals, movement, rest—as a stabilizing anchor while you build capacity to stay centered even as emotions shift.

The Balancer (When It's Working Well)

- You're grounded in your body and aware of your energy without overriding or neglecting it – Vital Self regulation.
- You're emotionally present, able to connect without merging and care without losing yourself – Heart Self clarity.
- You can hold your thoughts, emotions, and others' perspectives in the same space without collapsing into reactivity – Head Self integration.

Try This:

Keep nourishing your baseline. Even when things feel smooth, give your system regular anchors: a morning check-in, mindful transitions between roles, short breath breaks. And when stress hits, trust that returning to balance doesn't require perfection—just noticing, pausing, and realigning with what matters.

These aren't boxes to put yourself in—they're patterns to recognize and reflect on. The goal isn't to stay fixed in one category, but to develop the ability to move between self and other fluidly, depending on the moment.

Less Common Self-Other Patterns

While these patterns are common, they are anything but the rule. In many people, the Heart and Head Selves tend to lean in the same direction as the Vital Self—mirroring its inward, outward, or balanced orientation. This is because the Vital Self forms first and sets the foundational tone for how the child experiences energy, safety, and self-in-relation to the body and environment.

If the child learns early on that their internal sensations are safe and trustworthy, the Heart and Head Selves are more likely to develop in alignment with that internal orientation. If safety is found only through outer scanning or performance, the other Selves may follow that pull.

However, this is not always what happens. The Heart or Head Self may split off or compensate, developing a different orientation based on the child's specific environment, relationships, or coping strategies during key developmental windows.

For example, a child with an inward-leaning Vital Self—quiet, sensitive, and easily overstimulated—might naturally tend toward inwardness across the board.

However, if they grow up in an environment that values outward performance, emotional expressiveness, or physical toughness, the Heart Self may adapt by shifting outward.

In some cases, this may look like becoming socially charming, eager to connect, or emotionally expressive to compensate for the physical withdrawal.

In other cases, especially in more threatening or high-pressure environments, the outward shift may take the form of aggression, bravado, or emotional defensiveness as a survival adaptation.

In both versions, the child learns to perform outward engagement—whether through warmth or toughness—while remaining energetically self-contained or internally dysregulated.

This creates a split where the outer presentation masks the true internal experience, making self-connection and relational authenticity more difficult over time.

Similarly, a child with an outward-leaning Vital Self—energetic, expressive, constantly in motion—might be expected to act and engage constantly. However, if they experience emotional invalidation, authoritarian parenting, or shame around vulnerability, the Head Self may swing inward in response.

Rather than becoming bold and verbal, it retreats into daydreaming, imaginative isolation, or self-silencing. The result is a child whose body moves outward, but whose thoughts and emotions spiral inward, creating misalignment and internal confusion.

In this way, the Heart and Head Selves may either follow the Vital Self's orientation or diverge in a protective adaptation, especially if early caregiving was inconsistent, overcontrolling, or dismissive.

Understanding how each Self developed—and whether it leaned inward or outward in relation to the others—can be key to identifying what was adaptive, what was lost, and what's ready to re-align.

Layering Across the Selves

Let's look at how Self-Other Differentiation unfolds across the Three Selves and how early environmental influences shape each layer of development.

Vital Self (Early infancy)

This is where orientation begins. The infant's body is constantly signaling needs such as hunger, comfort, temperature, closeness.

- A child whose signals are consistently noticed and responded to may develop a flexible, self-regulating pattern, able to shift between inward awareness and outward attention as needed.
- But if care is inconsistent—such as in early hospitalization, adoption, or chaotic caregiving—the child may learn to amplify distress in order to be seen. This creates a high-arousal, externally focused orientation.
- Conversely, if the child is physically safe but overstimulated either due to excessive or intrusive interactions or a chaotic, overstimulating environment, they may withdraw and default to a low-arousal, internally focused orientation.

This early foundation doesn't lock in the child's personality, but it is one factor influencing how the Heart and Head Selves will later emerge.

Heart Self (Toddlerhood into early childhood)

As emotional connection becomes central, the child begins to learn how much space they can take up and how safe it is to express their needs.

- When caregivers are emotionally attuned and consistently available, the Heart Self forms a balanced relational orientation: capable of both receiving and offering connection, able to say yes and no, and resilient enough to navigate misattunement and repair.
- If the child is under-attended, they may default to being overly other-focused, developing people-pleasing patterns or hyper-attunement.

- If the child is over-attended or smothered, they may become emotionally self-focused, avoiding vulnerability or becoming boundary-pushing in search of autonomy.

As we mentioned, the direction this takes is strongly influenced by the underlying Vital Self pattern, but strong experiences such as neglect, over-control, or emotional inconsistency can override that early wiring and shape the Heart Self's orientation in new ways.

Head Self (Later childhood into adolescence)

Here the child begins building internal models of the world, including ideas about right and wrong, fairness, cause and effect, identity, and belonging.

- If the earlier Selves were supported and they experience a freedom to think and have their own views and opinions, the Head Self can begin from a place of curiosity and confidence, able to tolerate differing perspectives and engage in flexible, integrative thinking.

- But if the child experienced repeated relational misattunement, emotional volatility, or a feeling that their voice doesn't matter or is misunderstood, they may shift toward an Analytic Mode cognitive self-reliance: relying only on their own internal reasoning and dismissing external input. This can tilt toward logic, skepticism, and mental control as a protective strategy.

- Conversely, children raised in environments where authority was rigid or dismissive may instead develop a compensatory Holistic Mode tilt: rejecting structure in favor of intuition, symbolism, or abstract ideals, sometimes without grounding, and often with a susceptibility to taking on other people's views and reality.

In either case, the Head Self's differentiation becomes less about thinking freely, and more about protecting the system from further uncertainty.

As with the Heart Self, the direction this takes is strongly influenced by the underlying Vital Self pattern, but strong influences as identified above can determine the Head Self's overall orientation.

These patterns may linger, but they aren't permanent. With awareness and support, even longstanding imbalances can shift.

Example: A Layered Orientation

Imagine a child who begins life in an overstimulating environment—perhaps in a NICU or foster care system. Their Vital Self becomes high-arousal and other-focused, signaling loudly for needs to be met. Later, if they're adopted into a very attentive home, their Heart Self may shift to a more self-focused style, learning to protect their emotional space or regulate internally. Finally, in school, they may discover they are especially intelligent or perceptive and learn that others often don't "get it." Their Head Self becomes self-oriented, relying on their own analysis and perspective.

So we see a personality that appears highly independent (Heart Self Introversive Mode) and analytical (Head Self Analytic Mode), but underneath is a core Vital Self that's deeply environmentally reactive and over-adaptive (Vital Self High Arousal Mode).

This kind of layered pattern is very common, especially in people with early disruptions, asynchronous development, or high sensitivity.

It shows why no single Self-Other orientation defines the whole person—but also why the Vital Self remains the most influential "starting point" for how the system learns to balance self and other.

Everyday Examples of Self-Other Balance

When balance is working, daily life feels more easeful:

- Saying no without guilt, and respecting when someone else says no without taking it personally.
- Letting someone be upset without needing to fix it, and being able to share your own emotions without shame.
- Asking clearly for what you need, and listening openly when someone else shares theirs.
- Holding your ground in a disagreement while staying genuinely curious about the other person's perspective.
- Enjoying solitude without feeling alone, and being with others without losing your sense of self.

- Being with someone without merging with their emotional state, and being open to emotional support without making others responsible for regulating your feelings.

When balance is off, these same actions may feel overwhelming, aggravating or destabilizing. You might lose touch with your needs or become defensive. But when you are grounded in your own experience and recognize that others have their own emotional "weather," each interaction becomes an opportunity for clarity and growth.

Practices for Strengthening Self-Other Differentiation

Use these to reflect on how you relate to both your own experience and the experience of others:

- Where do I tend to over-identify with others, and where do I tend to shut them out?
- When do I lose track of my own needs or boundaries, and when do I override others' needs without realizing it?
- Which Self (Vital, Heart, Head) feels most stable in its Self–Other differentiation, and which one tends to collapse or overreach under stress?
- When I feel disconnected, do I retreat into myself or try to pull others in too close? What helps me come back to center?
- What does it feel like when I'm fully aware of both my own experience and someone else's without needing to change either?

These reflections help build awareness of when you're with yourself, when you're with others, and when you're able to be with both at the same time.

It can be helpful to add these to your journal so that you can look back at your earlier responses.

Guided Meditation: Centering the Selves

A practice for restoring balance in the Vital, Heart, and Head Selves, whether each tends to lean inward, outward, or fluctuate between the two.

Begin by sitting or lying down in a comfortable position.
Let your body settle—not into stillness, but into awareness.
Close your eyes or soften your gaze.

Vital Self

Bring your attention to your breath.
Don't try to change it.
Just notice how it's arriving.
Fast? Shallow? Slow? Deep?

Where does your breath live right now—high in your chest? Low in your belly?
See if you can move it downward as you relax.
Is your breathing even, or uneven?
Allow it to settle into deep, slow breaths.

Wherever it is, let it be. Let it tell you something about your State.

Now take a slow inhale…
And as you exhale, begin to let your attention move down into your body.
Down into sensation.
Into weight.
Into presence.

Say inwardly:

> "I am here in this body. In this breath. In this moment."

Now bring your awareness to your Vital Self—your energy, your body, your foundation.

Ask:

> *Do I feel more collapsed…more tense and overextended…or somewhere in between?*

If you feel collapsed—heavy, numb, or drained—let your breath gently rise with each inhale.
If you feel tense or overextended—tight, buzzy, overstimulated—let each exhale soften and sink your energy down.

Begin to imagine a State in the center for your Vital Self:
Relaxed, yet empowered. Rooted, yet alive.
Breathe into that possibility.

As you inhale, feel that balanced State entering your body.
As you exhale, let it spread through your limbs.

Now expand your awareness.
Become more present in your body and more aware of the space around you.

Imagine a field surrounding your body—your energetic boundary.
Breathe into it. See it glow.
Let it grow more stable as you inhale, more grounded as you exhale.
Let it become both deeply energizing and deeply settling.

Heart Self

Now shift your attention to your chest.
To the place where emotion lives, where connection forms, where boundaries are felt.

Ask:

> *Do I feel more fused with others…or more separated…or somewhere in between?*

If you feel over-merged—too attuned, emotionally tangled—use your breath to bring yourself back to center.
Feel your own pulse, your own emotional current.

If you feel closed or disconnected—tight, numb, or armored—breathe a little softness and expansiveness into your chest.
Imagine your heart is like a hot coal that you are blowing on with your breath, making it glow and radiate warmth.

Let warmth return to your emotional body.

Now imagine a balanced Heart State:
Open, but not porous. Available, but self-held.
Breathe into that.

With each inhale, feel your own feelings expanding out from your heart.
With each exhale, breathe out any heaviness in your heart.

Picture your heart field—your emotional presence—extending outward slightly, but only as far as feels true.
Let your breath infuse and nourish that field.
Let it hold both closeness and clarity.

Head Self

Now move your awareness up behind your forehead and your eyes.
To the space of thought, perspective, pattern, and meaning.

Ask:

> *Is my mind overactive… shut down… or somewhere in between?*

If your mind is in analytic overdrive—racing, planning, controlling—imagine giving it space.
Let thoughts drift like clouds. Let meaning emerge without effort.
Let your eyes and your vision soften and relax.

If your mind is foggy, detached, or scattered, let your breath become more defined and steady.
Bring shape back into your awareness—structure without force.

Now imagine a balanced Head Self:
Clear, calm, able to hold multiple truths without needing to control them.
Let your breath clear space around your thoughts and relax your head.
Let clarity return through stillness, not effort.

Picture your Head Self hovering gently above your Heart and Vital Selves.
Not in charge—just observing, integrating.
Let it rest for now.
Let it watch without rushing to explain.

Integration

Now return to your whole self.
Vital, Heart, and Head—each present. Each listened to. Each rebalancing.

Imagine your breath weaving the three together along your centerline.
Top to bottom, mind to heart to body.

Let your next few breaths be slow and complete.
You don't need to stay in balance forever.
You just need to return to it now.

When you feel ready, open your eyes.
Re-enter the outside world from your center.
With presence. With clarity. With choice.

Mind-Body Practices for Self-Other Repair

Support Differentiation and Balance Through the Three Selves

When Self-Other boundaries become blurred or brittle, your body often knows before your mind does. These mind-body practices help re-regulate, reconnect, and reclaim your space across the Vital, Heart, and Head Selves.

Vital Self: Grounding the Body and Reclaiming Space

When to use:

You feel overwhelmed by other people's energy or lose touch with your own body.

Questions to ask yourself:

- When you notice yourself shrinking back or dissociating, ask:
  "What's one sensation I can anchor to right now?"
- During a conversation, scan your body:
  "Can I notice my breathing, can I feel my feet on the ground while I listen?"
- At the end of the day, ask:
  "Did I abandon my body to get through the day or did I stay with it?"

Practices:

- **Weighted blanket or gentle pressure** to re-establish a physical boundary.
- **Shaking / bouncing** for 30–60 seconds to discharge sympathetic activation.
- **Boundary tapping**: Lightly tap around the outer edges of your body—shoulders, arms, legs—naming: *"This is me."*

Affirmation:

"I am here in my body. I know where I end and others begin."

Vital Self: Soothing Overdrive and Interrupting Overextension

When to use:

You feel driven, restless, tense, or find yourself overriding exhaustion to "push through." You're active but not present.

Questions to ask yourself:

- Mid-task, pause and ask:
  "What am I trying to achieve right now? Is it actually needed or am I avoiding a return to stillness?"

- Block off 10 minutes where nothing productive is allowed. Ask yourself and notice:
  What is rising up in me?
- When you feel urgency, ask:
  "Can I stay still and calm for three breaths without solving anything?"

Practices:
- **Still point lying pose:** Lie on your back with your legs up on a chair or wall. Place a light object (like a folded towel) on your belly. Let the weight settle you.
- **Breath deceleration:** Inhale for 3, exhale for 6. Emphasize the release. Repeat for 2–3 minutes until pace slows naturally.
- **Micro-freeze:** Stand still. Feel the floor. Count 5 breaths without moving at all. Allow your body to notice that nothing is required of it right now.

Affirmation:

"I am allowed to stop. I do not have to earn my right to rest."

Heart Self: Emotional Clarity and Relational Repair

When to use:
You feel enmeshed, reactive, ashamed, or disconnected from your feelings.

Questions to ask yourself:
- Before answering a request, pause and ask:
  "Is this yes coming from care or from fear of disconnection or being selfish?"
- When you feel someone else's emotion strongly, ask:
  "What's mine, what's theirs?"
- After a conversation, check in:
  "Did I disappear emotionally or did I stay present?"

Practices:
- **Hand-to-heart breathing**: Place your hand on your chest. Inhale for 4, exhale for 6. Say silently, *"I am here."*
- **Vocal boundary**: Practice saying *no* aloud in a calm tone when you're alone. Let the sound resonate within you and build a sense of calm, soft strength and confidence.

- **Loving-kindness phrases** (for self and other):
  "May I be clear and kind. May they be clear and kind. May we be free to be ourselves."

Affirmation:

"I can be with you without becoming you. I can love without losing myself."

Heart Self: Regulating Intensity and Relational Output

When to use:

You become reactive, controlling, emotionally intense, or use connection to direct, manage, or dominate.

Questions to ask yourself:

- The next time you feel a strong urge to correct, fix, or persuade, ask: *"Can I stay present without steering the moment?"*
- Let a conversation be incomplete. Ask yourself: *"Can I let someone have their own emotional truth, even if I don't agree?"*
- When expressing emotion, try this:
  "Am I sharing to connect, to show that I know something, or to control the outcome?"

Practices:

- **Hands-behind-heart pose:** Sit with your hands clasped behind your lower back and your chest open. Breathe slowly into the space behind your sternum. Practice emotional containment without collapse.
- **Non-response practice:** Imagine a conversation where you would normally interrupt, correct, or overreach. Instead, visualize letting the other speak while you simply hold your space inside.
- **Tone mirror check:** Record yourself saying something emotionally charged (*"I'm fine." "That's not true."*) and listen back. Can you hear an emotional strategy? Practice saying it again several times so that it's rooted in calm clarity.

Affirmation:

"I can feel deeply without reacting instantly. I can connect without controlling."

Head Self: Mental Boundaries and Cognitive Integration

When to use:

You're spiraling and losing touch with yourself in other people's stories, or you doubt your own reality, or you feel mentally scattered.

Questions to ask yourself:

- When you catch yourself looping, ask:
  "Whose voice is this? Is it mine?"
- Before offering your opinion, check in:
  "Am I speaking from clarity or from the need to soothe someone else's discomfort?"
- If you feel mentally foggy, ground with:
  "What do I see, hear, and feel right now?"

Practices:

- **Cognitive handoff**: Write down what's yours and what's theirs on opposite sides of a paper. Tear it in half. Keep yours. Burn or discard theirs.
- **Alternating logic + intuition journaling**: First list facts (what you know). Then write what you *feel or sense.* Notice how they interact.
- **Orienting practice**: Name 5 things you see, 4 you hear, 3 you can touch. Return to your own mind.
- **Allowing silences**: Practice not filling the space when there are silences in a conversation. Instead, focus on calming and slowing your breathing or noticing your body in relation to others.

Affirmation:

"I can think clearly. I am allowed to have my own perspective."

Head Self: Slowing Analysis and Releasing the Need to Know

When to use:

You're caught in overthink: problem-solving loops, over-researching, rationalizing emotions, or suppressing intuition.

Questions to ask yourself:

Pause mid-task and ask:
"What am I trying to control through this? What would happen if I paused instead?"

Let someone else lead for one hour. Ask:
"What's difficult about this? What's surprising about it?"

Practices:

- **Sensory override pause:** Choose one sensation (sound, scent, texture). Focus only on that for 20-30 seconds.
- **"I don't know" practice:** Write down something you've been spinning about. Then say aloud: *"I don't know."* Say it again, slower. See what happens when you allow that space.
- **Gaze widening exercise:** Stare at one object, then expand your visual field to take in everything in your peripheral vision. Hold that wide gaze for 30 seconds to shift your Head Self from narrow focus to relaxed awareness.

Affirmation:

"I do not need to figure it all out to be okay. I am allowed to rest inside uncertainty."

Real-Life Practice:

You don't need to overhaul your life to shift your Self-Other balance. In fact, small, repeated actions are what make the biggest difference.

Staying in yourself

The next time you're in a conversation, try focusing on slowing and deepening your breathing (grounding the Vital Self) then silently naming what's yours (your feeling, your thought, your response) and what's theirs. You don't have to fix, merge, or explain. Just observe the difference. With practice, this distinction becomes easier—and liberating.

Try a few of these:

- Observe a disagreement without rushing to fix it. Just notice what comes up inside you.

- Say no to a small request and let yourself feel the discomfort without immediately smoothing it over.
- Spend 30 minutes alone without a screen or task. Just be. Notice how your body and emotions respond.
- When you're upset, ask someone to simply listen. Make a point of asking them not to try to fix it, just to be present and witness you.
- Listen to someone else's emotions without absorbing or mirroring them, but just witnessing them with compassion. Stay grounded in your own experience.

Each one of these is a gentle repatterning. A small act of inner alignment. A way to remember: *I am here. I am me. I can be with you without becoming you.*

Workbook Reflection: Self-Other Exploration for Groups or Journaling

Use these prompts in group settings, dyads, or private reflection. Return to them over time to deepen insight and flexibility.

1. Your Default Mode

When I feel stressed, do I tend to collapse inward or reach outward?

Which Self (Vital, Heart, or Head) tends to dominate when I feel imbalanced?

2. Pattern Recognition

Which of the common patterns (Self-Leaner, Other-Leaner, Flipper, Balancer) do I relate to most? How am I different from them?

How does this show up in my body, my emotions, and my thinking?

3. Layered Influences

Was my early caregiving more under-attuned, over-attuned, or inconsistent, or was it relatively balanced?

Can I trace how my Vital Self patterns might have shaped my emotional and cognitive tendencies?

4. Boundaries in Action

> If I have a hard time saying no, where in my life does that show up?
>
> If I say no pretty easily, am I using that as a way to create separation?
>
> Where do I find it hard to *stay open* without collapsing into someone else's energy or separating from them?

5. Your Growing Edge

> What would a more balanced Self-Other relationship feel like in my body?
>
> What's one small practice I can commit to this week to support that balance?

A Note on Sensitivity and Identity

If you've ever asked yourself, *"Why is this so hard for me?"* you're not alone. People with sensitive nervous systems, a history of trauma, or emotionally inconsistent early experiences often find Self-Other boundaries especially challenging. This isn't a weakness. It's your system's way of trying to stay safe in a world that may not have always felt safe.

That kind of survival wiring runs deep. But it can also adapt.

With self-awareness, compassion, and practice, your system can learn new rhythms—ones that allow for connection *without collapse*, presence *without pressure*, and love that doesn't cost you yourself.

Final Thoughts

This chapter isn't about becoming perfectly balanced. The world outside and your inner world are constantly changing, so any one place won't stay balanced for long. It's about *dynamic balance*.

If you watch someone driving a car, they are constantly correcting even when driving on a straight section of road. Each turn of the wheel is in response to seeing that they are slightly off course, and they correct but then it goes to the other side. The more aware and present you are, the more quickly and subtly you correct.

You don't need to land in the center. You just need to keep seeking balance. Coming home to yourself, your breath, your body and the space around you. You can learn how to open the door to someone else without losing the thread of who you are or struggling to keep yourself safe.

That's the spiral of Self-Other Differentiation—layered, lived, and always evolving.

And as we'll explore in the next chapter, the way you express that differentiation in the world is through one of the most powerful tools you have: *boundaries*.

Chapter Nineteen
Setting Healthy Boundaries

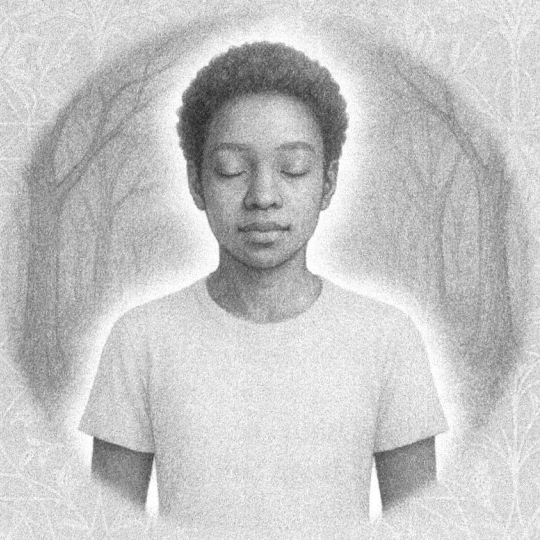

*I have built a sturdy fence
with a strong gate.
It keeps the garden safe
but doesn't keep me locked inside.*

*I welcome those who tread gently,
who wipe their feet before entering,
who don't mistake kindness
for collapse.*

*The ones who storm, push or trample
will meet the gate.
The ones who approach with care and respect
will find it open.*

~ Boundaries
  By Sam McClellan

Understanding Boundaries

Establishing healthy boundaries is crucial for maintaining emotional balance, nurturing relationships, and protecting yourself from overwhelm, burnout, and toxic relationships. Boundaries define your personal limits, helping you distinguish your needs, emotions, and responsibilities from those of others.

Boundaries are built on a strong sense of self and others. They are the invisible lines that define where *you* end and *others* begin. They create the necessary space for healthy connection, personal growth, and emotional safety.

- When boundaries are strong and clear, they protect your energy, clarify your values, and make your relationships safer and more sustainable.
- When boundaries are weak, porous, or overly rigid, that can lead to confusion, resentment, burnout, and even emotional harm.

In the Mind Matrix Model boundaries are not just about saying no, they are about balance. Each of the Selves has its own type of boundaries. **Vital Self** boundaries are physical and sensory. **Heart Self** boundaries are emotional and relational. **Head Self** boundaries are cognitive. They relate to your beliefs, values, inner clarity, and your ability to differentiate your thoughts and perspectives from those of others.

When boundaries across these Selves are respected, you're more likely to feel safe, emotionally regulated, and mentally clear. When they're violated, your system may shift into the Negative State—overwhelmed, anxious, reactive, or withdrawn.

Boundaries are not about making other people do what you want. They are about taking care of yourself and your relationships.

Good boundaries don't need to be held with anger. For some people, they can only get up the courage to hold a boundary if they are angry. But once you're angry you are triggered and dysregulated. And you can't stay angry forever. And then the boundaries fall and, often, you are left feeling shame and hopelessness.

This chapter is about working toward being able to keep clear boundaries and still stay in balance.

Types of Boundaries

There are a number of different types of boundaries to be aware of. Here are four important ones. Each Self experiences boundaries differently:

Physical Boundaries (Vital Self)

> These include your personal space, sensory preferences, privacy, rest needs, and sensory limits. Violations can feel intrusive or draining—like someone standing too close or touching without consent, something demanding your attention when your body is signaling the need for rest, or when your physical needs aren't being addressed.

Emotional Boundaries (Heart Self)

> These relate to how much emotional energy you give or receive in relationships. They help you hold your feelings as valid, separate from others' reactions or projections. Weak emotional boundaries often lead to people-pleasing, over-attunement, emotional flooding, or guilt for things outside your control. Too much control, while it may seem like good boundaries, is instead about protection through controlling others, or getting your own needs met ahead of theirs.

Time Boundaries (Heart + Head Self)

> Your time is one of your most valuable resources. Time boundaries include protecting your availability, pacing your commitments, and creating space for rest, reflection, or solitude. A lack of time boundaries can create exhaustion or resentment.

Mental Boundaries (Head Self)

> Mental boundaries allow you to think independently and maintain your inner clarity, even in the face of disagreement. They protect your values, beliefs, and cognitive space.
>
> When mental boundaries are weak, you may feel pressured to conform, doubt your perception of reality, or lose confidence in your voice. When excessive, you tend to value your own point of view and discount others'.

Example: Poor Boundaries

Elena is a compassionate, hardworking person who cares deeply about her friends, family, and coworkers. But lately, she's been feeling exhausted, emotionally overwhelmed, and resentful—and she's not quite sure why.

Vital Self (Physical Boundaries):

Elena's coworker often stops by her desk to vent for 30–40 minutes at a time. Even when she's visibly tired or hungry, Elena doesn't excuse herself. She skips lunch, ignores her body's tension, and pretends she's okay in order to be polite.

Inside, she feels drained and foggy, with mounting fatigue and a growing sense of irritability.

Heart Self (Emotional Boundaries):

A close friend frequently calls to talk about their latest crisis. Elena listens for hours, offering reassurance, even when she's feeling emotionally depleted. She feels guilty saying she's not available, even when her chest tightens just seeing the friend's name on her phone.

She begins to feel resentful and unnoticed, but she's afraid of confrontation. She tells herself she's just being "selfish" if she says no.

Head Self (Mental Boundaries):

In meetings, Elena often stays quiet when someone speaks over her or misrepresents her idea. She later replays the conversation in her head, unsure whether she's allowed to assert herself. She doubts her own clarity, especially when others are more vocal.

She second-guesses her perception, feeling increasingly uncertain and frustrated.

Example: Rigid or Overprotective Boundaries

Marcus is competent, efficient, and deeply values his independence. He's respected at work and seen as emotionally steady—but lately, his relationships have become strained, and he often feels misunderstood or burdened by others' needs.

Vital Self (Physical Boundaries – Overcontrolled)

Marcus has a strict routine and dislikes physical interruption. When a coworker approaches him unexpectedly at his desk, he responds curtly or with visible irritation. He avoids shared meals or casual contact and becomes agitated if someone touches his belongings.

He feels constantly overstimulated by others' presence, and responds by tightening control of his space and schedule. But underneath, his body feels chronically tense and hypervigilant.

Heart Self (Emotional Boundaries – Defensive)

When a friend tries to share something vulnerable, Marcus shifts the conversation, offers solutions, makes a joke, or makes an excuse to get away. He avoids emotional depth, believing it's messy or manipulative. If someone becomes upset with him, he quickly withdraws or frames them as overly emotional or unfair.

Inside, he feels safest when emotionally self-contained, but also increasingly isolated, misunderstood, and unseen. Perhaps even lonely.

Head Self (Mental Boundaries – Dismissive or Dominating)

In meetings, Marcus is quick to assert his viewpoint and often shuts down others' perspectives if they seem inefficient or emotionally charged, or because they threaten his dominance. He finds emotional nuance frustrating and prefers logic and action.

He frequently dismisses feedback as "subjective" or "not grounded in reality," and almost never admits to himself or others when his thinking might be limited by bias or defensiveness.

Identifying Your Boundaries

Many of us weren't explicitly taught how to notice, let alone communicate, our boundaries. Instead, we often discover them through discomfort. Feelings like irritation, resentment, anxiety, or emotional exhaustion are signals that something has crossed a line, whether spoken or unspoken.

Try reflecting on:

When do I feel drained or resentful in interactions?

When do I override my own needs to preserve harmony or avoid conflict?

Where do I feel tense or guarded around others, and why?

Reflect: Pay attention to physical and emotional cues that suggest a boundary has been crossed. Your body often knows before your mind.

Clarify Values: Boundaries arise from values. What matters most to you—honesty, rest, freedom, respect—should inform the lines you draw in relationships.

Communicating Your Boundaries

Even the clearest internal boundaries need to be communicated to be effective. Many people fear setting boundaries because they associate it with conflict, rejection, or seeming "selfish." But when done with clarity and respect, boundary-setting is a form of self-respect and a gift to others. It tells them how to relate to you honestly.

Be Direct and Calm: Use "I" statements to express what you need without blaming. For example:

> "I need to take some time for myself tonight."
>
> "I'm not comfortable discussing that right now."
>
> "I'm happy to help, but I'll need more notice next time."

Practice Assertiveness: Assertiveness is different from aggression. It's clear, respectful, and rooted in self-worth. You don't have to justify or overexplain your boundaries. If someone pushes back, that's a reflection of *their* discomfort, not your unkindness.

Maintaining and Reinforcing Boundaries

Setting a boundary once isn't always enough. Some people may push or test them especially if you've been more flexible in the past. Maintaining your boundaries is an ongoing practice that builds trust in yourself and teaches others how to treat you.

Stay Consistent: Repetition reinforces your limits. If you say no once and then say yes the next time, it sends a mixed message. You can adjust your boundaries as your needs change, but don't collapse them to avoid temporary discomfort.

Practice Saying No: "No" is not a rejection of others, it's a protection of your own capacity. *Sometimes no is a full sentence!* You don't have to explain your no unless you choose to. You can say:

> "That's not something I can commit to right now."
>
> "I need to decline, but I appreciate the invitation."
>
> "No, thank you."

Remember: Healthy boundaries are not walls. They are flexible, responsive, and allow for deep connection *without self-abandonment*.

As your Heart Self learns to trust that it can say yes or no from a place of grounded clarity, your relationships can become more honest, mutual, and nourishing.

Example: Holding Boundaries

After a period of burnout and reflection, Elena begins practicing small but consistent boundaries. She starts to notice how her body, emotions, and thoughts give her signals when something feels off, and she listens.

Vital Self (Physical Boundaries):

When her coworker drops by uninvited, Elena smiles and says warmly, "I want to hear how you're doing, but I'm in the middle of something. Can we catch up later?" She blocks out time for lunch and short walks to reset her nervous system.

She feels more grounded, energized, and in control of her own rhythm.

Heart Self (Emotional Boundaries):

When her friend calls again during a moment she needs rest, Elena replies, "Hey, I really care about you and want to be present when we talk. But I'm tapped out right now, can we talk tomorrow?" She stops overlistening in conversations and begins sharing her own needs, too.

She notices she feels less resentful and more authentic.

Head Self (Mental Boundaries):

In a meeting, when someone cuts her off, she says calmly, "Excuse me, I'd like to finish my thought. Then I'd love to hear yours." She reminds herself afterward: *"My ideas have value, even if others don't affirm them right away."*

She begins to trust her own thinking again, and her internal critic quiets.

Example: Practicing Strong Yet Flexible Boundaries

Marcus, after years of holding tight control over his space and emotions, begins to shift. He still values structure and clarity, but now makes space for connection, reflection, and emotional truth without sacrificing agency.

Vital Self (Physical Boundaries – Contained, Not Controlling)

When a coworker interrupts his workflow, Marcus pauses his task, looks up, and says clearly, "Give me five minutes to finish this and then I'm all yours." He resumes his task without guilt and meets the coworker afterward, fully present.

He still honors his need for control over his time, but now uses it to create rhythm, not rigidity. His body feels calmer, and his interactions feel more intentional than reactive.

Heart Self (Emotional Boundaries – Engaged, Not Defensive)

When a close friend shares something vulnerable, Marcus resists the urge to fix it. He listens, then responds, "I'm so sorry you're having to deal with that right now. Thanks for trusting me with that. I don't have a great answer, but I'm here with you."

He feels the instinct to pull away or take charge, but instead stays with the discomfort. He remains grounded in his own emotional field while being fully present with someone else's.

Head Self (Mental Boundaries – Clear, Not Dismissive)

In a meeting where a colleague challenges his idea, Marcus responds: "I hear where you're coming from. Here's why I still think this piece matters. Can we hold both perspectives for a moment to check them out?"

He doesn't collapse his thinking or bulldoze others. Instead, he uses structure and clarity to support mutual understanding. He trusts his thoughts and makes space for others' insights to refine them.

This version of Marcus shows that more dominant individuals can maintain strength, clarity, and efficiency—while developing discernment, flexibility, and relational depth. It's not about softening identity—it's about integrating it.

Before, During, and After: Building Healthy Boundaries

One helpful way to build better boundaries is to think in terms of before, during, and after. Boundaries aren't just something you set in the moment, they're a practice that develops across time, reflection, and experience.

- **Before** refers to moments when you're not currently in a boundary-challenging situation, but you're reflecting on patterns. This might include remembering times where you tend to give too much, avoid conflict, or shut down and thinking about how you could have acted differently but not out of a kind of judgment "if only," but rather out of discernment, "what would have worked better"?
  Reading this chapter is a perfect example. You're preparing your system with awareness and intention before stepping into a difficult interaction.
- **During** is often the hardest part. This is when you're in the moment—face-to-face with someone—and your boundaries are being tested. The key here is to *try to stay conscious and non-reactive*. If boundaries have been a challenge for you, don't expect perfection. It takes time, and you're not failing if it's hard.
  We get better through practice and self-reflection. Even a small step—pausing, naming your feeling, or choosing not to collapse—counts as progress.
- **After** is where integration happens. After a difficult interaction, the first step is to take care of yourself, to regulate. Then once you're grounded, review.

First, focus on regulation: ways to ground yourself physically, emotionally, and mentally. Give your nervous system a chance to settle and let the energy of the interaction move through you and drain away. Go for a walk, shake it off, breathe, cry—whatever helps bring you back into a calmer, more centered place.

As we discussed in the *Triggers and Overrides* chapter, the Head Self often tries to resolve boundary ruptures through overthinking, but this usually reactivates the wound rather than heals it.

Once you're grounded and clear, reflect briefly:

What happened?

What feelings came up?

How might I handle it differently next time?

If this is difficult, you can use the next section called Dipping Your Toe In to slow everything down so that you don't get overwhelmed.

Dipping Your Toe In

If you notice yourself becoming re-triggered just thinking about a boundary you need to set—or a time you didn't—you need to slow the process down and shift your focus to titrate it.

In Somatic Experiencing (SE), titration refers to the practice of gently and gradually processing traumatic or intense sensations by breaking them down into small, manageable pieces rather than confronting the full intensity all at once.

I like to call it "dipping your toe in," just like you do when you're checking to see if the water is too cold.

That means very briefly bringing the moment to mind, then immediately shifting your focus to your breath and your body.

- Be curious.
- Notice what sensations start to move through you.
- Does your breathing change—become shallow, tighten, or pause altogether?

Imagine your body as a still pool, and the memory or thought as a toe dipping into the surface. When you stir the water, just wait for it to calm again.

Watch your breath.

Let your body settle again.

When the pool feels calm—your breathing soft, deep, and steady—you can try again.

This process can be repeated as many times as needed, in one sitting or many, each clearing a bit more and going a little deeper, a layer at a time. You can use it directly after a difficult interaction, or (in the Before mode) thinking about types of interactions in general. The key is to slow everything down, rather than becoming immersed, to keep from being re-traumatized.

You're not trying to relive the event, you're learning how to be present with your own reactions without being consumed by them.

Each time you practice, you help your Monarch observe with discernment instead of judgment, and you give your Heart Self the safety it needs to become more resilient in future interactions.

Your Safe Place

If you find that the feelings are still too much and you can't settle, you can use a practice I call Your Safe Place.

Imagine being in a very safe, quiet place like in the woods, by a stream, on the beach, or in a field. You might also picture being with a very close friend or a beloved pet.

Close your eyes and try to really immerse yourself in all your senses—seeing, feeling, hearing, even smelling the place. The sound of a gentle breeze in the leaves of the trees. The feel of sunshine on your skin and the glow of it through your eyelids. Feel yourself there in your body. The more real you can make it, the better.

Allow yourself to relax and unwind, breathe slowly and deeply. Feel your muscles relax and your nervous system settling.

We call this Your Safe Place, and you can return to it as needed, any time you are triggered or if you are working through feelings and are getting overwhelmed.

Once you have settled, if you can, return to the process of very briefly thinking about what disturbed you and then going to your sensations to continue the process of dipping your toe in. Otherwise, take some time to calm and center, and perhaps return to it later.

Navigating Boundary Challenges

Boundaries can sometimes trigger discomfort, guilt, or resistance, especially if others are accustomed to different patterns.

Acknowledge Discomfort: Accept that discomfort may arise initially but remind yourself of your reasons and long-term benefits.

Self-Compassion: Offer yourself kindness if you get upset or triggered when setting boundaries, recognizing that your Sentries are going to push for you to feel guilty or unsure (pushback).

Reaffirm Your Right to Boundaries: Remind yourself regularly that boundaries support healthy relationships and personal growth.

Boundary Maintenance

Consistent reinforcement is crucial to maintaining your boundaries.

Regular Check-Ins: Periodically assess your boundaries, noticing if adjustments are needed based on changes in your life circumstances or relationships.

Self-Care Practices: Engage in regular self-care to reinforce your commitment to honoring your boundaries and nurturing your well-being.

By setting, communicating, and maintaining healthy boundaries, you empower yourself to foster relationships that respect your personal space and values, contributing to emotional clarity, resilience, and a stronger, healthier Vital Self.

The Boundaries Tripod

Your boundaries—and really, your entire approach to life—rest on three essential components. Think of them as the legs of a tripod: when all three are in balance, your stance is strong and steady. When one leg is missing or overextended, the whole structure tilts and becomes unstable.

Each leg corresponds to one of the Three Selves in the Mind Matrix Model:

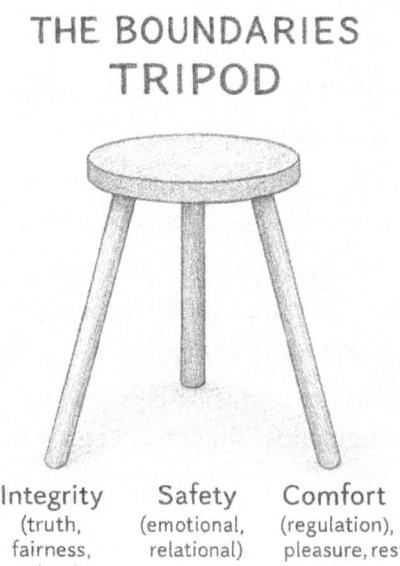

THE BOUNDARIES TRIPOD

Integrity (truth, fairness, duty)   Safety (emotional, relational)   Comfort (regulation), pleasure, rest

Integrity (Head Self): Doing what's right. Acting with honesty, fairness, respect, and personal responsibility—even when it's hard.

Comfort (Heart Self): Protecting your well-being—emotionally, relationally, energetically. Knowing what feels safe and when something feels off.

Safety (Vital Self): Seeking contentment, satisfaction, pleasure, and rest. Listening to your body's need for nourishment, rest, and regulation.

While balance is ideal, life often demands we shift emphasis based on the situation.

- If you're being chased by a tiger, your *Safety* is paramount. You're not going to worry about hurting your ankle (*Comfort*) or whether it's fair to the tiger that you're running away and not providing a meal (*Integrity*).
- If someone is in danger, your *Integrity* may compel you to act—even if it costs you some *Comfort* or carries a level of *risk (Safety)*. Ideally, you'll still keep your Vital Self in the loop to avoid reckless sacrifice.
- If you're stuck in a toxic workplace, *Comfort* and *Safety* may need to outweigh your sense of *responsibility (Integrity)* to the job or coworkers.

The key is not to sacrifice one leg permanently for another. Boundaries become distorted when one Self dominates at the expense of the others.

Examples of Imbalanced Boundaries

Here's a few examples of imbalanced boundaries:

Staying in a Draining Friendship:

You have a friend who always leans on you emotionally, but never shows up when you need support. You feel depleted every time you talk to them. Still, you keep answering their late-night calls, telling yourself it's the "right thing to do."

Here, *Integrity* (as loyalty) overrides both *Safety* (emotional well-being) and *Comfort* (rest and solitude), leaving your Heart and Vital Selves unsupported. Your stool is imbalanced.

Pushing Through Burnout at Work:

You've been working 12-hour days for weeks and your body is screaming for rest. But there's a big project deadline, and you pride yourself on being dependable. You tell yourself, "Other people are counting on me," and keep going despite mounting fatigue and brain fog.

Your Head Self is overriding your Vital Self, and ignoring your Heart Self's signals of stress and burnout. Long-term, this imbalance could lead to collapse.

Sacrificing Honesty for Harmony:

A family member repeatedly makes backhanded comments at dinner. You feel hurt but don't speak up, thinking, "It's not worth the conflict." You stay quiet to keep the peace.

Here, comfort and short-term emotional safety are prioritized, but integrity (truthfulness and self-respect) is sacrificed. It's really about what you feel is the best decision, but over time this kind of boundary collapse can create resentment and emotional suppression.

Postponing Your Wedding:

You're getting married in a week (comfort), but a coworker asks you to cover their shift so *they* can go on vacation. They plead, saying it's the only time they can get away. You feel bad for them, and you have a hard time saying no, so you agree—*and postpone your wedding*.

You've abandoned both comfort and safety in an attempt to follow a distorted version of integrity (over-responsibility to others). That's not sustainable or fair to yourself.

Questionnaire: Finding Your Boundary Imbalances

This questionnaire is designed to help you identify where your boundaries may be unbalanced between integrity (doing what's right), safety (ensuring your own well-being), and comfort (seeking enjoyment and ease).

You can also access a downloadable PDF version of the form as well as an interactive version by visiting the Mind Matrix Model website. You'll need to register if you haven't yet. You can sign up for free access by scanning the QR code or visiting this short link:

https://mmm.tips/boundaries

mmm.tips/boundaries

Answer the following questions honestly, selecting the response that best describes your tendencies.

1. When someone asks for your help but you're already overwhelmed, how do you respond?

A) I always help, even if it leaves me drained. (*Integrity imbalance—prioritizing others over personal well-being*)

B) I immediately say no, regardless of the situation. (*Safety imbalance—prioritizing protection over flexibility*)

C) I avoid the request entirely to prevent discomfort. (*Comfort imbalance—prioritizing ease over action*)

D) I assess whether I have the capacity before agreeing or declining. (*Balanced response*)

2. How do you handle conflict?

A) I avoid it at all costs, even if it means compromising my values. (*Safety/Comfort imbalance—prioritizing avoidance over integrity*)

B) I always stand my ground, even if it puts me in harm's way. (*Integrity imbalance—prioritizing principles over personal safety*)

C) I give in quickly to keep the peace. (*Comfort imbalance—prioritizing ease over self-advocacy*)

D) I engage when necessary but pick my battles wisely. (*Balanced response*)

3. At work, how do you react to an unfair request from your employer?

A) I comply, even if it crosses my limits. (*Integrity imbalance—prioritizing responsibility over well-being*)

B) I refuse immediately, even if it could affect my job security. (*Safety imbalance—prioritizing protection over compromise*)

C) I find ways to ignore or avoid it, hoping it resolves itself. (*Comfort imbalance—prioritizing ease over action*)

D) I assess my options, then set a boundary or negotiate. (*Balanced response*)

4. When making big life decisions, what do you prioritize most?

A) What I believe is the right thing to do, even if it's exhausting or difficult. (*Integrity imbalance—prioritizing duty over well-being*)

B) What feels safest, even if it limits my opportunities. (*Safety imbalance—prioritizing security over growth*)

C) What feels easiest or least uncomfortable, even if it lacks long-term benefits. (*Comfort imbalance—prioritizing ease over responsibility*)

D) A mix of all three—considering what's right, safe, and fulfilling. (*Balanced response*)

5. If a friend or family member repeatedly crosses your boundaries, for example is always taking your things without asking, how do you respond?

A) I tolerate it because I value the relationship. (*Integrity imbalance—prioritizing connection over self-respect*)

B) I cut them off entirely, regardless of the situation. (*Safety imbalance—prioritizing self-protection over communication*)

C) I avoid addressing the issue, even if it makes me unhappy. (*Comfort imbalance—prioritizing avoidance over resolution*)

D) I set clear boundaries and enforce them as needed. (*Balanced response*)

Interpreting Your Results

- **Mostly A's:** You may over-prioritize *integrity*, focusing on doing what's right even at the expense of your well-being. Learning to balance responsibility with self-care will strengthen your boundaries.

- **Mostly B's:** You may be overly focused on *safety*, avoiding risks and prioritizing protection. While self-preservation is important, finding flexibility can allow for healthier engagement with challenges.

- **Mostly C's:** You may prioritize *comfort*, avoiding discomfort even when it leads to longer-term issues. Practicing assertiveness and resilience will help you build stronger boundaries.

- **Mostly D's:** You have a relatively *balanced* approach to integrity, safety, and comfort. Keep refining your awareness to maintain this balance in different life situations.

Reflect on your answers and consider where you may need to adjust your boundaries. Are there areas where you tend to overextend yourself? Are there places where you retreat too quickly? Recognizing these patterns is the first step toward creating more sustainable and healthy boundaries in all aspects of your life.

Final Thoughts

Healthy boundaries are not fixed walls or rigid rules, they are dynamic expressions of our internal regulation, self-awareness, and capacity for connection. True boundaries emerge when we can differentiate between Self and Other across all three Selves: sensing where our body ends and another begins, knowing which emotions are ours to feel, and thinking our own thoughts even in the presence of strong external influence.

When boundaries are balanced, they provide safety without isolation, connection without fusion, and flexibility without collapse. This balance is not a permanent achievement, but a living process—one that shifts as our state changes, relationships evolve, and self-development deepens.

If your boundaries feel too porous or too rigid, it's not a sign of failure, it's a signal from your system. With care and practice, these patterns can be revisited, rebalanced, and gradually restructured.

Boundaries are not just about keeping things out; they are also about creating the conditions for something better to grow within.

In the next chapter, we'll reflect on what it means to live the Mind Matrix. Not as a concept, but as a living, breathing relationship with yourself and the world around you.

Let's bring it home.

Chapter Twenty

Conclusion
Living the Mind Matrix

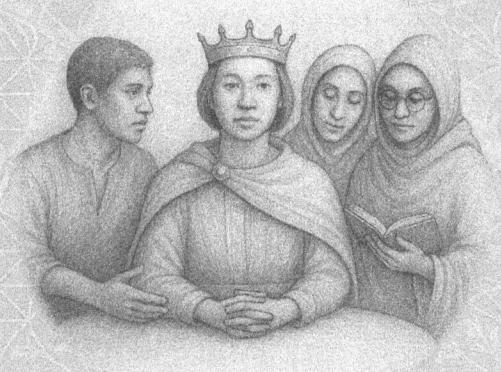

Henceforth I ask not good-fortune, I myself am good-fortune,
Henceforth I whimper no more, postpone no more, need nothing,
Done with indoor complaints, libraries, querulous criticisms,
Strong and content I travel the open road.

The earth, that is sufficient,
I do not want the constellations any nearer,
I know they are very well where they are,
I know they suffice for those who belong to them.

~ Excerpt from Song of the Open Road
  by Walt Whitman

The Kingdom Is Yours

You've made it to the final pages of the Mind Matrix Model core chapters, but really, this is just the beginning. The *Mind Matrix Model* wasn't written just to inform you. It was written to give you a map, a set of tools, and a compass for navigating your life with greater clarity, compassion, and power.

At the heart of the Model lies one core truth: your mind is a living system. It is shaped not only by thoughts or feelings, but by energy, environment, relationships, memory, and State. The Three Selves—Vital, Heart, and Head—are not abstract ideas. They are living aspects of you. Your Ministers of each Self are here to support your conscious self. Each one has its voice. Each one has its needs. And when they are balanced and in dialogue with themselves and with you, the Monarch, your inner world begins to move in harmony.

The Power of Awareness and State

Early in this book, you learned how each Self functions along its own axis: the Arousal Axis for the Vital Self, the Self-Other Axis for the Heart Self, and the Cognitive Axis for the Head Self. You saw how these axes operate independently, but also influence one another. And perhaps most importantly, you discovered the State Axis—the invisible tide that determines whether your Selves are acting in survive or thrive mode.

You learned to recognize the difference between the Positive State, where the system flows and you feel connected, curious, and resilient; and the Negative State, where old scripts, loops, and defenses can take over. You explored what happens when the system gets stuck, and how to shift it back using Override Strategies, from acupressure to movement, nutrition, reframing, and breath.

You've learned different therapies and modalities that can assist your particular issues and how the Mind Matrix Model can be a great adjunct to therapy.

You've begun to expand your State Range—not just trying to feel good, but becoming someone who can navigate more of life with more choice and less collapse.

The Three Selves: A Deeper Knowing

Along the way, you explored each of your Three Selves in depth:

The **Vital Self**, your body-based core, holds instinct, rhythm, and survival intelligence. You learned to listen to its messages through its path of communication, sensation—exhaustion, tension, hunger, pain, and pleasure—and how to bring it back into balance using tools like grounding practices, circadian rhythm care, diet, acupressure, adaptogens, and mindful rest.

The **Heart Self**, your relational and emotional center, has helped you understand patterns of connection, defense, and longing. You learned where you live within the introversive/extroversive spectrum. You saw how trauma, attachment, and early emotional imprinting can shape your Self-Other Range. You explored the difference between healthy inner awareness and echoism mode collapse, between external agency and narcissistic mode overdrive. You learned how to listen to the voice of the Heart Self, feelings. And to regulate the Heart Self through co-regulation, boundaries, gratitude, and emotional integration.

The **Head Self**, your cognitive and narrative mind, revealed your styles of thinking: Analytic and Holistic Modes—focused and diffuse, logical and symbolic. You discovered how the Head Self tries to protect you through Loops, planning, or disassociation, and how it can return to clarity through meditation, reframing, creativity, and rhythm. You learned to recognize the Critic and the Drifter, and how to support the Synthesizer within you.

The Monarch and the Ministers: Restoring Inner Leadership

By now, you've also gotten to know more about your Monarch—your conscious mind, your capacity for awareness, decision-making, and compassionate direction. The Monarch isn't a dictator. It's the integrator, the one who learns to listen to each Self, weigh their input, and guide your system toward coherence.

But the Monarch doesn't act alone. Each Self is overseen by its own Minister—an unconscious pattern manager who tries to keep you safe and functioning.

The **Minister of the Vital Self** manages survival: it controls your arousal level, energy, posture, tone, and the automatic responses of your body. It may push you to shut down when overwhelmed or surge into action when it senses threat, even if the Monarch isn't yet aware of it.

The **Minister of the Heart Self** manages relationships and emotions: it carries your attachment history, your relational strategies, and your sense of belonging. It's the one that activates old Scripts when connection feels at risk, sometimes playing the Echoist, the Narcissist, the Pleaser, or the Avoider to protect you.

The **Minister of the Head Self** manages thoughts, beliefs, and perspectives. It filters meaning, creates our reality, and chooses how to explain things to you. Under stress, it may hand you a Script filled with worst-case scenarios or tighten into rigidity. When integrated, it becomes the Synthesizer, helping you hold multiple truths and shift your mindset with grace.

When dysregulation occurs, it's often because the Ministers are trying to govern alone. They override the Monarch in the name of protection. They recycle old strategies because they don't yet trust that the Monarch is listening.

But as awareness grows, something shifts. The Monarch learns to recognize the Ministers' strategies. It learns to ask: *Is this protection still serving me?* And in that moment, something sacred happens: inner leadership returns to YOU.

> *The Monarch doesn't dominate—it listens, it integrates, it is guided by you, not through force, but through collaboration. No part of you is exiled. They are all brought to the table.*

This is the essence of the Mind Matrix: not a system of control, but a system of relationship.

Beyond the Selves: Loops, Scripts, Personas, and Overrides

We also explored how these Selves interact over time—how Loops form between them, how old Scripts can run without our permission, and how Personas get constructed to meet expectations, avoid pain, or survive complexity.

And we covered tools you can use—not just insights, but practical interventions—to shift these patterns.

We learned to track State Loops, recognize when one Self pulls others off course, and use targeted Override Strategies to intervene at the level of energy, emotion, or belief. You practiced Fast Overrides like sensory grounding and breathing techniques and explored Deep Overrides through lifestyle change, therapeutic modalities, herbs, nutritionals, and spiritual practices.

We also began to explore Self-Other Differentiation—the developmental path that forms your sense of identity, autonomy, and empathy. And you've seen how culture, media, and symbolic systems shape our internal landscape in ways both subtle and profound.

Integration Over Perfection

The goal isn't to "fix" yourself or always be in the Positive State. That's not how the system works. Growth happens through cycles. Through returning. Through noticing what shifts and responding wisely. The Monarch is not a tyrant who demands perfection. The Monarch listens, adjusts, and integrates.

Even dysregulation isn't failure—it's information. When one Self goes offline or takes over, it's a message from your system that something needs attention. And now, you have a language to understand those messages. You have Override Strategies to bring yourself back. You have the toolbox of a practice.

The Practice of Reconnection

If there is one thing to carry with you, it is this: *Healing is reconnection.* Reconnecting with your body, your feelings, your thoughts. Reconnecting with others, with the world, with the larger story of which you are a part. Whether you use movement, meditation, nutrition, therapy, journaling, or something entirely your own, the act of reconnection is sacred. It is the work.

Each time you pause to notice your breath, soothe your Heart Self, or invite your Head Self back from a spiral—each of these is a moment of reclaiming your agency. You are not broken. You are becoming more whole.

Next Steps: Living What You've Learned

So here you are—at the end of the last chapter of the main section. You've explored the landscape of the Mind Matrix: the Three Selves, the State Axis, the process of Self-Other Differentiation, the Monarch and Ministers, Override Strategies, and the art of setting boundaries that preserve your integrity while allowing for connection.

But really, this is just the beginning.

More than anything, this book is meant to be an ongoing resource. A companion for moments when you feel uncentered. A guide for helping your whole mind work in harmony. And a way to offer yourself choice, compassion, and clarity.

This isn't a checklist or a program to master, it's a way of seeing. A way of listening to your system. A way of always returning home to yourself.

So what comes next? You begin where you are.

Keep Listening

What are your Selves trying to tell you? How can you listen better?

What is your State in each moment? How can you keep returning to the Positive State?

Sometimes all it takes is a breath and a question:

> *What am I feeling?*
> *What do I need?*
> *Which part of me is speaking?*

You don't have to fix everything. Just begin listening.

Keep Practicing

Change doesn't happen all at once. It happens in spirals, moving through the same lessons again and again with new awareness each time.

So let the practices be small:

- One moment of grounding when you're overwhelmed.
- One "no" said without apology.
- One connection where you might have stepped back.
- One shift in State—just enough to notice the difference.

Don't wait until you feel perfect. Practice now, as you are.

Keep Reflecting

The Monarch learns by noticing. Each time you pause to ask how something affected you, you're building your ability to choose rather than react.

Maybe that means journaling. Maybe it's just thinking back after a conversation:

> *What worked?*
> *What didn't?*
> *What would I do differently next time?*

That's not judgment. That's discernment. That's learning.

Keep Connecting

Self-work doesn't mean isolation. In fact, the more clearly you know yourself, the more deeply you can connect.

When you meet others from your own grounded center, you model something powerful:

> *Presence without merging.*
> *Boundaries without aggression.*
> *Love without losing the thread of yourself.*

Keep Coming Back

You will forget. You will flip between Selves. You'll override yourself or others.

That's not failure, it's part of the rhythm.

I call it the aikido of the mind. In aikido, you learn how to fall gracefully and return to standing. In the Mind Matrix Model, you learn how to return to presence and to the Positive State when you get dysregulated.

What matters is how much you can remember to come back to yourself with as much self-compassion as you can.

Continuing Your Journey

The rest of the book—the Next Steps chapters—are here to support your ongoing practice as needed and you'll find a link to more Next Step chapters on the website. You'll find a number of practical chapters that address specific concerns through a Mind Matrix lens, ideal for when you're navigating particular challenges or seeking targeted guidance.

On the mindmatrixmodel.com website you'll find additional resources, some of which we've discussed:

- Additional Next Steps chapters and an Advanced section for more complex subjects or those that are more specific to a particular therapy. We'll be adding to these over time.
- Both downloadable and interactive questionnaire forms. The interactive forms calculate your results and offer suggestions of what to do next. You can also re-take the questionnaires over time and get reports on your progress and what you need to work on.
- A forum for asking and answering questions, reporting on findings and related research, making suggestions, interacting with other MMM users, etc.
- Social groups covering different interests related to the MMM that you can join or create.
- Private messaging for chatting with one or more individuals or within groups.
- There's also document uploads and downloads, news feeds, videos, photos, and we'll be adding more over time.

Final Thoughts

You've come a long way through this book, unpacking the structures of the mind, meeting the Three Selves, exploring States, and discovering how your inner world functions and adapts. At times, this journey may have felt like theory. At others, it may have touched something personal, raw, or even transformative.

The purpose of the Mind Matrix Model isn't to give you one more system to memorize. It's to offer a lens—a way of seeing—that brings clarity, compassion, and possibility to your inner experience. You now have tools not just for surviving, but for navigating life with greater awareness, choice, and integration.

And while understanding is powerful, it's only the beginning. Real change happens not just through insight, but through practice—through how you show up for yourself and others, day after day, moment by moment.

So as you close this book, take a moment. Breathe. Acknowledge everything in you that brought you here—the questions, the struggles, the strength.

You are now the steward of your inner kingdom. And that kingdom? It can be more resilient, more beautiful, and more whole than you could have imagined.

SECTION TWO

Next Steps

Additional content targeted at specific information and issues

Contents

Blocks & Procrastination: 389

Explores how internal resistance, emotional overwhelm, or trauma-based loops can lead to avoidance and inaction. Identifies which Self is typically involved in different types of blocks and offers targeted Override Strategies.

Dietary Guide 397

Outlines a Whole-Self approach to food and nourishment. Includes supportive dietary principles for State regulation, brain health, mood, and trauma recovery—tailored to each of the Three Selves when possible.

Acupressure For Yourself and Others..................405

Presents simple techniques for using acupressure. Includes practical guidance for self-application and offering acupressure to others in a safe, respectful way.

Essential Oils: 411

Introduces how to use essential oils as tools for shifting State, soothing Sentries, and supporting balance in the Vital, Heart, and Head Selves.

Homeopathy 415

Explores the principles and history of homeopathy, including how to use remedies safely and effectively. Covers commonly used remedies.

Nutritional Supplements & Adaptogens...............421

Covers vitamins, minerals, herbs, and adaptogens that help regulate stress, energy, and emotional stability. Organized by Self and State pattern, this chapter offers guidance on choosing and combining supplements safely and effectively.

Sleep Hygiene **431**

Explores the foundational role of sleep in regulating the Vital Self, emotional resilience, and mental clarity. Offers practical strategies for creating a sleep-supportive routine, troubleshooting common issues, and using holistic tools—from breathwork to herbs—to promote deep, restorative rest.

Mindfulness & Meditation **437**

Explores foundational mindfulness and meditation practices for regulating State, calming the mind, and cultivating emotional resilience. Covers Vipassana, moving meditation, mindfulness in daily life, and trauma-aware approaches. Includes techniques for distraction management, self-compassion, and supporting each Self through awareness and presence.

Online Resources

Online resources require that you sign up for a membership, which is free.

You can find additional Next Steps chapters on the website by using the QR code here or going to:

https://mmm.tips/next

You can also visit the Advanced section to explore the MMM theory paper, which explains the foundational theory behind the Model and how it connects with current understandings in neurology, psychology, cognitive science, and ancient mindfulness traditions.

Additional papers cover the Mind Matrix Model in relation to developmental stages, therapy models, Buddhism, autism, and other topics. This section will continue to grow as new insights and applications are added over time.

https://mmm.tips/advanced

Chapter Twenty-One

Blocks & Procrastination:
Understanding & Shifting Resistance

We've all felt it: the sluggish weight of a task we can't begin, the invisible wall that stops us from doing what we know we need to do.

In the Mind Matrix Model, these moments of stuckness are not laziness or failure—they are messages. Blocks and procrastination are signals from your Vital, Heart, or Head Self that something isn't aligned.

Understanding where the resistance comes from allows you to move through it skillfully.

Let's start by defining these within the Mind Matrix Model.

> A block is a frozen pattern in your Mind Matrix—a Script or Sentry that says: *"It's not safe to move forward."*
>
> Procrastination is the behavior that emerges when we heed that inner freeze.

Rather than seeing these as moral failings, the Mind Matrix helps us decode them as nervous system messages. Somewhere along the line, your nervous system learned that these were appropriate responses to keep you safe, whether physically, emotionally, or in your thoughts.

Each of the Three Selves experiences blocks differently. Let's explore your own.

Quick Quiz: Where Is Your Block Coming From?

For each statement, mark any that apply to what you're experiencing.

When facing a relatively normal task that brings up procrastination, avoidance or resistance:

Vital Self Block

- Do you feel physically heavy, tired, foggy, or drained when facing the task?
- Do you feel a strong urge to escape, sleep, eat, or go numb?
- Do you sense body-based resistance like stomach tension or shallow breath?

If yes, the block is likely coming from your Vital Self. The task may feel unsafe, overstimulating, or your body may be in freeze or fatigue.

Heart Self Block

- Do you fear failure or rejection? Does your mind jump to what others might think?
- Do you hear an inner voice saying you're not good enough or that someone will judge you?
- Do you feel shame or disappointment just thinking about trying?

If yes, the block is likely coming from your Heart Self. Relational pain, fear of judgment, or inner criticism may be keeping you stuck.

Head Self Block

- Do you feel overwhelmed by details or can't find a starting point?
- Do you get caught in planning, researching, or perfectionism?
- Does your mind spin in analysis or jump to distractions?

If yes, the block is likely coming from your Head Self. You may be stuck in overthinking, mental looping, or a collapsed sense of direction.

Working with Blocks

Each block is an attempt to *protect* you. When your Monarch is offline and the Selves sense danger, they activate old Scripts or Sentries. Procrastination becomes a survival strategy, not a logical choice.

The Monarch's job is not to shame or scold, but to act as the **Reflective Catalyst**, gently bringing awareness to the source of resistance.

Titrating the Task: How to Begin Gently

One powerful way to shift a block is to titrate your effort—break the task into smaller, safer parts. Ask:

> What is *one small thing* I can do that feels 5% uncomfortable, not 100% overwhelming?

> Can I move *toward* the task without committing to completing it?

For example:

> - Instead of writing the whole email, Open the email draft and type "Hi."
> - Instead of starting the project, Gather the materials or open the project folder.
> - Instead of committing to a hard decision, Spend 2 minutes breathing and imagining what a first step might look like.

This begins to unwind the Sentry activation and reactivates your Monarch's guidance.

Bring in the Reflective Catalyst

Here's how the Monarch can step in with compassion and strategy:

> **Name It Gently**
> "I'm noticing resistance. I wonder which Self is trying to protect me?"
>
> **Ask Questions, Not Demands**
> "What part of me is afraid? What would help me feel a little safer right now?"
>
> **Engage Curiosity Instead of Shame**
> "What's underneath this delay? Is there grief, fear, perfectionism, or exhaustion?"

Shift the State First, Then Act
Sometimes, action can't happen until your State changes. Try a short override first:

- 3 deep breaths with long exhales
- Pressing an acupressure point (like Pericardium 6 or Kidney 1)
- Drinking water, stretching, or grounding with your feet

Tools for Working with Procrastination

Block Type	Fast Overrides	Deep Strategies
Vital Self	Splash cold water, shake body, step outside	Somatic therapy, exercise routines, sleep rhythm repair
Heart Self	EFT tapping, co-regulation (call someone safe)	Journaling shame loops, inner child work, self-compassion therapy
Head Self	5-minute timers, Pomodoro technique, write "bad first draft"	Cognitive restructuring, guided meditations for clarity, DBT/CBT

Sample Override Sequence

Situation: You've been avoiding working on a project. You feel heavy, foggy, and ashamed.

Step 1 – Press Liver 3 acupressure point while breathing deeply
Step 2 – Say: "Some part of me is trying to protect me. That makes sense."
Step 3 – Set a 5-minute timer and say: "I don't have to finish it. I'll just *start*."
Step 4 – After the timer: celebrate. Even if you only opened the file.
Step 5 – Reflect: "What part of me softened? What helped shift my State?"

Case Studies

Here are some examples of how blocks can play out, and how you might address them. For further information, refer to the Balancing the Vital Self or whichever chapter for the Self you need to work with, as well as possibly the Working with Stress & Anxiety or Working with State chapters for working with the anxiety or depression blocks can bring up.

Vital Self: Sarah – "Everything Feels Heavy"

Profile:
Sarah is a yoga teacher and part-time writer who recently started a wellness blog. She has a backlog of half-written posts and keeps telling herself she'll finish them soon—but weeks go by. Every time she sits down to write, she feels an inexplicable heaviness and fatigue. Her body slumps, her mind goes blank, and she ends up napping or snacking instead.

Block Presentation:

    Sensations: Lethargy, shallow breath, heavy chest or limbs

    Avoidance Behavior: Sleeps, doom-scrolls, snacks

    Sentry Activation: "I don't have enough energy for this."

    Monarch Offline — Override by Minister of the Vital Self in a hypoaroused (shutdown) state.

Reflective Catalyst Question:
"What part of me feels unsafe to mobilize right now?"

Interventions Used:

    Fast Override: Stretch. Walk outside barefoot; press Kidney 1 (Yongquan) while breathing.

    Titration Strategy: Set a 2-minute "pulse" timer: write just one sentence each time the timer goes off.

    Long-Term: Began each morning with Pal Dan Gum to activate her system before creative work

Insight:
The act of "getting started" was experienced as a threat to rest—a leftover Vital Script from earlier burnout

Heart Self: Tasha – "What If I'm Not Good Enough?"

Profile:

Tasha is a graduate student preparing to submit her first article for publication. Though the topic excites her and her advisor is encouraging, every time she opens the document, an emotional wave crashes in. She begins editing obsessively, doubting every word, and eventually abandons the task entirely—then feels a pang of guilt and self-disappointment. Despite her talent, she dreads the moment someone else reads her work.

Block Presentation:

    Primary Emotions: Shame, fear of rejection, sadness

    Avoidance Behavior: Over-editing, self-censorship, emotional withdrawal

    Sentry Activation: "If people read this and don't like it, it means something is wrong with *me*."

    Dominant Scripts: "I have to be exceptional to be accepted." "I'll be rejected if I show up as I am."

    Monarch Overridden by Heart Minister, protecting against potential emotional pain by suppressing authenticity

Reflective Catalyst Question:

    "What part of me is afraid to be seen, and what does it need to feel safe?"

Interventions Used:

    Fast Override: Heart-centered journaling using compassionate prompts like "What am I afraid they'll feel about me?"

    Emotional Titration Strategy: Shared a rough paragraph—not for feedback, but simply for relational exposure—to a trusted classmate

    Heart Self Practice: Practiced inner dialogue between her Inner Critic and Inner Encourager, rewriting the critical voice with warmth and perspective

    Long-Term Shift: Created a small peer group where feedback began with appreciation before critique, to create safe relational mirrors

Insight:
Her procrastination wasn't about perfection—it was about emotional safety. Submitting the piece felt like submitting *herself.* By gently building her tolerance for emotional visibility, she began to show up with more courage.

Head Self: Diego – "I Don't Know Where to Start"

Profile:
Diego is a web designer freelancing on a new client website. He opens the project file, then gets distracted by reorganizing fonts, researching plugins, checking analytics... but never makes progress on the homepage design. His mind is constantly spinning with "what ifs" and vague pressure. "It's got to be amazing," he says. "But I don't even know what amazing looks like yet."

Block Presentation:

Sensations: Mental spinning, excessive or scattered focus

Avoidance Behavior: Research loops, perfectionist tinkering

Sentry Activation: "Don't start until you have the *right* idea, or you'll screw it up."

Monarch Pulled Offline by Head Self in analytic overdrive

Reflective Catalyst Question:
"Am I trying to **solve** my fear, or **feel** my fear?"

Interventions Used:

Fast Override: 5-4-3-2-1 sensory tracking grounding technique (bring attention to sensory input)

Titration Strategy: Used a timer to make a "bad first version" of homepage layout—no judgment, just action

Long-Term: Committed to morning body movement (Vital Self) before any screen time

Insight:
His mental loop was masking vulnerability—creating helped him reconnect to flow

Final Thoughts

Blocks and procrastination are not failures. They are invitations. Every delay holds a message about what needs soothing, clarity, or safety.

Instead of asking, "Why am I stuck?"
Try asking, "What part of me needs help moving forward?"

When your Monarch learns to ask this question often and kindly, the mind becomes a place of movement again—not just pressure or paralysis.

Chapter Twenty-Two

Dietary Guide

Understanding Your Body's Dietary Needs

Each person's body is unique, and our dietary needs can vary. Some people notice they feel more energized or fuller with protein-rich foods like beans, eggs, or lean meat, while others do better with more whole grains, fruits, and vegetables. Research shows that protein generally increases satiety more than carbohydrates or fat, helping you feel full longer.[1] The key is to listen to your body's signals: if you feel hungry soon after meals, try adding more lean protein or high-fiber foods to stabilize your blood sugar and keep energy levels steady.

Everyone's metabolism and lifestyle play a role. Athletes or active people often need more protein for muscle recovery, while others might thrive on slow-burning carbs (whole grains, starchy vegetables, legumes). Notice patterns: do you crash into fatigue after eating simple carbs (perhaps add some protein or healthy fat)? Or do you stay satisfied all day after a hearty bean soup or scrambled eggs? There's no one-size-fits-all rule—tracking how different foods make you feel is a practical way to identify the balance that works best for you.

Mediterranean Diet: A Time-Tested Foundation

The Mediterranean diet emphasizes whole, plant-rich foods and healthy fats. It includes lots of vegetables, fruits, beans, whole grains, nuts, olive oil, and moderate fish, while keeping red meat and sweets small. This way of eating is backed by decades of research. For example, the landmark PREDIMED trial in Spain found that people who ate Mediterranean-style meals with extra-virgin olive oil or nuts had about 30 percent fewer heart attacks and strokes than those who followed a low-fat diet.[2]

Studies also link the Mediterranean diet to better mood and cognition. A 2024 Harvard review reported that adults with depression who shifted to a Mediterranean diet saw a greater drop in symptoms than those in control groups.[3] In simple terms, eating meals rich in vegetables, whole grains, and healthy fats can reduce inflammation in the body and brain, which often shows up as clearer thinking and more balanced emotions. In Mind Matrix terms, choosing these foods soothes your Vital Self (keeping energy steady and body functions healthy), lifts your Heart Self (calming stress and improving mood), and nourishes your Head Self (supporting clear thought and focus).

Embracing Plants: Reducing Inflammation and Stress

Shifting toward more plant-based eating—focusing on complex carbohydrates like whole grains, vegetables, and legumes—can reduce bodily stress and inflammation. Plants are packed with fiber, vitamins, minerals, and antioxidants that help fight oxidative stress. A systematic review found that predominantly plant-based diets (including Mediterranean and DASH diets) are associated with lower levels of inflammation markers, whereas typical Western diets (high in processed meats and refined foods) raise them.[4]

Eating more vegetables, fruits, beans, and whole grains also feeds healthy gut bacteria, which in turn helps calm inflammation. For example, cultures that eat lots of beans, greens, and whole grains—such as some communities in India or Japan—tend to have less chronic inflammation and better overall health. In fact, research on the "Blue Zones" (areas with many centenarians) found that 95 percent of people over 100 ate a mostly plant-based diet rich in legumes and whole grains.[5] These plant-forward diets also tend to come with lifestyle habits (like moderate eating, communal meals, or regular physical activity) that researchers associate with longevity.

Global Dietary Wisdom

Healthy diets around the world share similar principles. The people of Ikaria (a Greek island in the Mediterranean) famously follow a diet rich in vegetables, olive oil, beans, and fish—and they live about seven years longer on average than Americans do.[5] In Okinawa, Japan, traditional diets focus on vegetables, tofu, and fish; in Latin America, long-standing cuisines center on corn, beans, squash, and chili peppers. These cultures often use healing spices (like turmeric, ginger, and garlic) and include fermented foods (like yogurt, kimchi, or sauerkraut) for gut health. Family meals or rituals (like communal dining) slow down eating, helping the Vital Self register fullness and nourishing the Heart Self through connection. Even in Nordic countries, researchers find benefits from their whole-foods traditions (rye breads, berries, and fish) that resemble aspects of the Mediterranean diet.

The lesson is that whole foods—especially plants—form the foundation of many healthy traditions worldwide. You can honor this wisdom by experimenting with dishes from different cuisines. Try a chickpea curry, a vegetable stir-fry, or a simple bean salad. These meals can satisfy your appetite and introduce your taste buds to healthier patterns. Each new healthy dish you enjoy is a step toward feeling vibrant and well.

The Gut-Brain Connection: Mood and Cognition

Your gut is often called your "second brain," and for good reason. The enteric nervous system in your digestive tract has millions of neurons and communicates constantly with your brain. This gut-brain axis works through nerves, hormones, and the immune system. In fact, the gut produces about 95 percent of the body's serotonin, a key neurotransmitter for mood [6]. Healthy gut microbes also produce short-chain fatty acids and other metabolites that benefit brain cells. Research shows that a balanced gut microbiome can improve emotional regulation and cognitive function.[6]

What you eat dramatically affects this system. A diet rich in fiber and fermented foods helps feed beneficial bacteria, which in turn support your Heart and Head Selves. Conversely, a high-sugar or high-fat diet can disrupt gut balance and lead to "brain fog," irritability, or even sleep issues. By choosing whole foods—prebiotics like oats and onions, probiotics like yogurt or kimchi, and plenty of vegetables—you literally nourish the cells that signal to your brain. Over time, you may notice that healthy changes can help your Head Self feel clearer and more focused, and your Heart Self feel more emotionally balanced.

Shifting Your Diet: What to Expect

Changing your diet can bring great benefits, but it often comes with temporary challenges. Physically, your body may need days or weeks to adapt when you add more fiber or cut back on sugar. You might feel hunger more intensely at first or have cravings for comfort foods. Some people report mild fatigue or headaches as their gut bacteria adjust. These symptoms usually fade as your body learns to use nutrient-dense foods efficiently and stabilizes blood sugar.

Emotionally and socially, expect some ups and downs too. If friends or family aren't changing their diet, you might feel left out at meals or tempted by familiar snacks. Others may question your choices, which can feel frustrating. It helps to remember why you're making changes in terms of the Mind Matrix: each nourishing meal is supporting your Vital Self's health, soothing stress for your Heart Self, and clearing the way for your Head Self to think clearly. For example, sometimes sharing your journey can bring support from others and strengthen your resolve.

Above all, progress is gradual. You will have days of strong success and days of slip-ups. This is perfectly normal. Even small steps—like adding an extra vegetable to your plate or choosing water instead of soda—add up over time. Each healthy choice feeds the Positive State of the Mind Matrix, where your Vital, Heart, and Head Selves all feel better. Give yourself credit for improvements, no matter how minor they seem. A compassionate mindset—reminding yourself that change is a process—will carry you farther than strict self-criticism ever could.

Mood-Supportive Foods: Nutrient-Rich Fuel for Resilience

To support stable mood, emotional flexibility, and energy balance, certain foods naturally enhance the production and function of **neurotransmitters** like serotonin, dopamine, and GABA.

Below is a breakdown by nutrient:

Omega-3 Fatty Acids

Fatty Fish (high EPA/DHA): Salmon (wild-caught is best), Sardines, Mackerel, Herring, Anchovies.
Plant-Based Sources (high ALA): Flaxseeds (ground), Chia seeds, Hemp seeds, Walnuts, Canola oil, Flaxseed oil.
Fortified Foods: Omega-3-enriched eggs, Algae-based DHA supplements (for vegetarians and vegans).

Note: EPA and DHA from marine sources have more direct anti-inflammatory and mood-regulating effects than ALA, though both are valuable.

Tryptophan-Rich Foods

Poultry: Turkey, Chicken.
Seeds and Nuts: Pumpkin seeds, Sunflower seeds, Sesame seeds, Almonds, Cashews.
Legumes: Soybeans (edamame, tofu, tempeh), Lentils, Chickpeas.
Whole Grains: Oats, Quinoa, Brown rice.
Dairy: Milk, Yogurt, Cheese.
Fruits: Bananas, Dates.
Other: Eggs.

Note: Pairing tryptophan-rich foods with moderate carbohydrates (e.g., sweet potatoes or brown rice) enhances serotonin synthesis by aiding transport across the blood-brain barrier.

Magnesium-Rich Foods

Leafy Greens: Spinach, Swiss chard, Kale, Beet greens.
Nuts and Seeds: Pumpkin seeds (very high in magnesium), Almonds, Brazil nuts, Sunflower seeds.
Legumes: Black beans, Kidney beans, Chickpeas, Lentils.
Whole Grains: Brown rice, Quinoa, Buckwheat.
Fruits and Vegetables: Bananas, Avocados, Dried figs.
Other: Dark chocolate (85%+ cocoa, in moderation—1 oz contains ~65 mg magnesium).

> **Note:** *Magnesium is especially important during stress recovery, and deficiencies are common in high-stress lifestyles or diets high in sugar and caffeine.*
>
> **Tip:** *Magnesium is depleted by stress, sugar, and caffeine. Eating magnesium-rich foods consistently can help rebuild your reserve.*

Practical Pairings

Here are examples of simple food combinations that support all three nutrients:

- Salmon with quinoa and steamed spinach
- Oatmeal topped with flaxseed, banana, and almonds
- Hummus (chickpeas + tahini) with whole grain pita and raw carrots
- Tempeh stir-fry with kale, bell peppers, and brown rice
- Hard-boiled egg with a side of walnuts and dark chocolate square

Practical Steps and Self-Compassion

Here are some practical ideas to ease into a healthier diet and practice self-kindness along the way:

Make Small Changes: Try one new swap per week. For example, have one meatless dinner (a bean chili or vegetable stir-fry) or replace sugary drinks with water or herbal tea.

Add, Don't Just Remove: Focus on adding nourishing foods. Fill half your plate with colorful vegetables, snack on nuts or yogurt, and add fruit to cereal or salads.

Meal Planning: Plan a few healthy meals each week. Batch-cook a soup or vegetable curry for quick meals.

Mindful Eating: Eat slowly and notice when you're full. This helps your Vital Self recognize satisfaction and supports your Heart Self through appreciation.

Stay Hydrated: Drink water or herbal teas throughout the day to support energy and digestion.

Celebrate Small Wins: Acknowledge every step forward. This builds encouragement and reinforces motivation.

Be patient with yourself. Each meal is a chance to support your Selves. Change is a process, not a test.

Intermittent Fasting: Supporting Your Body's Rhythm

Intermittent fasting (IF) means eating only during certain hours of the day or on certain days. Common methods include daily time-restricted eating (e.g., eating between 11 a.m. and 7 p.m.) or fasting for 24 hours once or twice a week.

Research shows IF can support fat metabolism, insulin sensitivity, and even mental clarity. After about 12–14 hours of fasting, your body starts burning fat for fuel and produces ketones, which many people find help with mental focus. Fasting also triggers cellular recycling processes (autophagy) and increases brain-derived neurotrophic factor (BDNF), a protein that supports memory and new brain connections[7,8]. Older adults who practice IF also report lower rates of depression and cognitive decline.[9]

If you try it, start gently—such as skipping breakfast and eating lunch and dinner within an 8-hour window. Drink water, broth, or herbal teas while fasting. As always, listen to your body. IF may not be right for everyone, particularly those with medical conditions or histories of disordered eating. Used wisely, it can be a tool to reset your system and strengthen your Vital and Head Selves.

Integrating Diet with the Mind Matrix

A healthy diet supports all Three Selves. The Vital Self benefits from physical stability and energy. The Heart Self calms when blood sugar is steady and inflammation is low. The Head Self thrives with consistent nourishment for focus, memory, and calm awareness.

Food is not just fuel—it's information for the body, mood, and mind. Every meal is an opportunity to support your inner kingdom and reinforce your Positive State. Choose meals that strengthen your Selves, and you will feel clearer, more resilient, and more connected to the life you want to live.

References

1. Paddon-Jones, D. et al. (2008). Protein, weight management, and satiety. *American Journal of Clinical Nutrition.*

2. Estruch, R. et al. (2013). Primary Prevention of Cardiovascular Disease with a Mediterranean Diet. *New England Journal of Medicine.*

3. Salamon, M. (2024). Mediterranean diet may help ease depression. *Harvard Health Publishing.*

4. Aleksandrova, K. et al. (2021). Dietary patterns and biomarkers of oxidative stress and inflammation. *Free Radical Biology & Medicine.*

5. Buettner, D. (2015). Lessons from the Blue Zones. *National Geographic Books / NCBI Bookshelf.*

6. Appleton, J. (2018). The Gut-Brain Axis: Influence of Microbiota on Mood and Mental Health. *Integrative Medicine: A Clinician's Journal.*

7. Monda, V. et al. (2022). Effects of Intermittent Fasting on Brain Metabolism. *International Journal of Molecular Sciences.*

8. Mattson, M. P. et al. (2017). Intermittent metabolic switching, neuroplasticity and brain health. *Nature Reviews Neuroscience.*

9. Wilkinson, M. J. et al. (2020). Ten-hour time-restricted eating reduces weight, blood pressure, and atherogenic lipids in patients with metabolic syndrome. *Cell Metabolism.*

Chapter Twenty-Three

Acupressure
For Yourself and Others

Acupressure is an ancient healing practice rooted in Traditional Chinese Medicine (TCM) that involves applying gentle, steady pressure to specific points on the body. This method helps regulate energy flow (Qi), alleviate discomfort, and promote overall balance in the body and mind. Practicing acupressure on yourself or others is a simple yet powerful way to support well-being.

Understanding Acupressure

Acupressure points are located along meridians, which are energy pathways in the body. Stimulating these points helps regulate the body's internal systems, reducing pain, stress, and emotional imbalances. Unlike acupuncture, which uses needles, acupressure relies on gentle finger pressure, making it accessible to anyone.

Basic Techniques for Acupressure

- Steady Finger Pressure: Use your thumb, index, or middle finger to apply firm but gentle pressure to the point.
- Circular Massage: Instead of holding pressure, you can also make slow, circular motions over the point.
- Breath Awareness: Take deep, slow breaths while applying pressure to enhance relaxation and effectiveness.
- Hold for 30 Seconds to 1 Minute: Apply pressure for at least 30 seconds and up to one minute, depending on the sensitivity and needs of the area.

Performing Acupressure on Yourself

Self-acupressure is a practical way to relieve tension, manage pain, and regulate emotions. Here's how to apply it effectively:

- Find a Quiet Space: Sit or lie in a comfortable position where you can focus on your body.
- Locate the Acupressure Point: Refer to an acupressure chart or guide to find the appropriate point for your concern.
- Apply Gentle, Firm Pressure: Press the point with consistent, steady pressure, adjusting intensity based on your comfort level.
- Massage Along the Meridian: The points are the most important areas on the meridians, but it's quite helpful to massage the meridians themselves. Once you've released a point, massage the neighboring meridian and points.
- Breathe Deeply: Slow, deep breaths, especially breathing out longer than breathing in, will calm your State.
- Repeat as Needed: Perform acupressure daily for lasting benefits.

Performing Acupressure on Others

When practicing acupressure on someone else, maintain a calming presence and ensure their comfort.

- Ask for Consent: Ensure the recipient is comfortable with acupressure and understands the process.

- Breathe Deeply: Slow, deep breaths will help to co-regulate the person you're working with.
- Find the Right Position: The recipient should be seated or lying down in a relaxed position.
- Use Gentle, Sustained Pressure: Adjust intensity based on the recipient's sensitivity. Communication is key.
- Encourage Deep Breathing: Guide them to inhale deeply and exhale slowly for a more effective session.
- Monitor Their Response: If any discomfort arises, adjust pressure or move to another point.

Common Acupressure Points and Their Uses

Listen to Your Body: If a point feels overly tender or painful, ease the pressure or choose another location.

Hydrate After a Session: Drinking water can help flush out toxins and support energy flow after acupressure.

Practicing acupressure regularly can enhance relaxation, improve circulation, and support overall well-being. Whether applied to yourself or shared with others, it's a simple, effective tool for physical and emotional balance.

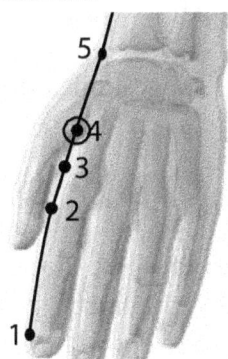

LI 4 (Hegu) – Located in the webbing between the thumb and index finger, pressing into the bone of the index finger (second metacarpal) as well as massaging all through the webbing.
Useful for headaches, stress relief, and general tension.

Pc 6 (Neiguan)
– Found four finger-widths below the wrist crease.

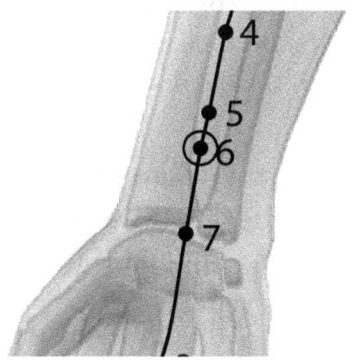

Helps with nausea, anxiety, and heart-related stress.

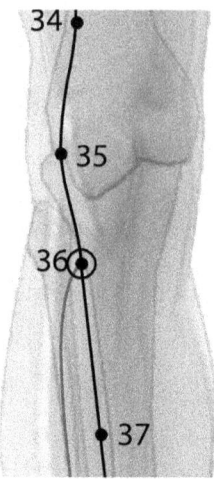

St 36 (Zusanli) Below the knee, about six finger-widths beneath the kneecap and three finger-widths beside the bone (tibia). Supports digestion, energy levels, and immune function.

GV 20 (Baihui) – On the top of the head in the center directly above the tops of the ears. Helps clear the mind and improve focus.

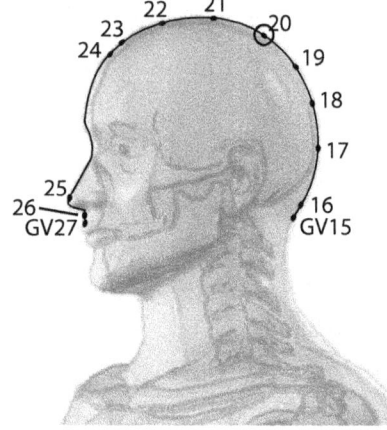

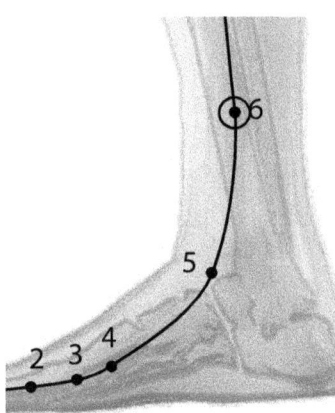

Sp 6 (Sanyinjiao) – Located six fingers above the inner ankle bump (medial malleolus)
Supports hormonal balance, digestion, and sleep.

Safety and Best Practices

Avoid Acupressure on Open Wounds or Inflamed Areas: Pressure should never be applied to broken skin or recent injuries. However, it can be very helpful to work around the area to increase Qi flow into and out of the area.

Pregnancy Considerations: Some acupressure points should be avoided during pregnancy unless guided by a professional. These include:

Sp 6 (Sanyinjiao) – Above the inner ankle, linked to uterine contractions (shown above).

LI 4 (Hegu) – Between the thumb and index finger, associated with labor induction (shown above).

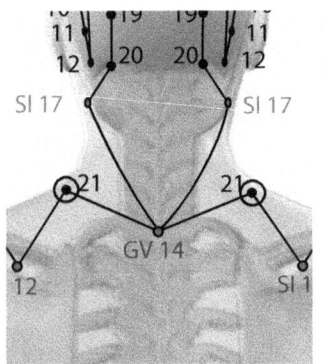

GB 21 (Jianjing) – On the top of the shoulders, may promote downward energy flow.

Bl 60 (Kunlun) – Behind the outer ankle bump (lateral malleolus), linked to labor stimulation.

Bl 67 (Zhiyin) – At the outer pinky toe, often used to turn breech babies.

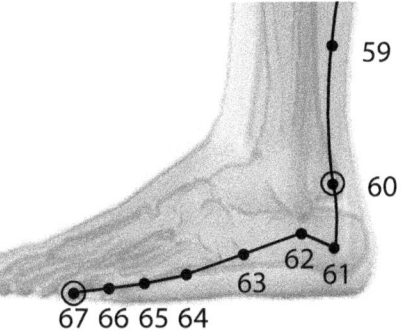

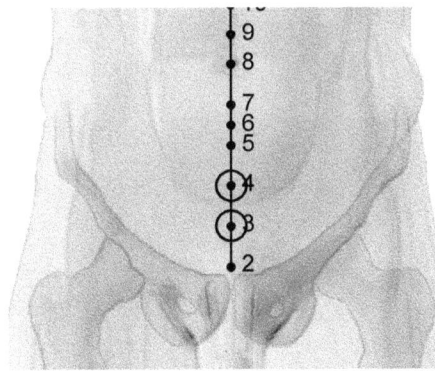

CV 3 (Zhongji) & CV-4 (Guanyuan) – Lower abdominal points that can stimulate the uterus.

Sp 10 (Xuehai) – Above the knee, traditionally avoided for its strong circulation effects.

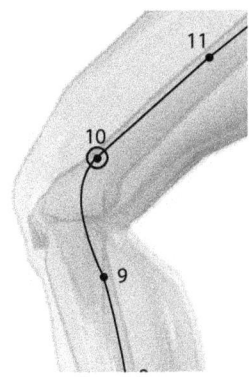

Best Practices for Pregnancy Acupressure: Always consult a qualified practitioner before using acupressure during pregnancy. If seeking relief for pregnancy-related symptoms, focus on gentle points such as Pc 6 (Neiguan) for nausea (shown above) or Yintang (Third Eye) for relaxation.

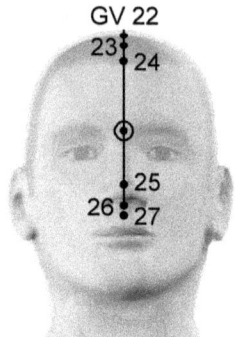

Chapter Twenty-Four

Essential Oils:
History, Use, and Safety

Essential oils have been used for thousands of years across different cultures for their therapeutic, medicinal, and spiritual properties. Their continued popularity today reflects their versatility and the growing body of evidence supporting their benefits.

Historical Background

Essential oils have a rich history, dating back to ancient civilizations:

Ancient Egypt: Egyptians used essential oils in embalming, cosmetics, and spiritual rituals.

Ancient China and India: Essential oils were integrated into traditional medicines, supporting physical and emotional health through aromatherapy, massage, and topical use.

Ancient Greece and Rome: Oils like lavender, frankincense, and myrrh were highly valued for health and ritual purposes.

Modern Research and Efficacy

Recent studies have validated several therapeutic properties of essential oils:

- **Lavender**: Clinically shown to reduce anxiety, stress, and improve sleep quality.
- **Peppermint**: Proven effective in enhancing alertness, relieving headaches, and improving cognitive performance.
- **Eucalyptus**: Demonstrated antimicrobial effects and support for respiratory health.
- **Frankincense**: Shown to have anti-inflammatory properties, potentially reducing stress and promoting emotional balance.

Though promising, research into essential oils is ongoing, and individual responses vary widely.

Methods of Use

Diffusion: Using a diffuser, essential oils are dispersed into the air, benefiting mood, stress relief, respiratory health, and overall well-being.

Topical Application: Diluting essential oils with a carrier oil (such as coconut, almond, or jojoba) allows safe application on the skin for localized therapeutic effects.

Inhalation: Direct inhalation (from the bottle or via a few drops on a tissue) provides quick emotional and respiratory benefits.

Bathing: Adding essential oils diluted with bath salts or carrier oils into warm baths promotes relaxation, reduces stress, and can ease muscle tension.

Safety Guidelines

Always dilute essential oils with a carrier oil (such as almond, jojoba, or coconut oil) before topical application to prevent skin irritation.

Conduct a patch test by applying a small amount to your skin to test sensitivity before extensive use.

Avoid ingesting essential oils unless under guidance from a qualified healthcare provider.

Keep essential oils away from children and pets.

Pregnant women, infants, and those with serious health conditions should consult a healthcare professional before use.

Be aware of oils that can increase sun sensitivity, such as citrus oils, and avoid sun exposure after application.

Using essential oils responsibly and knowledgeably can enhance your self-care routine, supporting physical health, emotional balance, and overall vitality.

Chapter Twenty-Five

Homeopathy
Gentle Remedies for Balance & Health

Homeopathy is a holistic healing modality developed over two centuries ago that uses extremely dilute natural substances to stimulate your body's own healing processes. It operates on the principle of "like cures like," meaning that substances causing symptoms in large doses can help alleviate those same symptoms in very small doses.

Homeopathy remains widely used across the world, even as it continues to face skepticism from much of the scientific and medical community. While some clinical trials and meta-analyses have found homeopathy to perform no better than placebo under randomized controlled conditions, it remains a central part of traditional and complementary medicine systems in many countries.

The global homeopathy market was valued at over $5 billion USD in 2023 and continues to grow—especially in Asia-Pacific and Latin America.

The World Health Organization (WHO) officially recognizes homeopathy as part of global traditional medicine practices.

Surveys consistently show high user satisfaction: between 60% and 80% of people who use homeopathy report being satisfied or highly satisfied with their experience.

Many describe meaningful improvements in chronic conditions, emotional stress, and hard-to-define physical symptoms—particularly in situations where conventional medicine may offer only limited relief or comes with side effects.

Even if its mechanism remains debated, homeopathy—at minimum—represents a skillful use of the placebo response, which Western medicine acknowledges as having a significant effect but often treats as a diagnostic nuisance rather than a therapeutic opportunity. While the placebo effect is well-documented in clinical trials, it is typically framed as a confounding variable, not as a tool to be deliberately cultivated for healing.

In the Mind Matrix framework, these symbolic processes are far from incidental—they are essential. The deeper the dysregulation or chronicity, the more likely it is that healing requires not just biological correction, but symbolic repair and felt internal safety. For many, homeopathy provides just that.

From my own experience, I was initially very skeptical of homeopathy because it seemed to either work or not work, with no clear indication why. But two events succeeded in changing my mind:

My first experience was in the mid- to late-1980's. I was a live-in caretaker for a woman with Alzheimer's Disease whose husband also died from the disease. Shortly after moving in, I got sick with a very high fever which was not typical for me.

Within a year, I started having health issues and getting weaker and over several years got so sick that I was unable to work more than a few hours a day. An NPR news report said that recent evidence had found that chlordane, the termite and ant treatment that came after DDT was outlawed, could cause Alzheimer's. I had the house tested, and they found extremely high levels of chlordane especially in the basement, where I was living.

My doctor at the time was training in homeopathy, and she recommended we try a 1M dose of sulphur, which is a very high dose. Within a few hours of taking it, I got a severe rash with itching all over my body very similar to poison ivy but I had not been exposed to poison ivy. I spent several nights trying to sleep in a cold bath, then the symptoms cleared and over the next few weeks, my chronic symptoms began to fade and my energy returned.

My second experience was in the 1988. I had moved into a new unfinished house I was building with my first wife and, shortly after, welcomed the birth of my daughter.

One night while we were sleeping, I heard my daughter start crying quite stridently. I jumped out of bed, started running to her…and promptly smashed my left pinkie toe into the leg of the bed. I fell back on the bed with intense pain (as you can imagine, I'm sure) and directed my wife to go after our daughter.

I stumbled my way downstairs in the dark, not wanting to turn on lights, to the bathroom and switched on the light. I looked down and my left toe was pointing west.

From the shock, I immediately became nauseous and dizzy and felt like I was going to faint. I fell into a chair, fervently praying "Please don't throw up…please don't pass out…" repeating this several times until it passed enough for me to make my way into the kitchen.

There, I grabbed a tube of homeopathic arnica, said to help with trauma, and downed a dose. An instant later, my dizziness and nausea passed and my feelings of shock and trauma passed. It was remarkable.

A Brief History of Homeopathy

Homeopathy was developed by German physician Samuel Hahnemann in the late 1700s as a response to the often brutal medical practices of his time, which included bloodletting, purging, and the use of toxic substances like mercury. Deeply dissatisfied with these methods, Hahnemann sought a gentler, more rational system of healing.

His breakthrough came when translating a medical text describing the use of cinchona bark (from which quinine is derived) to treat malaria. Curious, Hahnemann took cinchona himself and found that it produced malaria-like symptoms in his otherwise healthy body. This led him to propose the principle of "similia similibus curentur"—like cures like: a substance that produces symptoms in a healthy person can be used to treat similar symptoms in a sick person.

Over time, Hahnemann refined this idea into a complete medical system, introducing two additional key concepts:

- Potentization: The process of serial dilution and shaking (succussion) of a substance to enhance its healing potential while minimizing toxicity. He believed that the energetic imprint of the substance was retained, even when no measurable molecules remained.
- Individualization: Rather than treating a disease label, homeopathy emphasizes selecting a remedy based on the whole person—including their physical symptoms, emotional state, temperament, and personal history.

Homeopathy spread rapidly in the 19th century, especially in Europe, India, and the United States, where it offered a more humane alternative to the harsh treatments of conventional medicine. By the mid-1800s, it was widely practiced, with dedicated hospitals, medical schools, and professional societies. Although later marginalized by the rise of biomedicine and pharmaceutical science, homeopathy continued to thrive in many parts of the world, particularly in India, where it remains integrated into the national healthcare system.

Today, homeopathy is one of the most widely used systems of complementary medicine worldwide. Despite controversy and ongoing scientific debate, it is valued by millions for its gentle, individualized approach, especially in treating chronic conditions, emotional imbalances, and functional disorders.

How Homeopathy Works

Homeopathy remedies are created through a process of dilution and shaking (succussion), believed to enhance their healing properties while reducing potential side effects.

Individualized Treatment: Remedies are chosen based on detailed symptom profiles and the unique characteristics of each individual.

Energetic Healing: Remedies are thought to stimulate the body's vital force (your natural healing capacity), supporting recovery and balance without side effects common to conventional medicines.

Common Remedies for Everyday Issues

Below are some commonly used homeopathic remedies and their indications:

Arnica Montana: Bruises, physical trauma, muscle soreness, shock.

Aconitum Napellus (Aconite): Acute anxiety, panic attacks, sudden fear, emotional shock.

Ignatia Amara: Grief, emotional loss, acute sadness or disappointment.

Chamomilla: Calming irritability, teething discomfort in babies, emotional sensitivity.

Nux Vomica: Digestive discomfort, irritability, stress-related digestive symptoms, insomnia from overstimulation.

Pulsatilla: Emotional sensitivity, feelings of abandonment or loneliness, mood swings, and hormonal imbalances.

Safe and Effective Use of Homeopathy

To safely use homeopathic remedies:

- Match Symptoms Carefully: Choose a remedy that closely aligns with your specific physical and emotional symptoms.
- Dosage and Frequency: Typically, homeopathic remedies come as small pellets or tablets. Follow recommended dosage on the label or instructions provided by a practitioner.
- Avoid Strong Substances: Mint, strong coffee, or strongly aromatic substances may reduce the effectiveness of homeopathic remedies.
- Observe Response: Watch how your body responds. Stop or adjust dosage if you experience unexpected symptoms.

For chronic conditions, working with a homeopathic practitioner can offer more personalized, comprehensive treatment.

By thoughtfully integrating homeopathy into your wellness routine, you support your body's natural ability to maintain balance, fostering emotional, physical, and mental resilience.

When to Seek Professional Guidance

While homeopathy and other holistic methods can support healing, they are not a substitute for medical diagnosis or emergency care. If symptoms are severe, worsening, or persistent, it's important to consult a qualified healthcare professional. Always seek appropriate medical attention for acute or serious conditions, and use homeopathic remedies as part of a broader, informed care plan.

Chapter Twenty-Six

Nutritional Supplements & Adaptogens

Supporting Balance in the Selves

Your system—body, mind, and heart—is an ecosystem. When that system becomes unbalanced, the right supports can make a huge difference. Nutritional supplements, adaptogenic herbs, and gentle remedies offer ways to help bring your Three Selves back into harmony.

But not all supplements are created equal.

This chapter will guide you through the best and worst forms of commonly used nutrients, how to choose wisely based on your needs, and how specific combinations can support regulation across the Vital, Heart, and Head Selves.

The Basics: Why Supplement?

Modern life challenges the balance your body was built for. Stress, poor soil quality, processed foods, long-term medications, disrupted sleep, and environmental toxins can all deplete essential nutrients. Even if you're eating well, you may not be getting everything your system needs to stay stable—especially if your Vital Self is dysregulated or your stress has been long-term.

Supplements are not about fixing something broken. They're about restoring the system's ability to thrive.

How to Work with Supplements

When it comes to supplements, it's easy to think, "If a little helps, more must be better." But the truth is: **your body prefers clarity over complexity**. The most effective way to work with supplements is slowly, consciously, and with your own system in mind.

Here's how to do that.

1. Start Slow and Go One at a Time

Even if you're eager to feel better, don't start five new supplements at once. That makes it hard to tell what's helping—or what's causing side effects.

- **Choose one supplement to begin with.**
- **Start at a low dose**, even lower than the label recommends.
- Stay with that one supplement for **at least a few days to a week**, watching how your system responds.

This lets your body adjust and gives you a clear picture of its effects. Some people notice benefits within hours; for others, it's more gradual. If all goes well, you can either increase the dose slightly or add another supplement.

2. More Is Not Better

You don't need an overflowing supplement shelf. In fact, too many supplements at once can overwhelm your system, create side effects, or just be a waste of money.

What matters most is choosing the right support for your particular type of imbalance. A few well-chosen supplements will always work better than a kitchen-sink approach.

Ask:

> *What is my most pressing symptom or imbalance right now?*
>
> *Which Self (Vital, Heart, or Head) seems to be most affected?*
>
> *What supplement would support that Self's return to balance?*

Let your answers guide you.

3. Pay Attention to Your System's Cues

You are the best expert on your own body—if you learn to listen.

> If something makes you feel agitated, foggy, over-sedated, or jittery—it may not be the right fit.

> If you feel clearer, calmer, more stable, or simply "more like yourself," it's probably helping.

Sometimes what works great for one person might be too stimulating or too calming for another. That's okay. The key is **personalization**, not perfection.

4. Consider Timing and Synergy

When and how you take supplements can make a major difference in how well they work—and how well your system tolerates them. The same supplement can feel calming or overstimulating depending on the time of day, what it's taken with, or what else you've paired it with.

Think of it like tuning an orchestra: each instrument (or nutrient) plays a role, but it only sounds right when timed and balanced correctly.

Timing Matters: Morning, Midday, Evening

Morning – Activate and Energize

- **Stimulating adaptogens** like *Rhodiola Rosea, Asian ginseng*, or *Eleuthero (Siberian ginseng)* are best taken in the morning or early afternoon. They help boost mental clarity, motivation, and energy—but taken too late, they may disrupt sleep or cause restlessness.

- **B-complex vitamins** are also best taken early in the day. They support energy metabolism and brain function but can be too activating for some people at night.

- **Vitamin D3** (if supplementing) should be taken in the morning or with your first meal to align with your circadian rhythm and enhance mood and immune function.

Midday – Sustain and Stabilize

- **Omega-3 fatty acids (EPA/DHA)** can be taken with lunch or dinner. They help maintain emotional and cognitive balance throughout the day.

- **Adaptogen blends** that combine calming and energizing herbs (e.g., Reishi + Rhodiola) are often ideal for midday use, supporting endurance and mental resilience without overstimulation.

Evening – Calm, Restore, and Rebuild

- **Magnesium glycinate or threonate** is best taken in the evening, ideally 1–2 hours before bed. It helps quiet the nervous system, reduce muscle tension, and promote sleep. Threonate, in particular, can also enhance overnight brain repair.
- **Ashwagandha**, while technically an adaptogen, is calming and can be taken in the evening or at bedtime to ease stress and support sleep.
- **L-Theanine**, if being used for anxiety or restlessness, may be helpful either in the evening or situationally throughout the day.

> **Tip:** *If you're highly sensitive or have trouble sleeping, pay close attention to the timing of B vitamins and stimulating herbs—they may be better suited earlier in the day or at lower doses.*

Food Pairing for Better Absorption

Some supplements need food to work well. Others are best taken on an empty stomach. Here's how to pair them:

Fat-soluble nutrients like *Vitamin D, A, E, K* and *fish oil* should always be taken with food—especially a meal that includes healthy fats—to ensure proper absorption.

Magnesium, B vitamins, and **most adaptogens** can be taken with meals for better tolerance, especially if you have a sensitive stomach.

Iron (if you're using it) is best absorbed on an empty stomach with Vitamin C—but it often causes nausea. A light snack may help if this occurs.

When in doubt: *Taking supplements with a small meal or healthy fat source (like avocado, olive oil, or nut butter) is generally safe and well-tolerated.*

Smart Pairings (Synergy) to Maximize Benefits

Some supplements naturally complement each other to work even better:

Pairing	Why It Works
Magnesium + L-Theanine	Calms the nervous system without sedation. Great for anxiety, tension, or bedtime.
Omega-3s + B-complex	Supports emotional resilience, brain function, and cognitive clarity.
Rhodiola + Reishi	Energizing and grounding—boosts stamina while supporting stress recovery.
Ashwagandha + Holy Basil	Deep stress relief and emotional regulation, especially helpful for burnout and Heart Self overwhelm.
Magnesium + Zinc + B6	A classic trio for calming nervous system reactivity and supporting hormone balance.

Spacing and Splitting Your Dose

> - If a supplement gives you stomach upset or feels like "too much," try splitting the dose into two smaller amounts—one with breakfast, one with dinner.
> - For energy-based herbs or nutrients, spacing them helps avoid overstimulation while extending their effect.
> - For calming supplements, a larger dose in the evening may work better.

Balance is key. Don't be afraid to experiment gently. Your system will tell you what it likes, especially when you introduce supplements one at a time.

Final Word on Timing and Synergy

You don't need to get everything perfect. But a little attention to when and how you take your supplements can turn a "maybe it helps" into a "wow, I feel so much better."

Start simple. Build from there. And most importantly—listen to your system.

5. Less Is More When Your System Is Sensitive

If you're highly sensitive, anxious, or coming out of collapse, even small doses can feel like a lot. That's not a weakness—it's your system asking for gentle support.

> Cut capsules in half, or use a powdered or liquid version where you can control the dose more easily.
>
> Give yourself time to adapt.
>
> Track your reactions in a journal if needed.

The goal is not to find the "perfect" supplement plan. The goal is to build a supportive, ongoing relationship with your body—where supplements play a helpful but not overwhelming role in your healing.

Core Nutrients for Nervous System Support

Magnesium – The Mineral of Calm

Best forms: Magnesium *glycinate* and *threonate*

- Glycinate is gentle and well-absorbed. Ideal for stress, anxiety, and sleep support.
- Threonate crosses the blood-brain barrier and supports cognitive function.

Avoid: *Magnesium oxide* – poorly absorbed, often causes stomach upset or loose stools.

Helps with: Vital Self regulation, insomnia, tension, anxiety.

Omega-3 Fatty Acids – Brain and Mood Fuel

Best sources: Fish oil (EPA/DHA), especially from wild-caught salmon, sardines, mackerel, or algae-based options if plant-based.

Why they matter: Omega-3s support the brain's structure, stabilize mood, reduce inflammation, and help all Three Selves work better together.

Good for: Brain fog, depression, emotional volatility, systemic inflammation.

B Vitamins – Energy, Mood, and Resilience

Best forms: A methylated B-complex that includes methylfolate (B9) and methylcobalamin (B12).

Supports: Energy metabolism, adrenal resilience, mood regulation, and neurotransmitter synthesis.

Particularly important for Heart and Head Self under chronic stress.

Adaptogens: Herbs That Help You Adapt

Adaptogens are plant allies that help your system respond more flexibly to stress. They don't sedate or stimulate directly—instead, they support your body's ability to restore balance.

Calming Adaptogens (for anxiety, high stress, overarousal)

- **Ashwagandha**: Deeply grounding, reduces cortisol, supports sleep. Great for anxious Heart or hyperactive Vital states. May cause drowsiness in some.
- **Tulsi (Holy Basil)**: Calms without sedating. Supports Heart Self, relieves tension, and helps with mood swings or emotional reactivity.
- **Lemon Balm**: Soothes nervous agitation, helpful in both Heart and Vital dysregulation.
- **Reishi Mushroom**: Supports immune function, spiritual grounding, and Heart Self resilience.

Stimulating Adaptogens (for fatigue, collapse, hypoarousal)

- **Rhodiola Rosea**: Boosts physical and cognitive energy, especially helpful when the Head Self is foggy and the Vital Self is drained. ***Caution: Can be too stimulating for those prone to anxiety or overheating.***
- **Asian Ginseng**: Sharpens thinking and endurance. Better for Head-focused fatigue or performance stress.
- **American Ginseng**: Gentler and more calming; balances energy without overstimulation.

Pairing Tip: Use calming adaptogens (like Ashwagandha + Tulsi) for anxiety and overarousal. Use energy adaptogens (like Rhodiola + Reishi) for depression, collapse, or chronic fatigue.

Nutraceuticals and Other Helpful Compounds

- **L-Theanine**: An amino acid found in green tea. Calms without sedation. Works quickly (30–60 mins) and pairs well with magnesium.
- **Silexan (Lavender Oil Capsule)**: Clinically shown to reduce anxiety. Use only standardized oral forms, not essential oil.
- **Vitamin D3**: Supports mood, immune function, and hormone balance. Especially important in winter or for those with low sun exposure.
- **Zinc**: Supports immune health and neurological function. Often depleted under chronic stress.

Choosing the Right Support Based on Your Dominant Dysregulation

Dysregulation Type	Best Supports
Vital Overarousal (anxious, hyperactive, can't calm down)	Magnesium glycinate, Ashwagandha, Lemon Balm, Chamomile tea, Deep breathing practices
Vital Collapse (fatigue, low energy, shut down)	Rhodiola, Reishi, American Ginseng, B-complex, Vitamin D3
Heart Overload (over-attuned, overwhelmed)	Tulsi, Rose Petal tea, Magnesium, Pulsatilla or Ignatia (homeopathic)
Heart Numbness (shutdown, low affect)	Schisandra berry, Reishi, Milky Oat Seed, Emotional journaling + Co-regulation
Head Overthinking/ Looping	Magnesium threonate, L-Theanine, Silexan, CBT-based tools, guided journaling
Head Fog/Fatigue	Rhodiola, B12, Fish oil, Structured mental stimulation (games, puzzles)

A Word on Combinations

Sometimes supplements work better in synergy. A few combinations that pair especially well:

- **Magnesium glycinate + L-Theanine** - For calming anxious energy without sedation.
- **Omega-3s + B-complex** - For long-term cognitive and emotional stability.
- **Rhodiola + Reishi** - For depression with fatigue and low resilience.
- **Ashwagandha + Holy Basil** - For burnout with emotional depletion and stress sensitivity.

Safety & Sustainability

- Start small: Especially with adaptogens, see how your body responds before increasing the dose.
- Watch for overstimulation: If you feel jittery, agitated, or restless, reduce stimulating herbs or try a more calming one.
- Consult your provider: Especially if you're on medication or managing a health condition.
- Don't rely solely on supplements: They're support tools, not replacements for rest, nourishment, and emotional safety.

Final Thoughts

Your system is constantly trying to find its way back to balance. Nutritional support can give it a gentle nudge in the right direction. Whether your imbalance lives in the body, emotions, or mind, the right combination of nutrients and herbs can help your Three Selves feel steadier, more resilient, and more aligned.

As always, begin with awareness. Ask your Selves what they need. Then choose support that honors them all.

Chapter Twenty-Seven
Sleep Hygiene
Your Guide to Restful Sleep

Sleep is not just a physical necessity—it is a core function of the Vital Self and an essential foundation for emotional resilience, cognitive clarity, and State regulation. In the Mind Matrix Model, sleep is one of the most direct ways to restore balance across all Three Selves. Without it, your capacity for groundedness, connection, and reflective thinking deteriorates quickly.

Sleep hygiene refers to the practices and routines that support restorative, high-quality sleep. While many of these practices are familiar, they take on deeper meaning when understood through the lens of State, trauma recovery, and self-regulation.

Why Sleep Matters for the Mind Matrix

Sleep affects all Three Selves in distinct but overlapping ways:

Vital Self: Sleep restores the nervous system, regulates circadian rhythm, and supports immune and hormonal balance. Without enough sleep, the body can enter a state of chronic dysregulation—either hyperaroused or collapsed.

Heart Self: Sleep directly impacts emotional stability, social perception, and relational capacity. Sleep deprivation increases irritability, emotional reactivity, and sensitivity to rejection.

Head Self: Deep sleep is critical for memory consolidation, symbolic integration, and clear thinking. Lack of sleep makes abstract thought harder and fuels rigid, looping narratives.

When your State is unstable, sleep is often the first thing to suffer—and the most powerful lever for recovery.

System Effect of Sleep Loss

Sleep loss doesn't just cause tiredness, it dysregulates your entire Mind Matrix:

Vital Self: Increases sympathetic tone, impairs digestion, immunity, and hormonal regulation.

Heart Self: Heightens emotional reactivity, lowers empathy, and increases vigilance to perceived slights.

Head Self: Weakens memory, increases rumination, fuels black-and-white thinking.

State: Narrows your State Range, suppresses Reflective Catalyst function, increases vulnerability to Sentries and Loops.

Core Principles of Sleep Hygiene

Here are essential habits that support restful sleep and long-term nervous system health:

- Maintain a Consistent Schedule
- Go to bed and wake up around the same time each day—even on weekends—to align with your body's circadian rhythm.

- Establish a Pre-Sleep Wind-Down Routine
- Signal your system to shift gears with 30–60 minutes of low-stimulation activities: stretching, reading, journaling, breathwork, or taking a warm bath.
- Limit Screen Exposure Before Bed
- Blue light from phones, tablets, and computers suppresses melatonin. Try turning off screens an hour before bed and use warm-toned lighting in the evening.
- Optimize Your Sleep Environment
- Keep your bedroom cool (ideally 60–67°F / 15–19°C), dark, quiet, and free from distractions. Use blackout curtains, earplugs, or a white noise machine if needed.
- Monitor Food, Drink, and Substance Intake
- Avoid caffeine, alcohol, large meals, and high sugar intake within 3–4 hours of bedtime. These can disrupt blood sugar, digestion, and deep sleep cycles.
- Move Your Body During the Day
- Regular movement helps promote deeper sleep. Aim for 20–30 minutes of walking, stretching, or moderate exercise earlier in the day—not close to bedtime.
- Limit Naps
- If you nap during the day, keep it under 30 minutes and avoid late-afternoon naps that may interfere with nighttime rest.

When the Body Doesn't Feel Safe

Many people struggle with sleep not because they lack discipline, but because their nervous system doesn't feel safe enough to let go. This is especially common in trauma survivors, or anyone whose Vital Self has become dysregulated.

You may notice:

- Dread or anxiety increasing at bedtime
- Racing thoughts or emotional spirals when lying down
- Physical tension that won't release

- Waking suddenly at 2–4am with a sense of alarm

In these cases, it's important not to force sleep, but to build trust and rhythm in the body first. Try adding one or more of the following:

Vital Self Soothers (Bedtime Override Strategies)

- **5-Minute Body Scan:** Bring attention to each part of your body, slowly scanning from head to toes.
- **Legs-Up-the-Wall Pose (Viparita Karani):** A deeply calming inversion that helps lower arousal and shift into parasympathetic tone.
- **Weighted Blanket or Chest Pressure:** Gentle pressure across the body can support safety and containment (only if it feels comforting).
- **Butterfly Hug Tapping:** Cross arms over the chest and tap alternately on the shoulders while breathing slowly. Helps with self-soothing and bilateral regulation.
- **Warm Herbal Foot Soak or Foot Massage:** Pulls energy downward, especially helpful for those stuck in "head buzz" or emotional overload.

Acupressure Points for Sleep Support

Use gentle pressure or slow circular massage on the following points before bed. These support Vital Self regulation and help calm the Heart and Head.

Heart 7 (Shenmen): On the wrist crease, in line with the pinky. Calms the mind and relieves anxiety.

Pericardium 6 (Neiguan): On the inner forearm, three finger-widths above the wrist crease. Eases agitation and helps emotional release.

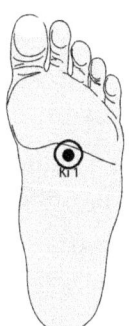

Kidney 1 (Yongquan): On the sole of the foot, in the depression just behind the ball. Grounds energy and quiets mental overstimulation.

Other Approaches

Difficulty Falling Asleep

- Try progressive muscle relaxation, guided visualization, or alternate nostril breathing to calm the nervous system.
- A warm bath 60–90 minutes before bed—especially with a few drops of lavender essential oil—can help lower core body temperature and promote melatonin release.
- Drink a small cup of warm milk or tart cherry juice, both of which contain natural sleep-supporting compounds like tryptophan or melatonin.
- Consider gentle herbs or supplements such as magnesium glycinate, lemon balm, or L-theanine to ease the transition into sleep.
- Avoid stimulating activities and devices, and instead create an environment of emotional and sensory spaciousness.

Nighttime Waking

- If awake for more than 15–20 minutes, get out of bed and do something calming. Avoid screens, overhead lights, or cognitive stimulation.
- Gentle movement (like swaying or rocking), listening to soothing ambient music, or drinking a few sips of chamomile tea can help reset the nervous system.
- If nighttime blood sugar dips are suspected, a small protein-rich snack (like a spoonful of almond butter) before bed may help maintain stability.

Early Morning Awakening

- Review your evening emotional state and reduce mental clutter before bed through journaling, meditation, or Heart Self check-ins.
- Use dim, warm light and soothing sounds (like soft music or a white noise machine) to ease any early reactivation of the stress response.
- Herbs like ashwagandha or holy basil may help regulate cortisol rhythms when taken regularly.
- Support your circadian rhythm with consistent exposure to natural morning light and a routine wake time, even if sleep was disrupted.

Final Note: Sleep as a Practice, Not a Test

Good sleep isn't a pass/fail event—it's a relationship. With your body. With your rhythm. With your Vital Self. Like any relationship, it takes attention, care, and consistency. You don't have to get it perfect. You just have to keep showing up—with softness, curiosity, and a willingness to rest.

Chapter Twenty-Eight
Mindfulness & Meditation
Finding Calm and Clarity

I remember when I first started trying to meditate. It wasn't exactly intentional—I had just moved to San Francisco and hadn't yet found a full-time job. I had plenty of time on my hands, and no money left over after rent and food.

I'd sit in my bedroom, playing my guitar until I got bored. Then I'd just sit. That's when I began noticing a stream of inner voices:

"I'm hungry."

No, I'm not.

"I should get some exercise."

I just finished exercising an hour ago.

"It's not good to just sit around."

There's nothing else to do.

"I should clean the apartment."

It's clean.

Over time, the voices got more insistent—until one popped up that made me laugh:

"What would your mother think if she could see you right now?!"

Eventually, I realized: I was meditating.

Of course, then came the judgmental voices.

"You're doing this all wrong. Meditation is supposed to feel blissful—and this sucks."

"You're not supposed to get distracted!"

At one point, my housemate mentioned that meditation wasn't supposed to be blissful all the time, that it's normal to get distracted, and that the key is to be kind to yourself. So the next time I sat down, I heard:

"You're not supposed to get distracted!"

Then a second voice:

"You're not supposed to beat yourself up for getting distracted!"

It was just as aggressive as the first.

Then a third voice emerged—more of a feeling than a thought:

"This is hopeless. I'll never be good at this."

And that was the moment something changed. I stopped engaging with the voices and moved my attention to my breath, to my body, to the space around me.

Everything softened. It wasn't bliss—but it was relief. And it was real.

I think of it like flying through a storm: it's chaos inside the clouds, but just above them, the sky is calm and blue. Shifting awareness into the Vital Self—into sensation, breath, grounding—isn't always dramatic, but it's the way out of the chatter of the Head Self. No wonder so many mindfulness practices start there.

Mindfulness and meditation play a vital role in calming the mind, balancing emotions, and restoring the nervous system. In the Mind Matrix Model, these practices help your Head Self become quieter, your Heart Self more steady, and your Vital Self more regulated. They are not quick fixes, but powerful tools for deepening awareness, cultivating self-compassion, and widening your State Range over time.

Foundations of Mindfulness and Meditation

Mindfulness is the act of bringing full attention to the present moment without judgment. Meditation is the structured practice that strengthens this capacity—like building a mental muscle. Together, they help you move out of autopilot and into conscious connection with your body, thoughts, and emotions.

In Mind Matrix terms, they bring your Reflective Catalyst online, increase the coherence between your Selves, and allow you to observe Scripts and Sentries without immediately acting on them.

A Variety of Traditions

Meditation has roots in many cultures and spiritual systems. Here are some commonly practiced forms:

Vipassana (Buddhist Insight Meditation)

As described earlier, Vipassana involves observing bodily sensations and mental events as they are—without clinging or resisting. It's excellent for building Heart Self emotional resilience and Vital Self interoceptive clarity.

Samatha (Calm Abiding, Buddhist)

This form focuses on a single object, often the breath, and trains the mind to remain steady. It's especially helpful when your Head Self is overactive or the system feels scattered.

Metta (Lovingkindness, Buddhist)

Involves repeating phrases like "May I be safe. May I be well." and then extending those wishes to others. This directly supports Heart Self healing, especially for people prone to harsh self-talk, shame, or emotional withdrawal.

Mantra Meditation (Hindu/Vedic)

Repeating sacred sounds or words (like "Om" or "So Hum") either silently or aloud. This builds focus and taps into the rhythmic, energetic balance of the Vital Self, while also calming mental chatter.

Yoga Nidra (Guided Rest Meditation)

A deep relaxation practice that helps guide awareness through the body. It is excellent for trauma-informed Vital Self regulation, especially for people who feel unsafe in stillness.

Zazen (Zen Buddhist Sitting Meditation)

A form of "just sitting" with awareness of posture, breath, and thought. This often highlights the relationship between State shifts and the thinking mind.

The Science of Mindfulness: How It Heals Mind and Body

Mindfulness and meditation aren't just spiritual practices, they are also powerful, evidence-based tools for improving physical, emotional, and cognitive health. Over the last two decades, a growing body of research has confirmed what many traditions have taught for centuries: quieting the mind can transform your health.

Mental and Emotional Benefits

Regular meditation has been shown to:

- Reduce anxiety and depression by calming the amygdala (the brain's alarm system) and enhancing emotion regulation via the prefrontal cortex.
- Improve attention and working memory, especially through practices like focused attention and breath awareness.
- Increase emotional resilience, helping you recover faster from stress or emotional upsets.
- Strengthen self-awareness and reduce reactivity, allowing more thoughtful responses instead of habitual reactions.
- Foster compassion and empathy, particularly through loving-kindness (Metta) and self-compassion practices.

Example: A 2014 meta-analysis published in JAMA Internal Medicine found that mindfulness meditation can significantly reduce symptoms of anxiety, depression, and pain, with effects comparable to antidepressants in some cases.[1]

Physical and Neurological Benefits

Meditation doesn't just calm your thoughts—it changes your brain and body:

- Reduces inflammation and cortisol (the stress hormone), which is linked to everything from heart disease to autoimmune issues.
- Improves immune function by supporting parasympathetic (rest-and-repair) tone.
- Lowers blood pressure and heart rate, particularly through practices that emphasize breath and body awareness.
- Increases gray matter in areas related to memory, empathy, and emotional regulation (e.g., hippocampus, insula, anterior cingulate cortex).
- Enhances sleep quality, particularly in people with insomnia or racing thoughts.

Example: A Harvard study in 2011 found that just 8 weeks of mindfulness meditation led to measurable increases in brain gray matter density, particularly in regions associated with self-awareness and stress regulation.[2]

Meditation and Trauma Recovery

For those dealing with trauma or chronic stress, meditation offers a gradual way to rebuild trust in the body and increase State stability. Mindfulness-based therapies like MBSR (Mindfulness-Based Stress Reduction) and MBCT (Mindfulness-Based Cognitive Therapy) have been shown to help reduce symptoms of PTSD, depression, and somatic distress.

Example: Research published in Psychological Trauma (2017) found that veterans with PTSD who engaged in mindfulness practices showed reductions in symptoms and improvements in emotional regulation and quality of life over 8–12 weeks.[3]

Why It Works

From a Mind Matrix Model perspective, meditation strengthens the Reflective Catalyst—the conscious aspect of the Monarch that allows you to observe your inner world without being overtaken by it. Over time, this cultivates:

- Vital Self stability (by calming the nervous system)
- Heart Self compassion and awareness
- Head Self clarity and spaciousness

It isn't about escaping life—it's about becoming more present to it.

How to Start (and Keep Going)

Start small. A 5–10 minute practice is enough to begin. Over time, as the mind and body learn to feel safe in stillness, you may increase duration. Use the following guidelines as a foundation:

> Sit or lie down comfortably, with your spine supported if possible.
>
> Begin with awareness of your breath, especially the feeling of it entering and exiting your nose or chest.
>
> Gently scan your body, noticing any areas of tension, heaviness, or numbness.
>
> Expect distraction—this is normal. Each time you return to your focus, you are building strength.
>
> Treat each interruption as a messenger, not a failure. Gently say "thank you" to the part of you that noticed.

The Meta of Meditation

It's common to experience meta-judgments during meditation—getting frustrated at yourself for being distracted, then criticizing yourself for getting frustrated. This inner loop is a Head Self Script, often echoing old patterns of self-criticism. Watch it with curiosity. Humor helps. You can think of it like watching puppies tumble—it's messy, but also a sign of life.

Moving Meditation

If seated meditation feels difficult, try a movement-based practice that keeps your awareness anchored in the body:

Walking Meditation:

Choose a safe, quiet space.

Walk slowly, tuning into each footstep.

Breathe in sync with your steps (e.g., 4 steps inhale, 4 steps exhale).

If the mind wanders, return attention to your feet and breath.

Other Options:

- Slow, mindful yoga
- Qigong or Tai Chi
- Washing dishes or folding laundry with attention to rhythm, sound, and sensation

Mindfulness in Everyday Life

You don't need a cushion or a quiet room to practice. Mindfulness can happen in transitions, during routine tasks, and in moments of tension:

- Pause between tasks: Take 3 breaths before switching activities.
- Check in during frustration: Notice your body—shoulders tight? Jaw clenched? Use that as a signal to reset.
- Micro-meditations: Place one hand on your chest and one on your belly for 30 seconds. Breathe. Feel. Return.

Mindfulness for Stress and State Repair

Meditation is not about escaping stress—it's about meeting it differently. Stressful moments can become cues for mindfulness. When you notice yourself getting anxious, shut down, or overwhelmed:

- Label what's happening ("I feel tension rising.")
- Connect with the body (feet on floor, air on skin, breath in belly)
- Name the State ("I may be sliding into a Negative State.")
- Choose an Override—touch, breath, mantra, movement.

Trauma-Aware Considerations

For people with unresolved trauma, stillness can sometimes feel unsafe. In these cases:

- Use shorter meditations with movement breaks
- Avoid lying down unless it feels secure
- Use external anchors (sound, candlelight, or touch)
- Start with guided meditations to avoid getting trapped in inner loops

Your system may resist dropping its guard at first. That's okay. Be patient and persistent, like you would with a scared animal. With time, your body will learn to trust the pause.

Final Thoughts

Meditation isn't about perfection or bliss, it's about building your relationship with yourself, gently, moment by moment. It sharpens your ability to notice your State, regulate it, and come home to your Vital, Heart, and Head Selves.

You don't need to do it every day for an hour. You just need to keep returning. Each breath is a new beginning.

References

1. **Goyal, M., Singh, S., Sibinga, E. M. S., et al.** (2014). *Meditation programs for psychological stress and well-being: A systematic review and meta-analysis.* JAMA Internal Medicine, 174(3), 357–368. https://doi.org/10.1001/jamainternmed.2013.13018

2. **Holzel, B. K., Carmody, J., Vangel, M., et al.** (2011). *Mindfulness practice leads to increases in regional brain gray matter density.* Psychiatry Research: Neuroimaging, 191(1), 36–43. https://doi.org/10.1016/j.pscychresns.2010.08.006

3. **Polusny, M. A., Erbes, C. R., Thuras, P., et al.** (2015). *Mindfulness-based stress reduction for posttraumatic stress disorder among veterans: A randomized clinical trial.* JAMA, 314(5), 456–465. https://doi.org/10.1001/jama.2015.8361

Annotated Bibliography

Introduction

The Mind Matrix Model was developed by Sam McClellan based on nearly fifty years of clinical practice, personal exploration, and investigation into how to optimize the body–mind. This has included deep explorations of neurology, psychology, alternative health, and contemplative traditions, most notably Buddhism.

Along the way, concepts from other fields have enriched this perspective, such as Dr. Craig Malkin's framing of echoism alongside narcissism, Peter Levine's observation of animals discharging acute trauma through shaking, the principles of Buddhist Psychology, and the holistic systems of Chinese medicine to name a few.

The sources listed here are included because their findings or frameworks validate, parallel, or converge with specific elements of the Mind Matrix Model (e.g., Three Selves; State/State Axis; Self–Other Differentiation; Axes of Vital/Heart/Head; Override Strategies; Sentries/Scripts), and/or as suggested works for further study.

Human Development

Ainsworth, M. D. S., Blehar, M. C., Waters, E., & Wall, S. (1978). *Patterns of Attachment: A psychological study of the strange situation*. Hillsdale, NJ: Lawrence Erlbaum Associates. (Reprinted 2015 by Psychology Press)
Seminal evidence linking caregiver attunement with secure vs. insecure attachment styles. Validates the Mind Matrix Model's claim that early relational safety scaffolds Heart Self regulation and later Self–Other balance. *(See also: Heart Self; Self–Other Development.)*

Bowen, M. (1993). *Family Therapy in Clinical Practice*. New York, NY: Jason Aronson.
"Differentiation of self" in family systems theory parallels the Mind Matrix Model's Self–Other Differentiation: maintaining self while staying connected. *(See also: Self–Other Differentiation; Boundaries.)*

Bowlby, J. (1988). *A Secure Base: Parent-Child Attachment and Healthy Human Development.* **New York, NY: Basic Books.**
Attachment as a foundation for exploration and autonomy. Corroborates the Mind Matrix Model's observation that safety (Vital Self) enables healthy differentiation and later Heart Self and Head Self-level integration. *(See also: Heart Self; Vital Self; Self–Other Development.)*

Decety, J., & Sommerville, J. A. (2003). Shared representations between self and other: a social cognitive neuroscience view. *Trends in Cognitive Sciences, 7*(12), 527–533.
Neural mechanisms for self–other distinction/empathy. Correlates with the Mind Matrix Model's Self–Other axis and the Heart/Head interplay in social understanding. *(See also: Self–Other Differentiation; Heart Axis.)*

Loevinger, J. (1976). *Ego Development: Conceptions and Theories (Jossey-Bass Behavioral Science Series).* **San Francisco, CA: JosseyBass.**
Stage model of ego maturity (increasing perspective-taking and integration). Parallels the Mind Matrix Model's Head Self growth and Self–Other Differentiation across adulthood. *(See also: Head Self; Self–Other Development.)*

Mahler, M. S., Pine, F., & Bergman, A. (1975). *The psychological birth of the human infant: Symbiosis and individuation.* **New York, NY: Basic Books.**
Separation–individuation phases (practicing, rapprochement) align with the Mind Matrix Model's spiral of safety → exploration → reintegration in early Vital/Heart development. *(See also: Vital Self; Heart Self; Self–Other Development.)*

Stern, D. N. (1985). *The Interpersonal World Of The Infant (View from Psychoanalysis and Developmental Psychology).* **New York, NY: Basic Books.**
Emergent → core → subjective → verbal self. Validates the Mind Matrix Model's view that Self–Other awareness is relational and pre-verbal before cognitive narrative forms. *(See also: Self–Other Development; Heart Self.)*

Neuroscience

Barrett, L. F. (2017). *How Emotions Are Made: The Secret Life of the Brain—How We Create Emotions Through Brain, Body, and Culture.* **Boston, MA: Mariner Books.**
Constructed emotion and interoception/allostasis. Supports the Mind Matrix Model's emphasis on the Vital Self, body-based signals, and state-dependent emotion. *(See also: Vital Self; State; Interoception.)*
Note: Barrett's constructionist view of emotions aligns more fully with the Mind Matrix Model's integration of body, relationship, and cognition, while Panksepp's primal affect (noted later) maps primarily onto the Vital Self as foundational but incomplete—useful for grounding, but not sufficient to explain Heart and Head layers.

Craig, A. D. (2009). How do you feel—now? The anterior insula and human awareness. *Nature Reviews Neuroscience, 10*(1), 59–70.
Interoception and the insula's role in subjective feeling validate the Mind Matrix Model's body-anchored model of State and awareness, with the anterior insula serving as a key neural gateway for the Monarch's integration of Vital, Heart, and Head signals. (See also: Vital Self; State Axis; Monarch.)

Fox, M. D., Snyder, A. Z., Vincent, J. L., Corbetta, M., Van Essen, D. C., & Raichle, M. E. (2005). The human brain is intrinsically organized into dynamic, anticorrelated functional networks. *Proceedings of the National Academy of Sciences, 102*(27), 9673–9678.
Classic evidence that the Task Positive Network (TPN—actually a set of task-focused networks, TPNs) works in opposition to the Default Mode Network (DMN). Supports the Mind Matrix Model's view of balance between reflective/internal and task/external modes. (See also: Head Axis—analytic/holistic; State; "modes.")

Gazzaniga, M. S. (2000). Cerebral specialization and interhemispheric communication: Does the corpus callosum enable the human condition? *Brain, 123*(7), 1293–1326.
Lateralization and integration across hemispheres. Parallels the Mind Matrix Model's *Head Axis* (analytic ↔ holistic) and the need for crosstalk. *(See also: Head Axis; Monarch.)*

McGilchrist, I. (2009). *The Master and His Emissary: The Divided Brain and the Making of the Western World.* **New Haven, CT: Yale University Press.**
Classic synthesis on hemispheric styles (contextual/holistic vs. abstract/analytic). Aligns with the Mind Matrix Model's Head Axis modes and the need for integration. (See also: Head Axis; Monarch.)
Note: While highly influential, the broad cultural and historical conclusions drawn from McGilchrist's hemispheric model are considered speculative by some critics and are a subject of ongoing debate.

Menon, V. (2011). Large-scale brain networks and psychopathology: a unifying triple network model. *Trends in Cognitive Sciences, 15(10), 483–506.*
Interactions among the Default Mode Network (DMN), Salience Network, and Central Executive/Task Positive Networks (TPNs) support the Mind Matrix Model's view of dynamic State shifting, with salience signals helping the brain move between internal and external modes. (See also: State Axis; Override Strategies.)

Noë, A. (2009). *Out of Our Heads: Why You Are Not Your Brain, and Other Lessons from the Biology of Consciousness.* **New York, NY: Hill and Wang.**
Argues consciousness is relational and world-embedded. Parallels the Mind Matrix Model's view of the Monarch as a field across Selves, not reducible to neural circuitry. (See also: Conscious Self/Monarch; Head Self; Heart Self.)

Panksepp, J., & Biven, L. (2012). *The Archaeology of Mind: Neuroevolutionary Origins of Human Emotions (Norton Series on Interpersonal Neurobiology).* **New York, NY: W. W. Norton & Company.**
Primal affect systems (FEAR, RAGE, CARE, etc.) support the Mind Matrix Model's Vital Self/Heart Self foundations for emotion/attachment. *(See also: Vital Self; Heart Self.)*
Note: See the above note within the Barrett (2017) entry concerning the conflict between these two views, and how each correlates with the Mind Matrix Model.

Raichle, M. E. (2015). The brain's default mode network. *Annual Review of Neuroscience, 38*, 433–447.
DMN as internally focused/self-referential baseline. Correlates with the Mind Matrix Model's Reflective Catalyst, State, and integration. *(See also: Head Self; State; Reflective Catalyst.)*

Thayer, J. F., & Lane, R. D. (2009). Claude Bernard and the heart–brain connection: Further elaboration of a model of neuro-visceral integration. *International Journal of Psychophysiology, 73*(2), 118–124.
HRV as an index of flexible regulation linking heart and prefrontal control. Supports the Mind Matrix Model's State regulation via body/brain coordination. *(See also: Vital Self; State; Override Strategies-breath.)*

Walker, M. (2017). *Why We Sleep.* New York, NY: Scribner.
Sleep's role in emotion regulation/memory consolidation. Corroborates the Mind Matrix Model's State hygiene (sleep) and Vital Self maintenance. *(See also: Working with State; Sleep Hygiene.)*

Psychology

Cain, S. (2012). *Quiet: The power of introverts in a world that can't stop talking.* New York, NY: Crown.
Cultural over-valuation of extroversion and strengths of introversion. Aligns with the Mind Matrix Model's Heart Self axis (introversion–extroversion) as a normal spectrum. *(See also: Heart Axis; Modes.)*

Cozolino, L. (2014). *The Neuroscience of Human Relationships: Attachment and the Developing Social Brain (Norton Series on Interpersonal Neurobiology)* (2nd ed.). New York, NY: W. W. Norton.
Relational safety as neural scaffolding. Validates the Mind Matrix Model's Heart Self and co-regulation emphasis. *(See also: Heart Self; Self–Other Development.)*

Depue, R. A., & Collins, P. F. (1999). Neurobiology of the structure of personality: Dopamine, facilitation of incentive motivation, and extraversion. *Behavioral and Brain Sciences, 22*(3), 491–517. https://doi.org/10.1017/S0140525X99002046
Annotation (unchanged in intent):
Dopaminergic sensitivity underlying extroversion. Correlates with the Mind Matrix Model's Heart Self axis and Vital Self arousal interplay. (See also: Heart Self Axis; Vital Self Axis.)

Eysenck, H. J. (1967). *The Biological Basis of Personality.* **Springfield, IL: Charles C. Thomas.**
Early biological model for introversion–extroversion (arousal thresholds). Parallels the Mind Matrix Model's Heart Self/Vital Self axes and modes. *(See also: Heart Axis; Vital Axis; Modes.)*

Kahneman, D. (2011). *Thinking, fast and slow.* **New York, NY: Farrar, Straus and Giroux.**
Dual-process (fast vs. slow) aligns with the Mind Matrix Model's automatic Ministers/Scripts vs. reflective Monarch. *(See also: Scripts; Monarch; Head Self.)*

Malkin, C. (2016). *Rethinking Narcissism: The Secret to Recognizing and Coping with Narcissists.* **New York, NY: Harper Perennial.**
Spectrum view of narcissism; introduces **echoism** which is a key component of the Mind Matrix Model. Validates the Model's echoism as Heart Self axis Negative State affect and Self–Other imbalance. *(See also: Heart Axis; Negative State; Self–Other Differentiation.)*

Siegel, D. J. (2001). *The Developing Mind: How Relationships and the Brain Interact to Shape Who We Are.* **New York, NY: The Guilford Press.**
Mind as embodied and relational; integration as well-being. Corroborates the Mind Matrix Model's Three Selves integration and Self–Other development. *(See also: Integration; Heart/Vital/Head Selves.)*

Relational & Self-Help

Bancroft, L. (2003). *Why Does He Do That?: Inside the Minds of Angry and Controlling Men* **New York, NY: Berkley Books.**
Explores patterns of coercive control. Useful alongside the Mind Matrix Model's framework for Negative State Heart Self dynamics and relational imbalance. (See also: Heart Self; Negative State; Boundaries.)

Biddulph, S. (2024). *Wild Creature Mind: The Neuroscience Breakthrough that Helps You Transform Anxiety and Live a Fierce and Loving Life.* **London, UK: Bluebird (Pan Macmillan).**
Explores an "animal/right-hemisphere" mode for regulating anxiety and recovering vitality. Useful complement to the Mind Matrix Model's Vital and Heart Selves work and practical State-range tools. (See also: Vital Self; Heart Self; State Range.)

Evans, P. (2010). *The Verbally Abusive Relationship : How to recognize it and how to respond.* (3rd ed.). Avon, MA: Adams Media.
Identifies patterns of verbal abuse and responses. Correlates with the Mind Matrix Model's descriptions of destructive Heart Self scripts and Self–Other imbalance. (See also: Heart Self; Scripts; Boundaries.)

Kaufman, S. B. (2021). *Transcend: The New Science of Self-Actualization.* New York, NY: TarcherPerigee.
Modern update of Maslow's hierarchy, emphasizing growth, creativity, and wholeness. Parallels the Mind Matrix Model's focus on integration across the Three Selves. (See also: Integration; Head Self; Heart Self.)

Quaglia, J. (2025). *From Self-Care to We-Care: The New Science of Mindful Boundaries and Caring from an Undivided Heart.* Boulder, CO: Shambhala Publications. (Foreword by Daniel J. Siegel.) Shambhala Publications
Proposes a science-based "we-care" framework and practical boundary skills. Connects with the Mind Matrix Model's Heart Self balance, Self–Other Differentiation, and compassion practices. (See also: Heart Self; Self–Other Differentiation; Compassion.)

Trauma

Felitti, V. J., et al. (1998). Relationship of childhood abuse and household dysfunction to many of the leading causes of death in adults: The Adverse Childhood Experiences (ACE) Study. *American Journal of Preventive Medicine, 14*(4), 245–258.
Dose–response link between early adversity and later mental/physical health. Validates the Mind Matrix Model's developmental roots of Negative State patterns. *(See also: State Axis; Trauma.)*

Lanius, R. A., Harricharan, S., Kearney, B. E., & Pandev-Girard, B. (2025). *Sensory Pathways to Healing from Trauma: Harnessing the Brain's Capacity for Change.* New York, NY: The Guilford Press.
Highlights how trauma alters all eight sensory systems (including interoception and vestibular) and offers "Bridging to Practice" sections for clinicians. Corroborates the Mind Matrix Model's emphasis on Vital Self regulation, sensory integration, and co-regulating practices; aligns with Override Strategies and State Range work.

LeDoux, J. (2015). *Anxious*. New York, NY: Viking.
Distinguishes fast fear circuits from conscious anxiety. Parallels the Mind Matrix Model's Vital vs. Head distinctions in threat processing. *(See also: Vital Self; Head Self; Sentries.)*

Levine, P. A. (1997). *Waking the Tiger*. Berkeley, CA: North Atlantic Books.
Somatic completion of defensive responses. Supports the Mind Matrix Model's bottom-up Vital Self interventions and discharge. *(See also: Vital Self; Override Strategies—movement, breath.)*

Porges, S. W. (2011). *The Polyvagal Theory: Neurophysiological Foundations of Emotions, Attachment, Communication, and Self-regulation*. New York, NY: W. W. Norton.
Autonomic states (ventral vagal, sympathetic, dorsal vagal) as safety/defense modes. **Correlates** with the Mind Matrix Model's State Axis and co-regulation focus.
Note: Polyvagal theory has proven to be a clinically influential model that maps well onto The Mind Matrix Model's understanding of State and safety/defense responses. Elements of the theory (e.g., distinctions within vagal pathways and the interpretation of heart-rate variability as a direct index of "vagal tone") are contested and show mixed empirical support. Even so, polyvagal-informed approaches are in regular clinical use and many practitioners report benefit.

van der Kolk, B. A. (2014). *The body keeps the score*. New York, NY: Viking.
Mind–body trauma mechanisms; supports movement, yoga, EMDR, neurofeedback. Validates the Mind Matrix Model's whole-system healing and body-anchored state work. *(See also: Working with State; Override Strategies.)*

van der Kolk, B. A., et al. (2016). A randomized controlled study of neurofeedback for chronic PTSD. *PLOS ONE, 11*(12), e0166752.
Neurofeedback improves PTSD symptoms. Corroborates the Mind Matrix Model's neurofeedback-informed view of arousal and Vital regulation. *(See also: Vital Self; State Range.)*

Therapeutic Modalities

Brown, R. P., & Gerbarg, P. L. (2005). Sudarshan Kriya yogic breathing in the treatment of stress, anxiety, and depression. *Journal of Alternative and Complementary Medicine, 11*(4), 711–717.
Breathwork improves stress/anxiety. Validates the Mind Matrix Model's breath-based Override Strategies. *(See also: Override Strategies—breath; Vital Self.)*

Corrigan, F. M., & Christie-Sands, J. (2020). Deep Brain Reorienting: A new trauma psychotherapy with a neurobiological foundation. *Medical Hypotheses, 142,* **109790.**
Targets brainstem orienting/shock responses. Parallels the Mind Matrix Model's focus on pre-affective Vital responses. *(Developing modality.) (See also: Vital Self; Sentries; Trauma.)*

Gilbert, P., & Simos, G. (Eds.). (2022). *Compassion focused therapy: Clinical practice and applications.* **Abingdon, UK: Routledge.**
Soothing system cultivation to counter threat. Aligns with the Mind Matrix Model's Heart Self and compassion-based Override Strategies. *(See also: Heart Self; Override Strategies.)*

Ogden, P., & Fisher, J. (2015). *Sensorimotor psychotherapy* **(2nd ed.). New York, NY: W. W. Norton.**
Embodied processing of trauma and attachment. Validates the Mind Matrix Model's bottom-up plus relational approach. *(See also: Vital/Heart Selves; Trauma.)*

Schwarz, L., Corrigan, F., Hull, A., & Raju, R. (2016). *The Comprehensive Resource Model.* **New York, NY: Routledge.**
Layered resourcing while processing trauma. Corroborates the Mind Matrix Model's multi-level resourcing across Three Selves. *(See also: Override Strategies; Trauma.)*

Schwartz, R. C., & Sweezy, M. (2020). *Internal Family Systems therapy* **(2nd ed.). New York, NY: The Guilford Press.**
"Parts" work aligns with the Mind Matrix Model's Ministers and Scripts under Monarch leadership. *(See also: Monarch; Ministers; Scripts.)*

Shapiro, F. (2018). *Eye Movement Desensitization and Reprocessing (EMDR) Therapy: Basic Principles, Protocols, and Procedures.* **(3rd ed.). New York, NY: Guilford.**
Bilateral stimulation for adaptive reprocessing. Supports the Mind Matrix Model's integration across states/networks. *(See also: State Shift; Working with State.)*

Sherlin, L., et al. (2011). Neurofeedback and basic learning theory: Implications for research and practice. *Journal of Neurotherapy,* **15(4), 292–304.**
Mechanisms and outcomes in neurofeedback. Corroborates the Mind Matrix Model's arousal training view of Vital Self regulation. *(See also: Vital Axis; State Range.)*

Contemplative Traditions & Integrative Health

Goldstein, A. N., & Walker, M. P. (2014). The role of sleep in emotional brain function. *Annual Review of Clinical Psychology, 10,* **679–708.**
Sleep as regulator of affective circuits. Supports the Mind Matrix Model's State hygiene and Vital-Heart Selves regulation. *(See also: Working with State; Sleep Hygiene.)*

Goleman, D., & Davidson, R. J. (2017). *Altered traits.* **New York, NY: Avery.**
Long-term meditation produces durable trait changes (attention, compassion). Supports the Mind Matrix Model's practice-driven trait growth across Selves. *(See also: Reflective Catalyst; Heart/Head Practices.)*

Kabat-Zinn, J. (2013). *Full Catastrophe Living (Revised Edition): Using the Wisdom of Your Body and Mind to Face Stress, Pain, and Illness.* **New York, NY: Bantam.**
Mindfulness-based stress reduction; body scans and yoga for regulation. Validates the Mind Matrix Model's grounding and present-moment tools. *(See also: Working with State; Monarch.)*

Kaptchuk, T. J. (2000). *The Web That Has No Weaver : Understanding Chinese Medicine.* **New York, NY: McGraw-Hill.**
Traditional Chinese Medicine (Qi, Five Elements) as holistic systems view. Parallels the Mind Matrix Model's integrative mind-body framing. *(See also: Vital Self; Acupressure.)*

Khalsa, S. S., et al. (2018). Interoception and Mental Health: A Roadmap. *Biological Psychiatry: Cognitive Neuroscience and Neuroimaging, 3(6), 501–513.*
Interoceptive accuracy/awareness and psychopathology. Validates the Mind Matrix Model's interoceptive training emphasis. *(See also: Vital Self; State.)*

Kornfield, J. (2009). *The Wise Heart: A Guide to the Universal Teachings of Buddhist Psychology.* **New York, NY: Bantam.**
Buddhist psychology on compassion and wisdom. Aligns with the Mind Matrix Model's inherent goodness and compassionate stance toward Sentries. *(See also: Heart Self; Monarch.)*

McClellan, S., & Monte, T. (1998). *Integrative Acupressure: A Hands-On Guide to Balancing the Body's Structure and Energy for Health and Healing.* **New York, NY: Perigee Trade.**
Foundational text outlining Integrative Acupressure as a synthesis of meridian theory with structural and emotional work.
Used as reference for: Working With the Vital/Heart/Head Self chapters; Working With State; Stress, Anxiety & Depression; Sleep Hygiene.

McClellan, S. (2022). *Acupressure Meridian Atlas: Integrative Acupressure.* **Finger Press Publishing.**
Comprehensive point atlas covering all twelve organ meridians and the eight extraordinary meridians, with locations and indications.
Used as reference for: Working With the Vital/Heart/Head Self chapters; Working With State; Stress, Anxiety & Depression; Sleep Hygiene.

Stux, G., & Pomeranz, B. (1991). *Basics of Acupuncture* **(2nd rev.). Berlin, Germany: Springer Verlag.**
Intro to acupuncture mechanisms and applications. Provides context for the Mind Matrix Model's acupressure protocols. *(See also: Acupressure; Override Strategies.)*

Thich Nhat Hanh. (1999). *The Heart of the Buddha's Teaching: Transforming Suffering into Peace, Joy, and Liberation.* **New York, NY: Harmony Books.**
Non-self, interbeing, mindfulness as practical ethics. Corroborates the Mind Matrix Model's non-pathologizing, relational view. *(See also: Heart/Head Selves; Reflective Catalyst.)*

Additional Cross-Domain References

Giedd, J. N., et al. (1999). Brain development during childhood and adolescence: a longitudinal MRI study. *Nature Neuroscience, 2*(10), 861–863.
Longitudinal MRI findings of cortical pruning and white matter growth is consistent with the Mind Matrix Model's two-spiral view of Self-Other Development, where each Self—Vital, Heart, and Head—re-emerges during adolescence at a higher level of complexity. *(See also: Head Self; Self–Other Development.)*

Grossman, P., & Taylor, E. W. (2007). Toward understanding respiratory sinus arrhythmia: Relations to cardiac vagal tone and physiological regulation. *Biological Psychology, 74*(2), 263–285.
Methodological cautions about vagal indices. Included to note debates relevant to Polyvagal Theory. *(See also: State Axis; Vital Self.)*

Libet, B., Gleason, C. A., Wright, E. W., & Pearl, D. K. (1983). Time of conscious intention to act in relation to onset of cerebral activity (readiness-potential). The unconscious initiation of a freely voluntary act. *Brain, 106*(3), 623–642.
Pre-conscious initiation of action supports the Mind Matrix Model's Ministers/Scripts preceding Monarch awareness. *(See also: Monarch; Scripts.)*

Menon, V., & Uddin, L. Q. (2010). Saliency, switching, attention and control: a network model of insula function. *Brain Structure and Function, 214*(5–6), 655–667.
Salience network in switching between the Default Mode Network (DMN) and the Task-Positive Networks (TPNs). Corroborates the Mind Matrix Model of State Shift/override. *(See also: State Shift; Override Strategies.)*

Shin, L. M., & Liberzon, I. (2010). The neurocircuitry of fear, stress, and anxiety disorders. *Neuropsychopharmacology, 35*(1), 169–191.
Threat circuitry maps to the Mind Matrix Model's Vital Self, Sentries and Head Self worry loops. *(See also: Sentries; Vital/Head Selves.)*

Index

Symbols

3-breath integration, 280
5-4-3-2-1 sensory tracking, 307, 309, 395
5-minute body scan, 434

A

ACC (anterior cingulate cortex), 25, 26, 142, 441
aconite (aconitum napellus), 129, 419
acupressure
　overview, 60, 405–407
　common points for, 407–408
　Head Self and, 221–222, 225–226, 229–232
　Heart Self and, 177–179, 181–183, 188–190
　Kidney Yin and Yang and, 129–130
　pregnancy and, 408–410
　sleep support and, 434–435
　State Shifts and, 271–272, 277–278, 284–285
　techniques for, 406–407
　Vital Self and, 129–137
adaptogens (herbs)
　overview, 427
　Heart Self and, 175–176, 180, 185
　pairings for, 428–429
　State Shifts and, 270, 276, 281–282
　timing and synergy of, 423–425
　Vital Self and, 123–124, 125
addictions, 87–88, 320
advance, recede, hold. *See* Sentries
advertisements, 319–320
agony advertising, 319–320
aikido of the mind, 381
ambiverts, 145–146
American ginseng (panax quinquefolius), 124, 185, 427
amygdala, 24, 100, 107, 108, 142
Analytic-Dominant dysregulation, 199–200, 202, 206–207
Analytic Mode (Head Self)
　overview, 196–197, 212, 289–290
　axis and, 9–10, 26–27, 197
　balance in, 220–223
　defined, 4, 26
　grounding of, 212–213
　healing, 209
　Self-Other Differentiation and, 336–337
　symbols and, 317
　trauma and, 204–205
ANS (autonomic nervous system), 4, 23, 100
anterior cingulate cortex (ACC). *See* ACC (anterior cingulate cortex)
antioxidants, 229

anxiety. *See* stress, anxiety and depression
appeasement, 38
argentum nitricum, 129
arnica montana, 419
arousal axis. *See* Vital Self Axis
art therapy, 175, 269
ashwagandha, 123, 175, 424, 427
Asian ginseng (panax ginseng or siberian ginseng). *See* ginseng
assertiveness, 362
attachment styles, 161
"Auguries of Innocence" (Blake), 315
authenticity, 162, 164
autism spectrum, people on, 35, 147, 156, 206
autonomic nervous system (ANS). *See* ANS (autonomic nervous system)
avoidance, 291
awareness
   "The Path of Awareness", 83
   practice needed for, 59
   proprioceptive awareness, 34–35, 98–99
   rituals and reminders for, 55–59
   State Magnets and, 250–255
axes, 8–11, 23, 25–27. *See also* Head Self Axis; Heart Self Axis; State Axis; Vital Self Axis

B

Baihui (Governing Vessel 20), 136–137, 225, 230, 272, 408
balance/regulation issues, defined, 3
Balancers, 339
banana, as having three parts, 5
"Barter" (Teasdale), 141
baryta carbonic, 176, 270
basal ganglia, 108
B-complex vitamins, 269, 276, 423, 427
BDNF (brain-derived neurotrophic factor), 403
behavioral disruption, 305
bell apps, 57
bergamot, 127, 176
Berry, Wendell, 65
bilateral stimulation, 310
black-and-white thinking, 289
Bladder 10 (Tianzhu), 231
Bladder 23 (Shenshu or Kidney Shu), 132
Bladder 60 (Kunlun), 409
Bladder 67 (Zhiyin), 409
Blake, William, 315
blocks, 389–396
Blue Zones, 398
body language, 160–161
body scans, 434
boundaries
   overview, 358

balance in, 368–369, 373
　　before, during, and after and, 364–367
　　challenges to, 367–368
　　communication of, 362–364
　　digital boundaries, 274
　　during, 364–367
　　examples of, 359–361
　　Heart Self and, 154
　　Holistic Mode imbalance and, 290
　　identification of, 361
　　imbalances in, 369–373
　　issues with, examples of, 359–361
　　maintaining and reinforcing of, 362–364
　　questionnaire for, 370–373
　　Self-Other Differentiation and, 336
　　setting as Override strategy, 312
　　tripod, as, 368–369
　　types of, 359
　　vocal boundaries, 349
"Boundaries" (McClellan), 357
boundary reset touch, 274
boundary tapping, 348
box breathing, 60, 274
bracelet method, 57
brain, 3–4. *See also* specific parts of the brain
brain-derived neurotrophic factor (BDNF), 403
brainstem, 22, 100
brainwave training, 224
Breath as Bridge meditation, 272–273
breath deceleration, 349
breathwork. *See also* mindfulness and meditation
　　overview, 60–61
　　breath deceleration, 349
　　cognitive reset breath, 233
　　conscious breathing, 114
　　fight or flight and, 310
　　Sighing Out Breath + Stretch, 267
　　State and, 267, 274, 280
Buddhist insight (Vipassana), 439
Butterfly Hugs, 300, 434
B vitamins, 123, 175, 282

C

calcarea carbonica, 128, 283
calcarea phosphorica, 228
calm abiding (Samantha), 439
Cascading Loops, 266
catastrophizing, 290
CBT (Cognitive Behavioral Therapy), 175, 224
cedarwood, 177, 283
Celestial Chimney (Conception Vessel 22), 178

central nervous system (CNS), 4, 321–322, 426–427. *See also* stress, anxiety and depression
cerebellum, 22, 100, 108
cerebral cortex, 26, 198
cerebrum, 24
chamomile, 127
chamomilla, 419
change, gradual, 400
change the frame (reframing), 233, 305, 311
check-ins with self, 126, 312
Chest Center (Conception Vessel 17), 190, 278, 284
choline, 229
chronic distress, 68
chronic illness, 103
cinnamon, 270
clary sage, 127, 181, 220, 283
CNS (central nervous system). *See* central nervous system; *See also* stress, anxiety and depression
codependency, 147
cognitive axis. *See* Analytic Mode (Head Self); Head Self Axis
Cognitive Behavioral Therapy (CBT), 175, 224
cognitive defusion, 308
cognitive flexibility training, 227–228, 312
cognitive handoff, 351
cognitive reframing, 233, 305, 311
cognitive reset breath, 233
cognitive restructuring, 224
cognitive Self. *See* Head Self
coherent breathing, 60
comfort, boundaries tripod and, 368–370
compartmentalization, 151
compassion for self, 161
Conception Vessel 3 (Zhongji), 409
Conception Vessel 4 (Guanyuan or Gate of Origin), 132–133, 409
Conception Vessel 6 (Qihai or Sea of Qi), 136
Conception Vessel 17 (Chest Center or Shanzhong or Sea of Tranquility), 190, 278, 284
Conception Vessel 22 (Celestial Chimney or Tiantu), 178
conflict resolution style, 160
connection pings, 268
conscious breathing, 114
conscious mind. *See* Monarch
consistency, 46, 314
consolidation of memory, 107
conspiratorial Loops, 307, 308, 313
containment practices, 274, 316, 348, 434
contentment, source of, ii
Contextual Personas, 156
CoQ10, 269
co-regulated contact, 268, 311
corpus callosum, 197
The Council Within meditation, 294–295
craniosacral therapy, 281

creative practices. *See also* journaling
  Head Self and, 220, 227
  interruption of obsessive Loops with, 313
  State and, 254, 268
creativity. *See* Holistic Mode (Head Self)
critical thinking exercises, 227, 313
criticism, self, 162, 163, 206
Critic, The, 202
cue languages, 59
culture, symbols changing of, 323
cypress, 187

D

Dabao (Spleen 21), 182
DBT (Dialectical Behavior Therapy. *See* Dialectical Behavior Therapy (DBT)
decision-making style, 160
Deep Brain Reorienting (DBR), 123
Default Mode Network (DMN), 107, 199
depression. *See* stress, anxiety and depression
detached survival, 292
development. *See* Self-Other Development/Differentiation
  Heart Self and, 146, 150, 152–153, 155
  trauma and, 104–105, 106, 155
  Vital Self and, 102
Dialectical Behavior Therapy (DBT), 179, 275
Dickinson, Emily, 257
dietary guide, 397–404
diffusion of essential oils, 127, 412
digital boundaries, 274
dipping your toe in. *See* titration
disconnection, 206
dis-ease (dukkha), 242
dissociation, 36, 86–87
distortion, 289
distraction, 38, 86–88
distress, 68
DMN (Default Mode Network). *See* Default Mode Network (DMN)
dominance, 38
Drifter, The, 202
drop the anchor, 274
"Dual" (McBain), 167
dukkha (dis-ease), 242
Dyer, Edward, 1–2
dynamic reading, 45
dysregulation, defined, 13

E

ease (sukha), 242
Echo, 149
Echoist Mode, 149–152, 153, 158, 335
economic insecurity, 104

eleuthero. *See* ginseng
EMDR (Eye Movement Desensitization and Reprocessing), 122
emergent properties of the mind, 16
emotional overwhelm, 207
emotional Self. *See* Heart Self
emotional sensitivity, 204
emotional suppression, 147
emotions. *See also* State
   overview, 256
   Head Self and, 246–247
   Heart Self and, 244–245
   interplay of Selves in, 247
   physical sensations and, 248
   State Axis and, 248–249
   State Magnets and, 250–255
   Vital Self and, 243–244
empathy, 160, 291
Empty Basin (Stomach 12, Quepen), 183
empty boat parable, iii
enmeshment, 205
enteric nervous system (ENS), 4, 23, 100, 399–400
environment
   mapping of, 327
   Self-Other Differentiation and, 15–16
   sounds in, 326
   State Shifts and, 280
   supportive symbols in, 325–326
   Vital Self and, 103, 126
equanimity, i–ii, 249–250, 251, 253
essential oils
   overview, 61, 411–414
   Head Self and, 220, 226, 229
   Heart Self and, 176–177, 181, 187–188
   State Shifts and, 270–271, 277, 283
   Vital Self and, 127–128
eucalyptus, 412
eustress, 67
evening routines, 212
evening transitions, 58
exercise/movement
   as foundation, 62
   freeze Loops and, 311
   inward-focused State and, 268
   movement memory, 98
   stress relief from, 69
   Vital Self and, 124
expressive art therapy, 269
extended exhale, 61
external changes, peace and, 249–250
externalize it (thought sorting), 233
Extroversive Mode (Heart Self), 10, 25, 143–145, 164. *See also* Heart Self Axis

Eye Movement Desensitization and Reprocessing (EMDR), 122

F

fasting, 403
fawn, 38, 306, 308, 312
fear, 69–70
fearful avoidance, 291
feelings, as not enemy, 91
Fengchi (Gallbladder 20), 232
Fengfu (Governing Vessel 16), 226, 230
ferritin, 269
fight or flight, 23, 36, 37–38, 307, 310
Fiji television study, 323
Flippers, 338–339
focused attention meditation, 224–225, 228
focus, State and,, 250–255
foot soaks/massages, 434
forgetting, reasons for, 56
frankincense, 127, 176, 220, 277, 283, 412
freeze Loops, 310–311
Fulio (Kidney 7), 131

G

GABA precursors, 276
Gallbladder 20 (Fengchi), 232
Gallbladder 21 (Jianjing), 409
gaslighting, 204
Gate of Origin (Conception Vessel 4), 132–133, 409
Gate of Origin (Pericardium 4), 182
gaze widening, 352
gelsemium, 128, 228, 277
genetics, 15, 103
Genetic Scripts, 37
geranium, 127, 188
ginger, 127, 270
ginseng, 124, 185, 270, 423, 427
  eleuthero (siberian ginseng), 185, 270
glycine, 276
good distraction level, 86
Governing Vessel 16 (Fengfu), 226, 230
Governing Vessel 20 (Baihui or Hundred Meetings), 136–137, 225, 230, 272, 408
Governing Vessel 24 (Shenting), 231
gratitude practices, 213, 251, 254
Great Abyss (Lung 9), 137
Great Embracement (Spleen 21), 182
Great Stream (Kidney 3), 131, 133, 135, 271
Great Surge (Liver 3), 135
grounded empathy, 291
grounding. *See also* adaptogens (herbs); breathwork; essential oils; mindfulness and meditation
  as symbol, 316
  grounded empathy, 291

of Head Self, 212–213
of Heart Self, 164
of Vital Self, 89–90, 110, 114
group therapy, 269
Guanyuan (Conception Vessel 4), 132–133, 409
guided meditation, 62
guided rest (Yoga Nidra), 440
Gushing Spring (Kidney 1), 134, 221–222, 278, 435
gut biome, 100, 399–400
gut brain. *See* enteric nervous system (ENS)

H

hafiz, 211
Hahnemann, Samuel, 417
Hakomi Therapy, 281
hand on heart, 274, 349
hands-behind-heart pose, 350
happiness versus equanimity, ii
harmonizers, 148
Head-Dominant Personas, 157
Head Loops, 266
Head Self. *See also* Analytic Mode (Head Self); Holistic Mode (Head Self); Ministers
 overview, 7, 26–27, 196, 210, 236, 377
 acupressure and, 221–222, 225–226, 229–232
 Analytic Mode, balancing of, 220–223
 balanced people, maintaining, 227–232
 balance in, 198, 202, 236, 291
 boundaries and, 359, 368–370
 chronic dysregulation of, 199–202
 cues from, 296–297
 defined, iv, 54
 emotions and, 246–247
 essential oils and, 220, 226, 229
 fear and, 70
 grounding of, 212–213
 healing, 209
 Holistic Mode, balancing of, 224–226
 homeopathy and, 228
 imbalances in, 289–290
 Loops and Overrides, 306–307, 308, 312–313
 meditation and, 213, 220, 224–225, 228, 234–235
 mental models and, 208–209, 333
 mindful engagement and, 85
 neurological basis of, 198–199
 nutritional strategies for, 229
 Override plan for, 300
 Override Strategies for, 232–233
 pushback and, 48, 49
 questionnaire for, 213–219
 rebalancing modalities generally, 294
 Self-Other Differentiation and, 15, 331, 332–333, 334, 336–337, 342–343, 351–352
 sleep and, 432

   State and, 12, 202–203, 246–247
   stress, anxiety, and depression and, 71–72, 77–78, 90–91
   supports for, 428
   symbols and, 317–318
   therapies for dysregulation in, 224
   trauma and, 204–208
Head Self Axis, 9–10, 26–27, 196–197. *See also* Analytic Mode (Head Self); Holistic Mode (Head Self)
Head Self Scripts, 37
Head Self Sentries, 38, 39–40
healing
   depression as, 75–77
   Head Self and, 209–210
   Heart Self and, 154–155, 161–162
   interconnection of Three Selves and, 78, 379
   layers of, 53
   personas and, 157
   stress, anxiety, and depression. *See* stress, anxiety and depression
   Vital Self trauma and, 105
Heart 1 (Supreme Spring or Ji Quan), 177
Heart 3 (Lesser Sea or Shao Hai), 183
Heart 5 (Penetrating Inside or Tong Li), 189
Heart 7 (Shenmen or Spirit Gate), 134, 189, 221, 271, 434
Heart-Dominant Personas, 157
Heart Loops, 266
Heart Self. *See also* Ministers
   overview, 7, 24–25, 142, 165, 168, 193, 377
   acupressure and, 177–179, 181–183, 188–190
   balanced people, maintaining, 184–190
   boundaries and, 359, 368–370
   chronic dysregulation of, 146–147
   cues from, 296
   defined, iv, 54
   emotions and, 244–245
   essential oils and, 176–177, 181, 187–188
   fear and, 70
   grounding of, 164
   healing, 154–155, 161–162
   homeopathy and, 176, 180–181, 185–187
   inward-focused people, balancing of, 175–179
   Loops and Overrides, 306, 307–308, 311–312
   meditation and, 184, 191–193
   mindful engagement and, 85
   neurological basis of, 24–25, 142–143
   nutritional strategies for, 175–176, 179–180, 184–185
   outward-focused people, balancing of, 179–183
   Override plan for, 299
   personas and, 155–158
   pushback and, 47, 48–49
   questionnaire for, 168–174
   rebalancing modalities generally, 294

Self-Other Differentiation and, 15, 158–159, 331, 332, 333–334, 335–336, 341–342, 349–350
signs of, 159–161
sleep and, 432
State and, 12, 148–152, 245
stress, anxiety, and depression and, 71–72, 77–78, 90
supports for, 428
symbols and, 317
systems used by, 24–25
trauma and, 152–153, 155, 159
Heart Self Axis
  overview, 8, 10, 25, 143–146
  State and, 148–152
Heart Self Scripts, 37
Heart Self Sentries, 38, 39
Heavenly Palace (Lung 3), 179
heaven versus hell, 254
Hegu (Large Intestine 4), 225, 230, 407, 409
herbs. *See* adaptogens (herbs)
High Arousal. *See* Vital Self Axis
hippocampus, 24, 26, 107, 142
hold, advance, recede. *See* Sentries
Holistic-Dominant dysregulation, 200–201, 202, 207
Holistic Mode (Head Self)
  overview, 196–197, 212, 290–291
  axis and, 9–10, 26–27, 197
  balance in, 224–226
  defined, 4, 26
  grounding of, 212–213
  healing, 209
  Self-Other Differentiation and, 336
  symbols and, 318
  trauma and, 205–206
holy basil (tulsi), 123, 175, 180, 185, 270, 276, 282
homeopathy
  overview, 61, 415–420
  effectiveness of, 415–417
  Head Self and, 228
  Heart Self and, 176, 180–181, 185–187
  history of, 417–418
  State Shifts and, 270, 276–277, 283
  use of, 419–420
  Vital Self and, 128–129
honesty, 164
"'Hope' is the thing with feathers" (Dickinson), 257
Hundred Meetings (Governing Vessel 20), 136–137, 225, 230, 272, 408
hydration, 125
hyperarousal, 102, 306, 307. *See also* Vital Self Axis
hypervigilance, 290, 335. *See also* Head Self Axis
hypoarousal, 102, 334. *See also* Vital Self Axis
hypothalamus, 24, 107, 142

I

idealization, 290
"I don't know" practice, 352
IF (intermittent fasting), 403
IFS (Internal Family Systems). *See* Internal Family Systems (IFS)
ignatia, 176, 270, 283
ignatia amara, 129, 185–186, 419
imagination, 205–206
individualization, 418
inflammation, 103, 398–399
Inner Gate (Pericardium 6), 133, 189, 231, 272, 278, 284, 407, 410, 434
"inner stillness" blend, 181
insula, 142
integration, 293, 297, 301. *See also* Three Selves
integrity, 155, 368–370
intermittent fasting (IF), 403
Internal Family Systems (IFS), 269
intrinsic self-worth, 161–162
Introversion Mode (Heart Self). *See* Heart Self Axis
intuition. *See* Holistic Mode (Head Self)
"The Inward Morning" (Thoreau), 95
i Quan (Heart 1), 177
iron, 269, 424
"I" statements, 362

J

jasmine, 187
Jianjing (Gallbladder 21), 409
journaling
  dynamic reading and, 45
  Head Self and, 209, 213, 220, 227
  Heart Self and, 179
  integration and, 301
  inward-focused State and, 268
  logic, alternating with, 351
  purposes of, 46, 49–50
  topics for, 50–51

K

Kidney 1 (Yongquan or Gushing Spring), 134, 221–222, 278, 435
Kidney 3 (Taixi or Great Stream), 131, 133, 135, 271
Kidney 7 (Fuliu or Returning Current), 131
Kidney 23 (Spirit Seal or Shenfeng), 178–179
Kidney 25 (Spirit Storehouse or Shencang), 182
Kidney 27 (Shufu or Shu Mansion), 284
Kidney Shu (Bladder 23), 132
Kidney Yin and Yang, 129–130
kingdom, mind as, 1–2, 17, 19–22, 29–32
Kunlun (Bladder 60), 409

L

lachesis, 180, 276

Large Intestine 4 (Hegu), 225, 230, 407, 409
last-resort distraction level, 86–88
lavender, 127, 188, 220, 229, 283, 412
lavender oil capsules, 428
learned scripts, 37
learning, 107, 228
left hemisphere, 198. *See also* Analytic Mode (Head Self)
left-right polarity, 9, 196. *See also* Analytic Mode (Head Self); Holistic Mode (Head Self)
legs-up-the-wall pose (Viparita Karani), 434
Leg Three Miles (Stomach 36), 132, 221, 285, 408
lemon balm, 175, 187, 282, 427
Lesser Sea (Heart 3), 183
Letters to a Young Poet, Letter Four (Rilke), 303
lifestyle. *See also* exercise/movement; mindfulness and meditation; nutrition
   foundations of, 62
   sleep and, 62, 125, 431–436
   Vital Self and, 103, 124
limbic system, 24–25
linden flower, 185
Listening Palace (Small Intestine 19), 178
Liver 3 (Taichong or Great Surge), 135
logic. *See* Analytic Mode (Head Self)
logic puzzles, 226, 227
Longfellow, Henry Wadsworth, 237
Loops
   overview, 266
   anxiety, 73
   defined, 2, 14, 304
   depression, 75
   experience by each Self of, 310–313
   general Loops, 304–306
   mental replay and, 252
   name the Loop strategy, 232–233
   State flexibility and, 314
   trauma-based loops, 306–309
   Vital Self in, 110
love, 253
loving-kindness phrases, 350
L-theanine, 175, 276, 424, 428
L-tyrosine, 282
Lung 1 (Middle Palace or Zhongfu), 190
Lung 3 (Heavenly Palace or Tian Fu), 179
Lung 9 (Taiyuan or Great Abyss), 137
lycopodium, 228
lycopodium clavatum, 130

M

magical thinking, 207, 290
magnesium, 123, 185, 401–402, 424, 426
magnesium glycinate, 270, 276, 282, 424, 426
magnesium oxide, 426

magnesium threonate, 270, 370, 376, 382, 424, 426
Malkin, Craig, 149, 150
mantra meditation, 439
MBCT (Mindfulness-Based Cognitive Therapy), 209, 275, 281
MBSR (Mindfulness-Based Stress Reduction), 122, 175
McBain, Alison, 167
McClellan, Sam, 113, 287, 357
media, 318–324
media diet, 322–324
meditation. *See* mindfulness and meditation
Mediterranean diet, 398
Melissa (lemon balm), 175, 187, 282, 427
memory, consolidation of, 107
memory training and enhancement, 226–227
mental models, 208–209, 333
mental replay, 252
microaggressions, 147
micro-freeze, 349
micro-no's, 312
Middleman illusion, 249–250
Middle Palace (Lung 1), 190
milky oat seed, 175, 270, 283
mind. *See* State; Three Selves
  aikido of, 381
  brain versus, 3–4
  emergent properties of, 16
  as a kingdom, 1–2, 17, 19–22, 29–32
  mental model constructed by. *See* mental models
mindful eating, 125, 402
mindful engagement level, 85
mindfulness and meditation
  bell apps, 57
  benefits of, 440–441
  defined, 439
  experience of, 437–438
  forms of, 439–440
  guided meditation, 62
  Head Self and, 213, 220, 224–225, 228, 234–235
  Heart Self and, 184, 191–193
  starting and continuing, 442–443
  State Shifts and, 254, 272–273, 279, 285
  Three Selves, rebalancing of, 294–295, 344–347
  trauma and, 441, 444
  Vital Self and, 125–126, 137–139
Mindfulness-Based Cognitive Therapy (MBCT), 209, 275, 281
Mindfulness-Based Stress Reduction (MBSR), 122, 175
mindful transitions, 58, 126
Mind Matrix Model. *See also* Ministers; Monarch; Scripts; Sentries; State; Three Selves; tools
  overview, 10–11, 18, 40–41, 376–379
  emergent properties of the mind and, 16
  navigation of book, 44–45

therapy with, 51–55
website for, 63, 382, 387
Mind Matrix Model Theory Paper, v, 387
Ministers
  overview, 33
  balance with Monarch, 36, 377–378
  defined, 17, 55
  of Head Self, 35, 378
  of Heart Self, 35, 157, 378
  Negative State and, 35–36, 41
  of Vital Self, 35–36, 378
Monarch
  overview, 33
  as Reflective Catalyst, 14, 33, 38, 40, 49, 442
  balance with Ministers, 36, 377–378
  blocks and, 391
  defined, 17, 54
  role of, 19–21, 288, 293
  State and, 41
Monarch mantras, 59
"Mont Blanc" (Shelley), 195
morning routines, 212, 268
motherwort, 180
motivation, 246
motor cortex, 108
movement. *See* exercise/movement
movement memory, 98
moving meditation, 443
"My Mind to Me A Kingdom Is" (Dyer), 1–2
myrrh, 181, 277

N

NAD+, 269
name the Loop strategy, 232–233
Narcissistic Personality Disorder (NPD), 152
Narcissist Mode, 149–152, 153, 158, 335–336
Narcissus, 150
narrative therapy, 275
natrum muriaticum, 128, 176, 186, 283
nature, exposure to, 126, 154, 209–210, 275, 327
navigation of the book, flexibility in, 44–45
Negative State. *See also* State; State Axis; State Shifts; stress, anxiety, and depression
  overview, 239
  Heart Self and, 149–152
  Ministers and, 35–36, 41
  Monarch role and, 41
  Positive State versus, 13, 240, 251
  qualities of the Three Selves in, 289
  triggers and, 14
Neiguan (Pericardium 6), 133, 189, 231, 272, 278, 284, 407, 410, 434
nettle leaf, 185
neurodivergence, 35, 147, 156, 206

neurofeedback, 122, 224
news, 320–321
non-response practice, 350
"Now is the time to know" (Hafiz), 221
NPD (Narcissistic Personality Disorder), 152
nutraceuticals, 428
nutrition. *See also* adaptogens (herbs)
   dietary guide for. *See* adaptogens (herbs)
   as foundation, 62
   Head Self and, 229–230
   Heart Self and, 175–176, 179–180, 184–185, 229
   State Shifts and, 269–270, 275–276, 282
   supplements, 421–427
   Vital Self and, 123–124, 125
nux vomica, 129, 181, 276, 419

O

object focus externalization, 267
obsessive Loops, 306, 308, 312–313
OFC (orbitofrontal cortex), 142
omega-3 fatty acids, 123, 175, 229, 276, 401, 423, 426
One Insult, a Thousand Echoes, 252
open monitoring meditation, 228
"open presence" blend, 177
opinion-based news, 321
orbitofrontal cortex (OFC), 142
other-focused. *See* Heart Self Axis
Other-Leaners, 338
over-association, 290
over-attunement to others, 147
Overrides, 292, 304
Override Strategies
   5-4-3-2-1 sensory tracking, 309
   blocks and, 392
   cues matched with, 298
   defined, 14, 55
   effectiveness, increasing, 314
   fast versus deep, 258
   for general Loops, 305–306
   Head Self and, 232–233, 300, 312–313
   Heart Self and, 299, 311–312
   as invitations, 286
   journaling and, 50–51
   selection of, 313
   sleep and, 434
   State and, 267–268, 274–275, 280–281
   State flexibility and, 314
   for trauma-based Loops, 307–309
   Vital Self and, 298, 310–311, 434
oversharing, 164
overthinking, 38, 206, 289

P

paranoia, 290
parasympathetic nervous system (PNS), 130
parasympathetic nervous system (PSN), 4, 23, 100
passionflower, 180, 276
patchouli, 127, 181, 277
"The Path of Awareness", 83
The Peace of Wild Things (Berry), 65
peace, State and, 249–250
Penetrating Inside (Heart 5), 189
peppermint, 127, 226, 229, 412
perfectionism, 205, 206, 380–381, 426
Pericardium 4 (Gate of Origin or Ximen), 182
Pericardium 6 (Neiguan or Inner Gate), 133, 189, 231, 272, 278, 284, 407, 410, 434
peripheral nervous system (PNS), 4
perseveration, 38
personalization, 423
personal tokens, 326
personas, 155–158
perspective widening, 308, 313
phosphoricum acidum, 128
phosphorus, 180, 186–187, 276, 283
physical Self. *See* Vital Self
placebo effect, 416
play, problem-solving and, 213, 222–223
PNS (parasympathetic nervous system), 4, 23, 100, 130
PNS (peripheral nervous system), 4
polyvagal-informed therapy, 275
Positive State. *See* State; State Axis; State Shifts
  overview, 239
  Monarch role and, 41
  Negative State versus, 13, 240, 251
  qualities of Three Selves in, 288–289
Post-it notes for the soul, 55–56
posture Override, 223
potentization, 418
practice, not perfection, 380–381
praise, 204
PREDIMED trial, 398
prefrontal cortex, 108, 198
probiotics, 184
problem-solving, play and, 213, 222–223
procrastination, 389–396
proprioceptive awareness, 34–35, 98–99
prosody, 197
protective personas, 158
Psychological Trauma research, 441
pulsatilla, 128, 176, 186, 270, 419
purposeful sacrifice, 291
pushback and, 47, 48
pushback/resistance, 47–49, 207

Q

Qihai (Conception Vessel 6), 136
Quepen (Stomach 12), 183

R

"The Rainy Day" (Longfellow), 237
RAS (reticular activating system), 22, 100, 107–109
rationalization, 289
rational override, 292
reactive state, empty boat parable and, iii
reality, creation of. *See* symbols
reality testing, 209, 308
recede, advance, hold. *See* Sentries
reflection. *See* journaling
  boundaries, 361, 365
  Head Self, 219
  Heart Self, 174
  learning from, 381
  Loops and Overrides, 314
  pushback and, 48–49
  Self-Other Differentiation, 344, 353–354
  State Shifts, 264
  symbolic mapping, 327
  tools, 47
  Vital Self, 121
Reflective Catalyst
  defined, 14, 33
  meditation and, 442
  pushback and, 49
  Scripts and, 38
  Sentries and, 40
reframing (change the frame), 233, 305, 311
reishi mushrooms, 180, 276, 427
relapse, 92
relational authenticity, 162, 164
relational intelligence, 301
relational stress, 147
relational therapy, 184, 282
Relational Therapy, 184
reminders, awareness and, 55–58
replay of events, 252
resentment tracking, 312
resistance/pushback, 47–49, 207
rest, Vital Self and, 114
reticular activating system (RAS). *See* RAS (reticular activating system)
Returning Current (Kidney 7), 131
Return to Center meditation, 279
"Return to Your Breath" (McClellan), 113
rhodiola, 270, 282
rhodiola rosea, 123, 124, 175, 427
rhythmic rituals, 280

Rhythm Within meditation, 285
right hemisphere, 198. *See also* Holistic Mode (Head Self)
rigid thinking, 208, 289, 336–337
Rilke, Rainer Maria, 81, 303
ritual corners, 58
ritual objects, 326
rituals
  awareness and, 55–59
  Head Self and, 212–213
  heart self and, 164
  morning activation, 268
  State Shifts and, 274, 280, 326–327
  symbols and, 326–327
rosemary, 127, 226, 229
rose otto, 176, 271
rose (petal or tincture), 176, 270
rose (Rosa damascena), 187

S

sacrifice, 291
Safe Place, 89, 367
safety. *See also* trauma
  boundaries tripod and, 368–370
  Head Self and, 313
  Heart Self and, 154, 162
  sleep and, 433–436
  symbols and, 316
  Vital Self and, 106–107
Samatha (calm abiding), 439
Samurai and the Monk, 253, 254
sandalwood, 127, 181, 220, 277
Sanyinjiao (Spleen 6), 134, 232, 277, 408
schisandra berry, 176
screen time, 324–325
Scripts. *See also* Sentries
  overview, 36–37
  blocks as, 389
  defined, 14, 55
  Head Self and, 442
  Heart self and, 158
  mindfuness and meditation and, 442
SE (Somatic Experiencing). *See* Somatic Experiencing (SE)
Sea of Qi (Conception Vessel 6), 136
Sea of Tranquility (Conception Vessel 17), 190
seasons, State and, 281
second brain. *See* enteric nervous system (ENS)
"The Self" (McClellan), 287
self-check affirmation, 280
self-compassion, 161, 311, 367, 402–403
self-containment, 154
self-critical voices, 162, 163, 206

self-destructive behaviors, as suppression, 86–88
self-esteem, 40, 163
Self-Leaners, 337–338
Self-Other Development/Differentiation. *See also* boundaries
   overview, 15–16, 355
   balance in, 343–344, 355
   defined, 330
   Head Self and, 15, 331, 332–333, 334, 336–337, 342, 351–352
   Heart Self and, 15, 158–159, 331, 332, 333–334, 335–336, 341–342, 349–350
   interruption of, 106, 347–350
   layering across the Selves and, 341–343
   meditation and, 344–347
   patterns in, 337–341
   sensitive people and, 354
   stages of, 15–16, 330–333
   strengthening and repair practices, 344, 347–353
   Vital Self and, 15, 110, 331, 332, 333, 334–335, 337, 341, 348–349
self-regulation, 224, 501
self-worth, 161–162
sensory activation, 311
sensory override pause, 352
Sentries
   overview, 37–38
   blocks as, 389
   communication by, 39–40
   defined, 14, 55
   journaling and, 50
   resistance from, 47
   self-critical voices and, 163
sepia, 129
septal nuclei, 142
shame
   Heart Self and, 151, 162
   Loops and, 306, 307, 311
   personas and, 157–158
Shanzhong (Conception Vessel 17), 190, 278, 284
Shao Hai (Heart 3), 183
shelf, placing things on, 73
Shelley, Percy Bysshe, 195
Shencang (Kidney 25), 182
Shenfeng (Kidney 23), 178–179
Shenmen (Heart 7), 134, 189, 221, 271, 434
Shenshu (Bladder 23), 132
Shenting (Governing Vessel 24), 231
shoulder reset + still point, 280
Shufu (Kidney 27), 284
Shu Mansion (Kidney 27), 284
shutdown Loops, 306
Siberian ginseng (eleuthero), 185, 270
Sighing Out Breath + Stretch, 267
silence, 351

silexan, 428
silicea, 176, 270
sitting meditation (Zazen), 440
skullcap, 180, 276
sleep, 62, 125, 431–436
Small Intestine 19 (Listening Palace or Ting Gong), 178
SNS (sympathetic nervous system), 4, 23, 100
Socratic questioning, 227
Somatic Experiencing (SE), 123, 269, 366
somatic reset, 306
"Song of Myself" (Whitman), 329
"Song of the Open Road" (Whitman), 375
"Sonnets to Orpheus" (Rilke), 81
Sp 10 (Xuehai), 409
spiral thinking, 207
Spirit Gate (Heart 7), 134, 189, 221, 271, 434
Spirit Seal (Kidney 23), 178–179
Spirit Storehouse (Kidney 25), 182
spiritual bypass, 290
Spleen 3 (Taibai or Supreme White), 136
Spleen 6 (Sanyinjiao or Three Yin Intersection), 134, 232, 277, 408
Spleen 21 (Great Embracement or Dabao), 182
stacking, 314
staphysagria, 186
State. *See also* Negative State; Positive State; stress, anxiety, and depression
  overview, 11–13
  blocks and, 392
  defined, iv, 55
  flexibility and, 314
  fluid nature of, 242, 286
  journaling and, 50
  media and, 321–322
  orientation and, 286
  positive versus negative orientation and, 254–255
  Three Selves and, 240–242
  triggers and, 241
State Axis. *See also* Negative State; Positive State; State Shifts
  overview, 238–240
  emotions and, 248–249
  Head Self and, 12, 202–203, 246–247
  Heart Self and, 12, 148–152, 245
  questionnaire for, 258–265
  Vital Self and, 12, 109–110, 244
State Magnets, 250–255
State Range, 110, 238, 265
State Shifts
  acupressure and, 271–272, 277–278, 284–285
  balanced orientation, maintaining, 279–285
  defined, 254
  essential oils and, 270–271, 277, 283
  homeopathy and, 270, 276–277, 283

    inward-focused State, balancing of, 267–273
    meditation and, 272–273, 279, 285
    mindfulness and meditation for, 443
    nutritional strategies for, 269–270, 275–276, 282
    outward-focused State, balancing of, 273–279
    rituals and, 274, 280, 326–327
    symbols and, 318
    therapies for, 269, 275, 281–282
staying in yourself, 352–353
stick programming, 320
stillness in motion, 274
still point lying pose, 349
stimulating breath, 267
Stomach 12 (Empty Basin or Quepen), 183
Stomach 36 (Zusanli or Leg Three Miles), 132, 221, 285, 408
strategic focus, 292
stress, anxiety and depression. *See also* mindfulness and meditation
    overview, 66, 79
    anxiety as second step in, 70–73
    depression as third step in, 74–77
    Heart Self and, 161
    impacts of, 17
    interconnectedness of, 66–67, 82, 92
    Loops and, 73, 75
    mental model building disrupted by, 208–209, 333
    plant-based diet to reduce, 398–399
    principles for healing, 91–93
    relational stress, Heart Self and, 147
    Self-Other Differentiation and, 15–16
    starting point to healing, 82–83
    stress as first step in, 67–69
    supporting each Self, 89–91
    three-level toolbox for, 85–89
    unreleased stress, 69, 71
    Your Safe Place and, 89, 367
structural oppression, 104
subconscious, 34
sukha (ease), 242
sulphur, 128, 180, 277, 283
supplements, nutritional, 421–427. *See also* adaptogens (herbs)
supportive symbols, 325–326
Supreme Spring (Heart 1), 177
Supreme White (Spleen 3), 136
Survive Mode, 11–12. *See also* Negative State
sweet orange, 177, 270
switch anchor, 280
symbolic anchors, 281
symbolic chaos, 205
symbolic field mapping, 327
symbolic input detox, 233
symbolic overload, 322, 324–326

symbolic play, 222–223
symbolic threats, 103
symbols
  overview, 316
  Head Sef and, 317–318
  Heart Self and, 317
  as keys to consciousness, 328
  mapping environment, 327
  media and, 318–324
  overload and, 322, 324–326
  trauma and, 318
  Vital Self and, 316
Symbols
  overview, 316
sympathetic nervous system (SNS), 4, 23, 100, 130
synthesizer, 202

T

Taibai (Spleen 3), 136
Taichong (Liver 3), 135
Taixi (Kidney 3), 131, 133, 135, 271
Taiyuan (Lung 9), 137
Task-Positive Networks (TPNs), 199
task switching exercises, 228
Teasdale, Sara, 141
techniques. *See* tools
temperature shift + movement, 268
thalamus, 24, 26, 142
therapy
  art therapy, 175, 269
  Cognitive Behavioral Therapy (CBT), 175, 224
  Craniosacral Therapy, 281
  Dialectical Behavior Therapy (DBT), 179, 275
  group therapy, 269
  Hakomi Therapy, 281
  Head Self dysregulation and, 224
  Mindfulness-Based Cognitive Therapy, 209, 275, 281
  Mind Matrix Model and, 51–55
  Narrative Therapy, 275
  Polyvagal-Informed Therapy, 275
  Relational Therapy, 184, 282
  State Shifts and, 269, 275, 281–282
  Vital Self dysregulation and, 122–124
Third Eye Point (Yintang), 222, 410
Thoreau, Henry David, 95
thought labeling, 312
thought records, 224
thought sorting (externalize it), 233
three-level toolbox for stress, anxiety, and depression, 85–89
Three Selves. *See also* Head Self; Heart Self; Vital Self
  overview, 6–7
  axes of, generally, 8–11, 23, 25–27

balance in, 293–302, 344–347
  collective wisdom of, 29–32
  cues from, 295–297
  cultural history of, 6
  defined, 54
  emotions and, 243–246
  in balance, 288
  interplay of, 27, 241–242
  Self-Other Differentiation and, 15–16
  State and, 240–242, 288–289
  two Selves overriding third Self, 291–292
Three Yin Intersection (Spleen 6), 134, 232, 277, 408
Thrive Mode, 11–12. *See also* Positive State
Tian Fu (Lung 3), 179
Tiantu (Conception Vessel 22), 178
Tianzhu (Bladder 10), 231
Ting Gong (Small Intestine 19), 178
titration, 86–88, 92, 154, 366, 391
tone mirror check, 350
Tong Li (Heart 5), 189
tools, 45–47, 60–62, 85–89, 392. *See also* acupressure; adaptogens (herbs); breathwork; essential oils; exercise/movement; homeopathy; mindfulness and meditation; nutrition; sleep
TPNs (Task-Positive Networks), 199
Traditional Chinese Medicine. *See* acupressure
transitional micro-practices, 58, 126
trauma
  defined, 13
  Head Self and, 204–208
  Heart Self and, 152–153, 155, 159
  Loops based on, 306–309
  mindfulness and meditation and, 441, 444
  Self-Other Differentiation and, 15–16
  symbols and, 318
  Vital Self and, 102, 104–107
trauma responses, defined, 3
triggers. *See also* Negative State
  defined, 14
  disruption of, 305
  process of learning new response to, 83–85
  State and, 14, 241
  symbols as, 317
tripod, boundaries and, 368–370
trust, 161
tryptophan, 401
tulsi (holy basil), 123, 175, 180, 185, 270, 276, 282, 427

U

unconscious, 34

V

vagus nerve, 100–101
vagus nerve stimulation, 311

valerian root, 180
veratrum album, 181
vetiver, 181, 188, 277
Viparita Karani (legs-up-the-wall pose), 434
Vipassana (Buddhist insight), 439
vision-boarding, 213, 222–223
visual arts. *See* creative practices
Vital-Dominant Personas, 156
Vital Loops, 266
Vital Self. *See also* Ministers
  overview, 6–7, 22–23, 96–99, 140, 377
  acupressure and, 129–137
  boundaries and, 359, 368–370
  chronic dysregulation of, 102–104
  cues from, 295–296
  defined, iii, 54
  emotions and, 243–244
  essential oils and, 127–128
  fear and, 70
  grounding of, 89–90, 110, 114
  homeopathy and, 128–129
  imbalances in, 101–102
  lifestyle changes for, 124–126
  Loops and Overrides, 110, 306, 307, 310–311
  media and, 321
  meditation and, 125–126, 137–139
  mindful engagement and,, 85
  neurological basis of, 22–23, 99–101
  nutritional strategies for, 123–124, 125
  Override plan for, 298
  pushback and, 47, 48
  questionnaire for, 115–121
  rebalancing modalities generally, 293
  Self-Other Differentiation and, 15, 110, 332, 333, 334–335, 337, 341, 348–349
  sleep and, 432
  State and, 12, 109–110, 244
  stress, anxiety, and depression and, 71–72, 77–78, 89–90
  supports for, 428
  symbols and, 316
  systems used by, 22–23
  therapies for dysregulation in, 122–124
  trauma and, 102, 104–107
Vital Self Axis, 8, 10, 23, 107–109
Vital Self Scripts, 37
Vital Self Sentries, 37–38, 39
vitamin B-complex, 269, 276, 423, 427
vitamin D3, 423, 428
vocal boundaries, 349
voice activation, 267
voice tone mirror check, 350

W

walking meditation, 443
weighted blankets, 274, 316, 348, 434
Whitman, Walt, 329, 375
window-gaze pause, 274
withdrawal, 38
wood betony, 180

X

Ximen (Pericardium 4), 182
Xuehai (Sp 10), 409

Y

yarrow, 188
Yintang (Third Eye Point), 222, 410
Yin/Yang, ii
ylang ylang, 127, 177, 220
Yoga Nidra, 440
Yongquan (Kidney 1), 134, 221–222, 278, 435
Your Safe Place, 89, 367

Z

Zazen (sitting meditation), 440
Zhiyin (Bladder 67), 409
Zhongfu (Lung 1), 190
Zhongji (Conception Vessel 3), 409
Zhuangzi, iii
zinc, 428
Zusanli (Stomach 36), 132, 221, 285, 408

About the Author

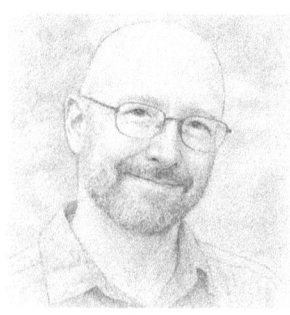

Sam McClellan is an integrative complementary health practitioner, educator, and author with nearly five decades of experience practicing and teaching health work. He is the creator of Integrative Acupressure (IA), a unique body-mind approach that combines Chinese medicine with Western and complementary practices to support well-being.

While attending Hampshire College, Sam developed and tested a form of music therapy called Music of the Five Elements, based on Chinese medicine and designed to evoke emotional states in a progression that harmonizes the mind. He recorded an album of the same name on Spirit Records—a musical guided meditation—recently remastered and re-released internationally as both a digital download and LP on the Séance Centre record label.

Sam has taught internationally, developed therapeutic programs for professionals, and worked with thousands of clients from diverse backgrounds to promote optimal health, trauma recovery, emotional balance, and personal growth. His work emphasizes State regulation and Self-Other Differentiation, bridging scientific insight with practical tools for everyday life.

In the 1990s, Sam trained as a neurofeedback clinician, an experience that deepened his understanding of brain function and later informed the Mind Matrix Model, his comprehensive framework for understanding and working to optimize the mind. The Model blends insights from neurology, psychology, and contemplative traditions such as Buddhism into an accessible system for transforming patterns of thought, emotion, and behavior.

Currently, Sam collaborates with innovators in psychology and neurology to further integrate somatic approaches into trauma and mental health work. The Mind Matrix Model represents the culmination of his lifelong commitment to making body-mind understanding accessible, actionable, and transformative for a wide audience.

He lives and works in Western Massachusetts.

www.ingramcontent.com/pod-product-compliance
Lightning Source LLC
Chambersburg PA
CBHW070605030426
42337CB00020B/3697